MW00449334

COCHLEAR IMPLANTS FOR kids

WARREN ESTABROOKS
Editor

Alexander Graham Bell Association for the Deaf and Hard of Hearing, Inc.
3417 Volta Place, NW, Washington, DC 20007-2778

Alexander Graham Bell Association for the Deaf and Hard of Hearing, Inc.
3417 Volta Place, NW
Washington, DC 20007-2778

Photo Credits
Cover kids: Eric Sieloff, Dara Keller, Katie Kilmartin, Kelvin Ko, Hunter Jackson, Kevin Kishore, Lauren Nayman.
Text photos courteously supplied by: Advanced Bionics Corp., Sylmar, CA: *4, 10, 51;* Cochlear AG, Basel, Switzerland: *39, 89;* Cochlear Corp., Englewood, CO: *13, 16, 25, 61;* Hospital for Sick Children, Toronto, ON, Canada: *64;* Med-El Corp., Innsbruck, Austria: *39, 89;* North York General Hospital, Toronto, ON, Canada: *1, 69, 257;* The Sieloff Family, *54;* The Zbikowski Family, *45.*

For information about cochlear implants, contact:
Cochlear Implant Club International
5335 Wisconsin Avenue, NW, Suite 440
Washington, DC 20015-2034, USA

Cover design: Nika Design
Editing/Desktop publishing: Francine Geraci

Printed in Canada
10 9 8 7 6 5 4 3 2

Dedication

Cochlear Implants for Kids is dedicated to the world's children who have cochlear implants, to their families and friends, and to the professionals whose privilege it is to work with them.

Acknowledgments

Cochlear Implants for Kids took more than two years from conception to completion. Many accolades are deserved, especially for:

Mary Woodburn, secretary extraordinaire, for typing the entire book and for pursuing the dream;

Karen MacIver-Lux and Jonathan Samson, former students and my friends, for hours of proofreading;

Professional and parent contributors, for graciously accepting the challenge;

John Kilmartin, for designing and donating the cover;

Advanced Bionics Corporation, Cochlear Corporation, and Med-El Corporation, for exceptional print and photographic material;

A.G. Bell Association for the Deaf, especially Donna Dickman and Elizabeth Quigley, for years of support, commitment, and advocacy;

Francine Geraci, for exceptional professional expertise, guidance, and attention to detail;

The Learning to Listen Foundation Board of Directors, for encouragement, dedication, and support;

John Craig and Ariella Samson, for their mentorship; and

Pierre-Roch Côté, for a wonderful life.

The Editor

WARREN ESTABROOKS, M.Ed., Cert. AVT, is Director of Auditory-Verbal Therapy, Learning to Listen Foundation (LLF), at the Phillips House, North York General Hospital in Toronto, ON, Canada.

Estabrooks is a Charter Director of Auditory-Verbal International, Inc., a member of both the Alexander Graham Bell Association for the Deaf and the Network of Educators of Children with Cochlear Implants.

Estabrooks has been honored for his work by the Alexander Graham Bell Association for the Deaf, Auditory-Verbal International, Inc., Learning to Listen Foundation, North York General Hospital, and Voice for Hearing-Impaired Children. He is a consultant in professional education and auditory-verbal practice, and lectures internationally.

Estabrooks has made numerous contributions to the literature, including: *Do You Hear That?* (1992), *Hear & Listen! Talk & Sing!* (1994), *Auditory-Verbal Therapy for Parents and Professionals* (1994), and *The ABC's of AVT* (1995).

Preface

*C*ochlear Implants for Kids is a labor of love and exemplifies the collaboration of state-of-the-art medicine, technology, research, and habilitation required to help children who have cochlear implants to maximize the potential for hearing and listening provided by cochlear implant surgery and habilitative follow-up. Parents and professionals from around the world have generously worked for countless hours to bring the gift of *Cochlear Implants for Kids* to all those who work with, live with, and love these special children.

It is my hope that *Cochlear Implants for Kids* will help to foster a deeper understanding of medical, technical, habilitative, educational, and family issues for future generations of children who have cochlear implants, their parents and caregivers, and the professionals who provide them with guidance and support.

Cochlear Implants for Kids is also intended to be a celebration — and everyone is invited.

Warren Estabrooks, M.Ed., Cert. AVT
Toronto, Canada
Spring 1998

Contributors

Editor
Warren Estabrooks, M.Ed., Cert. AVT
Director, Auditory-Verbal Therapy
Learning to Listen Foundation
North York General Hospital
Toronto, Ontario, Canada

Professionals
Jo Acree, M.S., CCC-A, Cert. AVT
Central Speech & Hearing Clinic
Winnipeg, Manitoba, Canada

Thomas Balkany, M.D.
Annelle V. Hodges, Ph.D.
Kenneth W. Goodman, Ph.D.
University of Miami
School of Medicine
Miami, Florida

Anne L. Beiter, M.S., CCC-A/S-LP
Cochlear Corporation
Englewood, Colorado

Nancy S. Caleffe-Schenck, M.Ed.,
    C.E.D., CCC-A, Cert. AVT
Private Practice
Evergreen, Colorado

Teresa Caruso, M.Sc.(A).,
    Aud.(C)., Cert. AVT
Central Speech & Hearing Clinic
Winnipeg, Manitoba, Canada

Noel Cohen, M.D.
Professor and Chairman
Department of Otolaryngology
NYU Medical Center
New York, New York

Stephen Epstein, M.D.
Director, The Ear Center
Wheaton, Maryland

Todd Houston, MSP, CCC-SLP,
    Cert. AVT
University of South Carolina
Columbia, South Carolina

Jan Hutchison, M.A., Cert. AVT
Private Practice
Denver, Colorado

Amy McConkey Robbins, M.S.
Communication Consulting
    Services
Indianapolis, Indiana

Tina Olmstead, M.Sc., Cert. AVT
Children's Hospital of Eastern
    Ontario
Ottawa, Ontario, Canada

Jon K. Shallop, Ph.D.
Director, Auditory Research,
    HealthONE
Denver, Colorado

William H. Shapiro, M.A.
Susan B. Waltzman, Ph.D.
Department of Otolaryngology
NYU Medical Center
New York, New York

Judith I. Simser, O.Ont.,
    B.Ed., Cert. AVT
Children's Hearing Foundation
Taipei, Taiwan

Pamela Steacie, M.Sc., Cert. AVT
Children's Hospital of Eastern
    Ontario
Ottawa, Ontario, Canada

Sally Tannenbaum, M.Ed.,
    C.E.D., Cert. AVT
Private Practice
Chicago, Illinois

Beth Walker, M.Ed., C.E.D.,
    Cert. AVT
Private Practice
Dadeville, Alabama

Carol Zara, M.A., CCC-SLP
League for the Hard of Hearing
New York, New York

Parents
Dianne Blair
Woodstock, Ontario, Canada

Gael Cole
Kanata, Ontario, Canada

Reba Demeter
La Canada, California, USA

Cheryl Exner
Regina, Saskatchewan, Canada

Glynis Kilmartin
Toronto, Ontario, Canada

Elaine Matlow Tal-El
Jerusalem, Israel

Joanna Nichols
Taipei, Taiwan

Eva Quateman
Chicago, Illinois, USA

Marta Salvucci
Rio de Janeiro, Brazil

Susan Schonfeld
Chicago, Illinois, USA

Mike Sieloff
Sarnia, Ontario, Canada

Theresa Spraggon
Sydney, Australia

Karen Sworik
London, Ontario, Canada

Gaby Thierbach
Meggen, Switzerland

Contents

IV Family Stories from Around the World

Appendices

Foreword

Stephen Epstein, M.D.

The most significant achievement in scientific technology of the 20th century designed to assist children who are profoundly hearing impaired since the advent of hearing aids and tactile devices is the *cochlear implant.*

The earliest cochlear implant, the single-channel implant, was approved by the Food and Drug Administration (FDA) in the United States in 1984 for use in adults only. The single-channel cochlear implant enabled adults who are profoundly hearing impaired to be aware of environmental sounds and to monitor their own voices. Even though a limited number of children received the single-channel cochlear implant during a clinical trial, it was not formally approved by the FDA for use by children at that time. Following the 1985 approval of a multichannel cochlear implant for use with adults who had postlinguistic deafness, a large-scale clinical trial with children was initiated, and, in 1990, the FDA finally approved one multichannel cochlear implant (Nucleus 22) for use in children aged two to 17 years.

Even though there is excitement and enthusiasm about the long-term benefits of the cochlear implant in children who are profoundly hearing impaired, there exists opposition from particular groups. This air of controversy adds to the natural concerns and anxieties that parents usually have when considering a cochlear implant for their child. A significant concern is the fact that the cochlear implant is a relatively new device. Parents usually know little about how the implant works, whether their child is a potential candidate, where to go for the implant, which steps are undertaken prior to the surgery, and what is involved in the surgery itself. There are questions about what happens after the surgery and what can be expected from a child in regard to the improvement of hearing and the development of speech and language. Perhaps the most difficult aspect of the decision is in choosing the appropriate time for the child to receive a cochlear implant and establishing what the parents' rights are in making this decision.

Cochlear Implants for Kids provides many answers about parents' concerns and about professional practice. In this book, Warren Estabrooks has assembled knowledge and guidance from world-class experts dealing with all aspects of cochlear implantation in children.

Assuming the child receives little or no benefit from hearing aids, one step in the decision process is to become familiar with the cochlear implant itself, how it works, and the many benefits it can provide. One of parents' major concerns is whether or not their child is a potential candidate for the implant and which steps must be taken to determine the child's eligibility. *Anne Beiter* and *Jon Shallop* have provided some answers in chapter 1, "Cochlear Implants: Past, Present, Future."

A further concern of parents of a child with profound hearing impairment is the recognition that they are facing one of the most important decisions that will affect their child for the rest of his or her life. What are the moral and ethical considerations in deciding whether a child should receive a cochlear implant? *Drs. Thomas Balkany, Annelle Hodges,* and *Kenneth Goodman* discuss them in chapter 2, "Cochlear Implants for Young Children: Ethical Issues."

Another area of concern is the surgery itself. What tests must be given, and how is the child prepared for the surgery? How is it performed? How many hours does it take, and how long will the child remain in the hospital? How will the child feel after the surgery? The more the parents are familiar with the surgical procedure, the better prepared both they and the child will be. *Dr. Noel Cohen,* writing especially with parents in mind, answers some of these questions in chapter 3, "What Parents Need to Know About Cochlear Implant Surgery."

What happens after the surgery when the child is ready to put the cochlear implant to use? What does it mean to program the implant, and what is involved in the programming? Perhaps the most anxiously awaited moment during the process is the child's reaction when the cochlear implant is first activated, approximately four weeks after the surgery. What will the child hear for the first time? What kind of reaction should be expected, and how can parents best prepare themselves and their child for this special moment? *William Shapiro* and *Susan Waltzman* cover these topics in chapter 4, "Cochlear Implant Programming for Children: The Basics."

In taking full advantage of the current technology of the cochlear implant, many children can hear speech and environmental sounds without relying on visual cues, touch, kinesthetic feedback, or sign language. In chapter 5, *Warren Estabrooks* discusses "Learning to Listen with a Cochlear Implant: A Model for Children." In preparation for the detailed habilitation in chapter 6, Estabrooks provides a model upon which therapists, teachers, and parents can base the development of the child's new listening potential after he or she has received a cochlear implant.

There are diverse approaches to therapy after cochlear implantation. One of the unique aspects of this book is that it provides detailed lesson plans from expert therapists and teachers who work with children who have cochlear implants. These dedicated professionals guide children who are enrolled in regular classrooms, auditory-verbal programs, oral programs, or total communication programs to hear, listen, talk, and communicate to the best of their abilities.

While life with children who have cochlear implants can be a challenge, it can also be a joy. With that in mind, the reader will be entertained and completely engaged by the family stories in part IV of *Cochlear Implants for Kids*.

Modern technology and advances in medical science have enabled the cochlear implant to develop at a rate no one thought possible. Progress doesn't stop there. Improvements in the implant itself, in the surgical techniques and procedures, and in post-implantation therapy are continuing, so that children can receive the maximum benefit from the cochlear implant.

Parents of children who may be potential candidates for the cochlear implant, or who have already received one, will find *Cochlear Implants for Kids* helpful in broadening their knowledge, clarifying their concerns, and alleviating their fears.

The cochlear implant has made a tremendous impact on the lives of children who are profoundly hearing impaired and their families. This book gives the reader a multidimensional insight into one of the most significant technological advances of the 20th century and into the lives of those it affects.

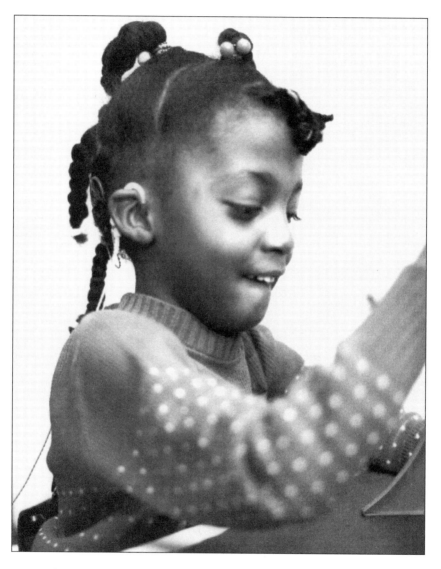

PART I

History and Ethical Issues

Overleaf: Elizabeth McBride, Denver, Colorado, USA

CHAPTER I

Cochlear Implants: Past, Present, Future

Anne L. Beiter, M.S.
Jon K. Shallop, Ph.D.

Cochlear implants are auditory prostheses that provide hearing to individuals who have severe-to-profound hearing impairments and cannot benefit from conventional amplification. These biomedical devices convert sound energy into low-level electrical currents that are used to stimulate the auditory or hearing nerve directly, thus bypassing the damaged inner ear or cochlea. Cochlear implants have become the medical treatment of choice for those adults and children who, because of the severity of their hearing impairment, cannot understand spoken language through amplified residual hearing. As noted in the 1995 National Institutes of Health Consensus Statement on Cochlear Implants in Adults and Children, "the multichannel cochlear implant has become a widely accepted auditory prosthesis for both adults and children." Almost all individuals with this degree of hearing impairment have sufficient auditory nerve fibers in their hearing nerve that can be stimulated electrically.

The Normal Hearing Process

In order to understand how cochlear implants work, it is useful to describe briefly the normal hearing process. In the normally functioning auditory system (Figure 1 on the next page), the outer and middle ears act as a bridge to transfer acoustic pressure changes (sound waves) to the fluids of the part of the inner ear known as the cochlea. This is accomplished by one of the three small middle-ear bones pushing into and out of the cochlea at a place called the oval window. The

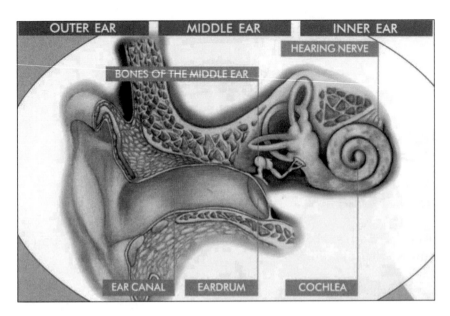

Figure 1   Structure of the outer, middle, and inner ear

vibrations that are set up in the fluids of the inner ear cause other structures within the cochlea to vibrate. This ultimately results in stimulation of the auditory sensory cells (the hair cells).

The cochlea is organized so that the highest-frequency or highest-pitch sounds cause maximum vibration or stimulation of the hair cells at the base of the cochlea (the end nearest to the middle ear). The lowest-frequency or lowest-pitch sounds cause maximum displacement and stimulation of the sensory cells at the other end, the apex of the cochlea. Therefore, the frequency or pitch of the sound determines which hair cells are stimulated maximally. In addition, the sensory hair cells are activated according to the frequency to which they respond best and also to their location along the cochlea where they connect with the fibers of the hearing nerve. In a similar manner to the hair cells, the individual nerve fibers respond best to a specific frequency. This organization by "best" frequency of the hair cells and auditory nerve fibers is referred to as *tonotopic organization*. Information about specific sounds is coded by the place in the cochlea at which the sensory cells are stimulated maximally and also by the timing patterns of how the nerve fibers respond to sounds. See Durrant and Lovrinic (1977) and Yost and Nielsen (1977) for detailed information on the anatomy and physiology of the auditory system.

Stimulation of the hair cells within the inner ear converts mechanical energy into the electrochemical activity that results in electrical responses of the auditory nerve, and these neural impulses are transmitted through the brainstem to the auditory centers of the brain for interpretation. When the hair cells of the cochlea are damaged or missing, the result is sensory hearing loss. However, in most cases, when the sensory cells are damaged, there is also some loss of individual nerve fibers. Therefore, this type of hearing impairment is typically called *sensorineural,* referring to damage to the sensory end organ and the nerve itself. In the case of profound deafness, almost all the sensory cells are missing or so severely damaged that sound cannot be converted into the electrical impulses that ultimately generate the sensations of hearing. Thus, the primary function of a cochlear implant is to stimulate the auditory nerve directly in the absence of functional sensory hair cells in the cochlea.

History of Cochlear Implants

The earliest known report of hearing sensations resulting from direct electrical stimulation has been attributed to Alessandro Volta. He connected a battery to two metal rods that were inserted into his ears and reported a "jolt" in the head and a boiling-type noise (Simmons, 1966). However, the first systematic investigation of the effects of electrical stimulation of the auditory nerve in a deaf person is usually attributed to two French surgeons, Djourno and Eyries, as described by Luxford and Brackman (1985). In 1957, they placed an electrode in a portion of the hearing nerve during an operation for facial nerve repair. Later, when they stimulated the nerve with various electrical currents, the patient discriminated different sounds and a few common words. Following this, pioneering researchers, such as Drs. William House, Blair Simmons, and Robin Michelson in the United States, and Prof. Graeme Clark in Australia, studied the effects of electrical stimulation on the auditory nerve in both animals and human adult research subjects.

Since these earliest studies on electrical hearing, research has continued with the aim of making implantable devices for the purpose of providing hearing on a long-term basis for individuals with severe-to-profound hearing impairments. These systems must provide safe and effective electrical stimulation. Various single-channel and multichannel cochlear implant systems have been developed in Europe, the United States, and Australia. Detailed accounts of the development of cochlear implants are available in a number of sources (Clark, 1997; Luxford &

Brackman, 1985; House & Berliner, 1991; Mecklenburg & Lehnhardt, 1991; Staller, 1985; Tyler & Tye-Murray, 1991).

Single-Channel Cochlear Implants

Some of the earliest cochlear prostheses were single-channel cochlear implant systems. These systems are less complex than multichannel systems and consist of a single electrode that is placed within or near the cochlea. All sound information that is processed and converted into electrical current is delivered to that single active electrode with a reference or ground electrode that may be either in or outside of the cochlea. Information conveyed about speech by such systems tends to be limited to loudness and timing; information related to the frequency or pitch of sounds is minimal. Most information about the frequency of speech sounds, which is critical for speech understanding, is generally conveyed by the area of stimulation within the cochlea.

The 3M/House single-channel cochlear implant is the best known and most used of the early systems. It was developed by William House, M.D. and colleagues in the early 1970s. This system used analog speech-processing technology, meaning that a continuously varying electrical voltage represented the ongoing changes in the sound waves. The processor amplified and bandpassed the acoustic signal, then changed it to an electrical signal that was used to modulate or vary the amplitude of a 16 KHz carrier signal by changing its voltage. This modulated electrical signal was sent across the skin via an external coil to an internal coil, which delivered the electrical signals to a single active electrode that had been inserted a short distance (approximately 6 mm) into the cochlea (Staller, 1985; Wilson, 1993).

In November 1984, the U.S. Food and Drug Administration (FDA) granted commercial use of this device in adults with profound deafness. Individuals who received this implant generally gained the benefits of sound detection, environmental sound awareness, and the perception of some speech cues, primarily timing and intensity, that aided them in speechreading. In general, recipients were unable to recognize or understand speech without visual cues. Although the 3M/House device was implanted in selected children with profound deafness under the jurisdiction of a multicenter clinical trial regulated by the FDA, it never gained the necessary U.S. regulatory approval for commercial use in children. In 1987, the 3M Company stopped manufacturing this system.

In 1998, Dr. House is manufacturing a single-channel implant that is based on the design of the previous 3M/House implant. This device is called the AllHear cochlear implant and consists of virtually the same implanted component with a single active electrode as the 3M/House device and an all-on-the-head processor (House, 1996). Currently in the United States, this device is available only to selected adults with profound deafness under the auspices of a multicenter clinical investigation regulated by the FDA.

Another single-channel system, developed in Vienna and Innsbruck, Austria by engineers Burian, Hochmair-Desoyer, and Hochmair, was supported in the United States by the 3M Company and was known as the Vienna/3M device. There were two configurations of this device; one was intracochlear, and the other extracochlear. The intracochlear system consisted of four electrodes that were implanted into the cochlea; however, electrical current was sent to only one of the electrodes, presumably the one that gave the recipient the best responses. The extracochlear device consisted of a single electrode that was placed just outside the cochlea near a structure called the round window. The Vienna device also used single-channel analog processing of sounds, but the processing was more sophisticated than that used in the 3M/House implant (Luxford & Brackman, 1985; Tyler & Tye-Murray, 1991; Wilson, 1993). The majority of individuals who received the Vienna device received their implant in Europe.

Speech perception results, as reported in the scientific literature, appeared better than those obtained with the 3M/House device, with a few implant recipients achieving speech understanding through the device without the aid of visual cues. However, most of these results came from non-English-speaking subjects, and this level of benefit could not be replicated with English-speaking adult subjects in the United States. The Vienna/3M device is no longer available; however, the Vienna group (now the Med-El company) has developed another single-channel system. This implant has both a body-worn and ear-level processor. It has been used in Europe, mainly in individuals whose cochlea may be filled with new bone growth following meningitis, thus making the insertion of a long, multichannel electrode array into the cochlea more difficult (Hochmair-Desoyer, Steinwender, Klasek, Sürth, & Kerber, 1994). Currently, it is not used in the United States.

Other single-channel systems have been developed for both clinical and research purposes in England, Switzerland, Germany, and France. However, none of these devices to date, other than the Vienna/3M device, has been used in the United States.

Multichannel Cochlear Implants

Multichannel cochlear implant systems have multiple electrodes that are placed within the cochlea and are stimulated independently. Each electrode receives different information about the sound signal. Electrical stimulation of different places or sites within the cochlea has the potential of producing different pitch sensations for the implant recipient that can provide important information for speech understanding. Multichannel devices attempt to preserve some of the normal tonotopic or frequency organization of the cochlea. In multichannel implants, specific electrode sites within the cochlea are stimulated to cause activation of focused groups of nerve endings that would attempt to mimic the patterns found in the normal auditory system. Thus, while single-channel implants provide some continuous information about the temporal (timing) and intensity (loudness) characteristics of speech, multichannel implants also provide this information, as well as important data about the frequency characteristics of the speech signal.

A number of different multichannel implant systems have been built in the United States and elsewhere. Eddington and colleagues at the University of Utah developed a six-electrode cochlear implant with reference electrodes that were placed outside the cochlea. The electrode array was inserted approximately 22 mm into the inner ear. This array was attached to a connector that came through the skin. The speech processor changed the incoming sound information from the ear-level microphone into an analog electrical signal and divided this signal into four separate channels. The output of each channel was sent simultaneously to a different electrode in the cochlea. Based on the testing of each individual's responses on the six electrodes, four of the six electrodes in the cochlea were chosen for receiving the electrical stimulation. Thus, this was a four-channel system. Information from the lowest-frequency channel was directed to the electrode placed deepest into the cochlea; progressively, each higher-frequency channel stimulated more basally placed electrodes, with the highest-frequency channel stimulating the electrode closest to the middle ear (Eddington, 1983; Dorman, Hamsly, Dankowski, Smith, & McCandless, 1989). In the United States, this system was studied only in adult subjects with profound deafness under the auspices of a multicenter clinical investigation regulated by the FDA. The technology was purchased by the Smith & Nephew Richards Company (and is known as the Ineraid device) with the intention of making it commercially available. However, it did not gain the necessary regulatory approval in the United States. This device is no longer available.

The research group at the University of California San Francisco (UCSF) also developed a four-channel system that included an electrode array with 16 electrodes placed on precurved silicone rubber material shaped like the turns of the cochlea. During surgery, the array was straightened temporarily for insertion approximately 24 mm into the cochlea. Once the array was inside, it resumed its original curved shape. The 16 electrodes formed eight electrode pairs, four of which were chosen for electrical stimulation. The speech processor divided the incoming sounds into four separate bands or channels. Analog electrical signals from the four channels of the processor were sent to four separate external coils that transmitted the signal across the skin by radio-frequency (RF) transmission to four individual implanted receiving coils connected to the array (Rebscher, 1985). Based on individual testing during the fitting process, four electrode pairs inside the cochlea were selected to receive electrical stimulation. Output from the lowest-frequency channel of the processor was sent to the selected electrode pair that was deepest in the cochlea, and each of the progressively higher-frequency channels of the processor was delivered to an electrode pair that was placed closer to the base of the cochlea. All four electrode pairs were stimulated simultaneously with analog waveforms.

Storz Instrument Company manufactured the UCSF device during the FDA-regulated clinical investigation in adult subjects. However, the clinical trial and manufacture of the device were suspended so that the system could be redesigned. The redesigned UCSF cochlear implant system has become the present-day Clarion Multistrategy Cochlear Implant, manufactured by Advanced Bionics Corporation (Figure 2 on the next page). This device, which will be discussed in more detail later, was implanted in adult subjects with profound deafness under the auspices of a FDA-regulated clinical investigation from 1991–1996, when regulatory approval was gained for commercial distribution. In the United States the device was under clinical investigation in children until June 1997, when regulatory approval was received.

At the University of Melbourne in Melbourne, Australia, Clark and associates focused their work on a system that delivered digitally controlled, electrical pulsatile stimuli to electrodes implanted in the cochlea. *Pulsatile stimuli* are a digitized series of pulses or square waves that are used to represent the original sound waveform. The height (amplitude) and the width (duration) of each pulse can be varied. These variations result in changes of perceived loudness. In addition, the rate can vary at which the pulses are sent to stimulate the

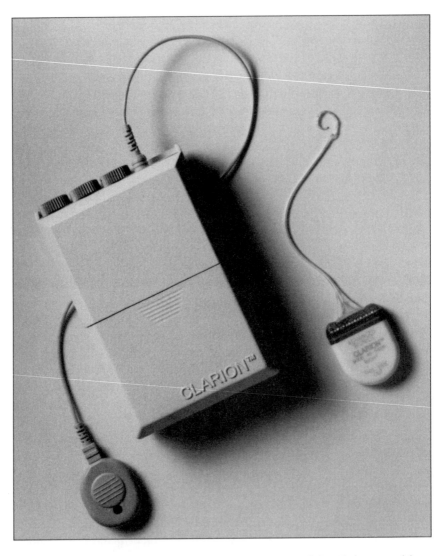

Figure 2   The internal and external components of the Clarion cochlear implant system. The implanted component, called the implantable cochlear stimulator (ICS), consists of the intracochlear electrode array, receiving antenna or coil, and the electronics package. As with the early UCSF implant, the 16 electrodes are placed on a precurved carrier and arranged as eight pairs in such a way as to bring them closer to the auditory nerve endings. The array is connected to the electronics, which are encased in a hermetically sealed ceramic case to keep out body fluids (Schindler & Kessler, 1993; Kessler & Schindler, 1994).

auditory nerve fibers. In the system developed by Clark and colleagues, pulsatile stimuli were delivered to electrode pairs sequentially (i.e., one at a time) as opposed to simultaneously (Patrick & Clark, 1991). An outcome of the original research was collaboration between the University of Melbourne and the company, Nucleus Limited (now Cochlear Limited), based in Sydney, Australia, that manufactured the device. This device is known as the Nucleus 22 Cochlear Implant System.

The device included an array with 22 banded electrodes placed on a flexible silastic carrier which could be inserted up to 25 mm into the cochlea. The array was connected to the implanted receiver/stimulator. Information about the incoming sound was analyzed, and specific features of the speech sounds, known to be important for speech understanding, were extracted and digitally encoded by the speech processor for delivery to the electrodes. The digital code was sent across the skin by RF transmission to the receiver, where it was decoded so that the hermetically sealed stimulator could send electrical pulses to specific electrode pairs along the array. Based on the frequency information extracted from incoming sounds, specific electrodes at specific locations within the cochlea were stimulated, one after the other, with electrical pulses. Again, an attempt was made to preserve some of the tonotopic organization of the cochlea. That is, each electrode was assigned a frequency band, with the electrodes deepest within the cochlea receiving low-frequency or low-pitch information and progressively higher-frequency information being assigned to electrodes at locations progressively closer to the base of the cochlea (Patrick & Clark, 1991; Brimacombe & Beiter, 1996).

In 1983, clinical studies regulated by the FDA began in the United States with adults who were postlinguistically deafened (deafened after learning language), and the FDA granted commercial distribution of the implant system for use in this population in 1985. Subsequently, clinical trials began in children aged two years and older, and the device became available on a commercial basis in 1990 for use with children who have profound hearing impairments.

Over the last 15 years, four speech-processing strategies have evolved for use with the Nucleus device. Each strategy became more complex and provided more information about speech and environmental sounds. To date, development of this system has resulted in the commercial introduction of four different speech processors. However, the internal components have remained the same. The latest and most advanced strategy, called Spectral Peak or the SPEAK strategy, is implemented in the Spectra 22 speech processor (Figure 3). In the SPEAK strategy, each of the active electrodes in the cochlea is assigned to one of the 20 digitally programmable bandpass filters. The filter outputs are scanned repetitively, and the filters with the greatest outputs (called maxima) are selected. During each cycle, an average of six (and up to 10) electrode pairs are stimulated. The electrodes that are chosen depend upon which filters contain the maxima at any given moment. This strategy emphasizes the spectral (pitch and intensity) aspects of speech sounds.

Recent research from the Austrian group (Med-El) has focused on an eight-channel implant system (the COMBI 40; Figure 4, page 14) that delivers sequential pulsatile stimuli at a very high stimulation rate to the electrodes implanted inside the cochlea. The speech processor divides the sound signal into eight frequency bands. The information in each of the bands is digitized and sent across the skin on an RF carrier. The electrical stimulation sent to the electrodes is a series of pulses. For each stimulation cycle, each of the eight electrodes is stimulated one at a time. The amount of electrical current sent to each electrode is proportional to the output (the amount of energy) from each of the eight bandpass filters (frequency bands) (Zierhofer, Peter, Brill, Czylok, Pohl, Hochmair-Desoyer, & Hochmair, 1994). This type of stimulation strategy, developed by Blake Wilson and colleagues, is called *continuous interleaved sampling* (CIS) (Wilson, Lawson, Zerbi, Finley, & Wolford, 1991; Wilson, Lawson, Zerbi, & Finley, 1994). The most recent system manufactured by the Med-El Company (the COMBI 40+) can stimulate up to 12 separate channels.

Chouard and colleagues in France worked on various multichannel designs, which culminated in a 12-channel electrode array in which the electrodes were placed in depressions along the carrier that was inserted into the inner ear. Later, this array included 15 separate electrodes. The most recent system uses digital signal-processing technology to divide sound information into 15 separate bands or channels. Each channel is assigned to one of the electrodes in the cochlea. Stimulation of the electrodes occurs sequentially with electrical pulses that vary in height and width according to the amount of current delivered to the nerve fibers. The amount of electrical current is directly related to the amount of energy in the original sound input. Like most of the present-day devices, the electrical signal is sent across the skin by RF transmission to the implanted receiver and electrode array (Mecklenburg & Lehnhardt, 1991; Beliaeff, Dubus, Leveau, Repetto, & Vincent, 1994).

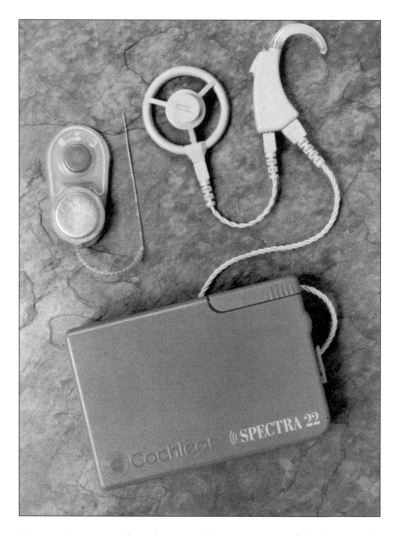

Figure 3   Internal and external components of the Spectra 22 cochlear implant system. The current version of the speech processor is powered by an AA battery.

The most recent version of the device, called the Digisonic DX10, is manufactured in France by the MXM Company and is not available in the United States.

Other multichannel systems have been developed in Germany, Belgium, and England. However, none of these systems have been used in the United States.

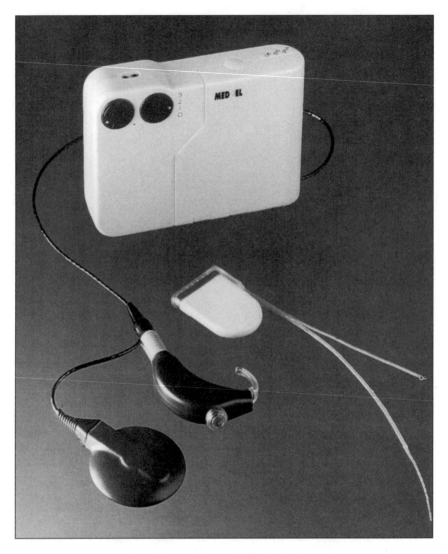

Figure 4   The internal and external components of the Med-El cochlear implant system.

How Cochlear Implants Work

Cochlear implants are designed to replace the sensory cells (i.e., the hair cells of the cochlea) of the auditory system. The hair cells convert the mechanical fluid motion of the inner ear into electrical impulses that are transmitted by the auditory nerve and interpreted by the brain as sound. Individuals with sensorineural hearing impairment have damaged or nonfunctional hair cells within the cochlea. When the hair cells are damaged or missing, sound cannot be converted into electrical impulses. In contrast to implants, hearing aids simply amplify the sound waves or pressure changes that reach the inner ear; they do not replace a nonfunctional part (in this case, the hair cells) of the system. Because the cochlea and its function are very complex, present-day cochlear implants are only a substitute and not a true replacement of the sensory cells.

Cochlear implants work by placing electrodes within or near the cochlea and applying an electrical current to the electrode site. This current spreads and, thus, stimulates the remaining neural tissue. The resulting electrical discharge of auditory nerve fibers proceeds up through the auditory neural tracks in the brainstem to the brain for interpretation. While each cochlear implant system has distinguishing characteristics, all systems share some basic components. All contain wearable, external, and implanted internal components. Sounds in the environment are picked up by a microphone, typically worn at ear level, and are changed into an electrical signal that is sent to the processor via thin cables. This ongoing electrical representation of the original acoustic signal is manipulated or processed. The processing of the original sound patterns into electrical patterns or code is specific to each system. The output from the external body-worn processor is sent to the implanted portion, called the cochlear implant. Present-day clinical systems (Figure 5 on the next page) use transcutaneous communication from the external to the internal coil, meaning that the skin is intact and coded electrical information is sent across the skin, often by radio-frequency (RF) transmission from a transmitting coil or antenna. The coded signal is picked up by an internal receiving coil, decoded, and sent to the stimulator portion of the implant. Based on the decoded information received, the stimulator delivers varying amounts of electrical current to specific electrodes that have been implanted within the cochlea. This current stimulates the auditory nerve fibers. The resulting neural impulses continue up the central nervous system to the auditory centers of the brain for interpretation.

Cochlear implants are individualized to the specific requirements of each recipient. In particular, each individual's settings are directly related to the amount of electrical energy (current) needed to generate a soft or "just hearing" response and a comfortably loud hearing level on each electrode pair that will be used. The difference between the amount of

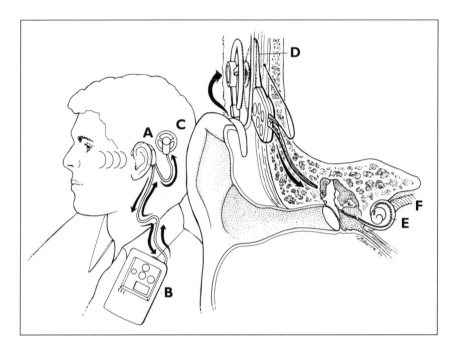

Figure 5 How cochlear implants work: Sound is picked up by a micro-phone (A) and sent to the processor (B) where the signal is manipulat-ed and coded. The output from the processor is sent to the transmitting coil (C), then this coded signal is sent across the skin to the receiving coil and stimulator portions of the cochlear implant (D). The stimulator delivers electrical current to the electrodes that have been implanted in the cochlea (E). The resulting neural activity travels up the hearing nerve (F) to the brain for interpretation.

electrical current that causes a comfortably loud hearing response and the amount of current to "just hear" (i.e., the threshold) is called the *dynamic range*. The dynamic range will vary from person to person and from electrode to electrode in the same individual. The fitting of multichannel devices may include place-pitch assessment (i.e., the ranking of the perceived sounds resulting from the stimulation of each electrode from lowest to highest pitch) and the selection of which elec-trodes will be used for stimulation. In multichannel systems, typically this individualized fitting or programming is accomplished with a com-puter, device-specific customized software, and an interface unit that is unique to each implant system. Today's speech processors are micro-computers that store in memory the specific electrical stimulation requirements for the individual recipient of a cochlear implant. The information stored in the processor can be updated easily through reprogramming. In chapter 4, Shapiro and Waltzman provide detailed information about programming each of the systems that is currently available for use in children.

Present Multichannel Cochlear Implant Systems

The Med-El COMBI 40 and the COMBI 40+
Cochlear Implant Systems

These systems, manufactured by the Med-El Company of Innsbruck, Austria, as described briefly above, are the outgrowth of research by the Austrian group in collaboration with various research institutions. The main differences between the COMBI 40 and the COMBI 40+ relate to the maximum number of channels available for electrical stimulation (eight in the COMBI 40 and 12 in the COMBI 40+) and to the thickness of the implanted receiver/stimulator portion. The thickness of the COMBI 40+ has been reduced to approximately four millimeters.

For both models, the implanted part consists of a small receiver/ stimulator, the electrode array, and the reference electrode. The electronic components of the receiver/stimulator are contained within a ceramic case. The integrated circuit that determines the stimulation can send out a total of over 18,000 pulses per second to the implanted electrodes. The electrode array of the COMBI 40+ has 24 electrodes that are arranged as 12 connected pairs. The COMBI 40 has 16 electrodes arranged as eight connected pairs. The reference or ground electrode is separate from the active electrodes and is placed outside the cochlea during surgery. Electrode pairs (between the intracochlear and the ground electrode) are stimulated with sequential pulses.

The external equipment includes an ear-level microphone, transmitter, body-worn processor, and cables. The processor uses two AA batteries. The processor codes sound information and sends this coded signal to the implant by RF transmission. The processor can store up to three different programs in its memory. Currently, the COMBI 40 and 40+ implement a continuous interleaved sampling (CIS) strategy (Med-El, 1997). CIS strategies emphasize the timing or temporal information contained in speech rather than the specific frequency information of the various speech sounds (Wilson et al., 1994).

At this time in the United States, the Med-El COMBI 40 is undergoing multicenter clinical investigation under the auspices of the FDA. The study is limited to adults with postlinguistic profound deafness. In Europe, adults and children have received this device. In addition, in Europe, some adults and children have received COMBI 40+ implants. The COMBI 40+ is not available for clinical trial in the United States currently (June, 1998).

The Advanced Bionics Corporation Clarion Multistrategy Cochlear Implant System

The Clarion cochlear implant system (Figure 2, page 10) became available on an investigational basis in 1991 for adults with postlinguistic profound hearing impairment. This device is now commercially available for use in adults and children with profound deafness. It utilizes earlier research from the University of California San Francisco group, in addition to collaborative efforts from the Neuroscience Program Office of the Research Triangle Institute (RTI) in North Carolina and MiniMed Technologies, a manufacturer of cardiac pacemakers.

The external portion of the system includes a speech processor and a headpiece. The headpiece consists of the microphone and RF transmitting antenna or coil worn on the head over the implanted part. The headpiece is held in place over the internal portion by a set of magnets, one located in the headpiece and the other in the implantable cochlear stimulator (ICS). The headpiece is connected to the processor by a cable. The processor receives sound, processes it into a maximum of eight filters or channels, and digitally codes the information. The processor receives power from a battery pack and sends the necessary power and coded information across the skin via the RF transmitter to the ICS. The speech processor can store up to three separate programs. This provides flexibility, especially when fitting the device in young children.

Processing of speech is accomplished through either an analog strategy, called simultaneous analog stimulation (SAS), or a pulsatile strategy, called continuous interleaved sampling (CIS). In the analog strategy, the eight electrode pairs are stimulated simultaneously with a continuous electrical current that represents the amount of energy in the input bands. In the pulsatile strategy, electrical pulses that vary in rate (pulses per second), amplitude (height of the pulse), and duration (total time of the pulse) are presented nonsimultaneously to the eight electrode pairs. Currently, children receive programming that uses only the CIS pulsatile strategy.

When using the CIS strategy, the maximum rate of stimulation for each channel depends upon the pulse duration, the pulse rate, and the number of channels used. The device has a moderate overall maximum rate of stimulation of 6,664 pulses per second when using all eight channels. The CIS strategy emphasizes the temporal, or continuously varying timing information in speech. Most users of the Clarion receive programming that employs the CIS strategy (Kessler & Schindler, 1994; Advanced Bionics, 1997).

The initial version of the system (version 1.0) became available for commercial distribution in adults in 1996. Shortly thereafter, version 1.2, using a slightly smaller implant and processor, also became commercially available for adults. Pediatric clinical trials with version 1.2 of the system began in March 1995, and regulatory approval for commercial distribution in children occurred in June 1997.

The Nucleus 22 Cochlear Implant System

Clinical trials with the Nucleus 22 system began in 1983 with adult subjects who were postlinguistically deafened. The device became available for commercial distribution in 1985. In 1986, pediatric clinical trials commenced with approval for commercial distribution in 1990. The electrode array is made up of 22 banded electrodes and 10 nonstimulating support rings that gradually decrease in diameter (as does the cochlea) along a flexible silicone rubber carrier. This array can be inserted up to approximately 25 mm into the cochlea. The receiving coil is located around the perimeter of the implant, and the integrated circuit is placed inside within a hermetically sealed titanium case. The entire receiver/stimulator package is covered with a biocompatible, flexible silicone rubber (Patrick & Clark, 1991; Brimacombe & Beiter, 1996).

The cochlear implant consists of the implanted receiver/stimulator package and the electrode array. The external components are the behind-the-ear microphone, the transmitting coil, the speech processor, and the connecting cables. The current version of the speech processor, the Spectra 22 (Figure 3, page 13), is powered by an AA battery. It receives continuously varying electrical signals from an ear-level microphone, divides this information into 20 programmable frequency bandpass filters, and continuously scans the outputs of the filters. The processor selects the six to 10 filters with the most acoustic energy (called maxima), digitizes the information, and delivers pulsatile stimulation that represents the strongest energy in the signal. Each of the 20 frequency filters is assigned to one of the 20 active electrode pairs (or channels) within the cochlea. The electrode pair deepest in the cochlea is assigned the lowest-frequency/lowest-pitch filter, and the electrode pair nearest the middle ear at the base of the cochlea is assigned the highest-frequency/highest-pitch filter. The integrated circuit scans the filter outputs, and up to 10 electrode pairs may be stimulated in quick succession to represent the speech signal at any given time. On average, six electrode pairs (or channels) are stimulated for each scan of the filters. The overall stimulation rate is approximately 2000 pulses per second. This strategy is known as Spectral Peak (SPEAK).

The SPEAK strategy is designed to represent the continuously changing frequency information that is inherent in speech and is critical for speech understanding. This speech-processing strategy continuously varies the rate of stimulation and the number of different channels stimulated at the 20 possible sites, based on the specific frequency and intensity information extracted from the ongoing speech signal. All the information is changed to a specific digital code and sent across the skin by RF transmission from the external transmitting antenna coil to the internal receiver. The digital stream of information is decoded, and the stimulator sends electrical pulses to the selected electrode pairs (Brimacombe & Beiter, 1996; Seligman & McDermott, 1995; Staller, Beiter, & Brimacombe, 1994).

Candidacy Issues of Children

The evaluation of potential pediatric cochlear implant candidates occurs most effectively within the framework of a team, consisting of the parents together with professionals from otolaryngology, audiology, speech-language pathology, auditory habilitation (auditory-verbal, where available), education, and psychology. Professionals from other disciplines may be invited onto the team as the need arises. Adolescent and teenage implant candidates also are included as part of their own team. Cowan and Clark (1997) and Caleffe-Schenck (1993) provide excellent reviews of the goals, objectives, and dynamics of a multidisciplinary cochlear implant program.

Table 1 summarizes the recommended pediatric selection criteria. These are guidelines to assist the team in selecting those children who are likely to benefit from a cochlear implant, and the guidelines apply regardless of which device is being used (Brimacombe & Beiter, 1996; Staller et al., 1994).

The family is vital to the team approach, providing information about the child's communication abilities through residual hearing as well as his or her use of other communication modalities. The family provides the necessary support structure for the child's development

Table 1. Preoperative Selection Criteria for Children

1.   Profound bilateral sensorineural hearing loss.

2.   Two years of age and older.

3.   Intact auditory nerve.

4.   Little or no benefit from hearing aids. For children whose hearing aids have not been previously or appropriately amplified, a minimum six-month trial with hearing aids or other sensory devices is recommended, in conjunction with appropriate intensive auditory therapy.

5.   No medical contraindications to undergoing surgery.

6.   No active middle-ear disease.

7.   An educational setting that emphasizes auditory therapy and communication.

8.   The family, and, if possible, the candidate should be highly motivated and have realistic expectations.

and use of either amplification or the cochlear implant. Thus, the parents must be well informed about their child's hearing loss and any special needs their child may have. This includes advocating for services, in partnership with professionals involved in the child's education and habilitation, and being fully committed to the long-term habilitation process (Beiter & Estabrooks, 1996).

Team professionals have the responsibility of explaining the results of all evaluation procedures to the family, using terms that are understandable. They provide information about the cochlear implant process, which includes the importance of commitment to auditory-oral or auditory-verbal habilitation in order to maximize outcomes. Professionals must explain how the cochlear implant works and detail the financial responsibility associated with long-term maintenance of the system. They explain alternative communication approaches that could be chosen and the long-term expectations that might be anticipated with each alternative available to the family. Arranging for families who are considering a cochlear implant for their child to talk openly with other families who have made the decision is valuable in uncovering potential misunderstandings and unrealistic expectations. Such issues should be resolved prior to implantation.

From an audiological perspective, children with bilateral, profound (>90 dB HL [Hearing Level]) sensorineural hearing loss who obtain minimal information about speech through well-fitted amplification may be considered for cochlear implantation. Present criteria stipulate that children should be two years of age or older. (In December 1997, the FDA approved lowering the age limit to 18 months for the Nucleus 22 system.) In order to assess benefit from amplification, pediatric cochlear implant candidates should undergo a trial period (typically, at least six months) with hearing aids, during which time they should receive very intensive auditory habilitation. The purpose of the trial is to determine whether they can obtain sufficient help from amplified residual hearing to develop speech and language through audition or audition and speechreading.

The surgeon and other medical professionals, as necessary, evaluate the child's overall physical condition, making sure that there are no contraindications to surgery. Preoperatively, high-resolution CAT scans are taken to examine the cochleae and assist in the selection of the ear for implantation. The surgeon's role and the surgery are discussed in detail in chapter 3.

The speech-language pathologist and/or therapist assess the child's overall communication abilities and may conduct a period of diagnostic teaching to determine the amount of information that the child receives through amplified residual hearing. Regardless of the child's primary communication mode, it is important to assess the child's speech production and oral language skills (both receptive and expressive). The educator and parents also provide important information about how the child communicates on a daily basis. The child's teacher reviews the child's academic, auditory, cognitive, linguistic, and social functioning in the school setting. The team psychologist may assist the parents with any behavioral issues and also can evaluate the child's cognitive, social, and emotional development. The psychologist along with other team members can discuss with the parents and, when appropriate, the candidate, their expectations regarding benefits from the device. The psychologist helps to make an assessment of whether these expectations are potentially realistic and whether the family is motivated to provide the long-term support needed for the child to maximize use of the device.

It is important that the entire team meet as a group to discuss their evaluations and final recommendations regarding implantation. The parents will play an integral role in this team meeting. The pediatric candidacy evaluation process is reviewed in detail in Brimacombe and Beiter (1996).

Results: Auditory Skill Development of Children Using Cochlear Implants

Multichannel cochlear implants are designed to provide important information about sound that will allow children to develop the basic auditory skills necessary to use hearing and speech for communication. These skills develop over time, and the rate of progress will vary from child to child. Thus, it is important that children's abilities are assessed periodically to measure progress and to assist in setting goals for auditory learning. Many variables can influence the amount of benefit an individual child receives. One important factor is the commitment of the family, therapists, and teachers to following a strong auditory habilitation program.

Typically, the evaluation of auditory skills in children has consisted of the assessment of speech perception abilities using the cochlear implant. These abilities range from the most basic — the detection of sound — to the most complex — the comprehension of spoken language. Audiologists and therapists favor the use of a battery of speech perception measures to evaluate more completely the skills the child is developing. It is important to choose tests that are appropriate for the child's chronological age, cognitive level, and language abilities. Tests may be either *closed set,* in which case the child chooses the response from a number of predetermined alternatives, or *open set,* in which case the child is not provided with any alternatives from which to choose. Researchers such as Geers and Moog (1987), Geers and Brenner (1994), Staller, Beiter, Brimacombe, Mecklenburg, and Arndt (1991), and Dowell and Cowan (1997) have proposed categorizing speech perception abilities as a method of summarizing children's performance on various tests. These categories may range from the simple detection of speech sounds to good open-set word recognition.

Studies have shown that children using multichannel cochlear implants demonstrate significant improvement in the identification of words within a closed set using hearing alone and in their lipreading abilities compared with their preoperative performance with hearing aids (Geers & Brenner, 1994; Staller, et al., 1994; Tyler, Fryauf-Bertschy, Kelsay, Gantz, Woodworth, & Parkinson, 1997). Also, many children develop some open-set word and/or sentence recognition, although this level of performance is reached over a period of time. Some researchers have reported very high levels of open-set speech recognition, especially in children who received their cochlear implant at an early age and are in auditory-oral communication settings. This research has shown that even children who are born with profound hearing loss or lose their hearing very early in life can reach high levels of performance. However, for these children, the age at implantation appears to be a significant factor in predicting performance (Staller et al., 1994; Waltzman, Cohen, Gomolin, Shapiro, Ozdomar, & Hoffman, 1994; Dowell & Cowan, 1997; Osberger, 1997).

Researchers have shown that young children can take advantage of more advanced speech coding strategies to improve their auditory skills even if they have learned most of their information about sound with a different, less sophisticated speech coding strategy. For example, after six to 12 months of use of the SPEAK strategy, the majority of children who change to SPEAK achieved open-set speech recognition. In contrast, a much smaller proportion (20%) of these children achieved this level of performance with the earlier multipeak speech coding strategy, even with extended experience (Staller, Menapace, Domico, Mills, Dowell, Geers, et al., 1997).

Children's speech production skills and general speech intelligibility improve with cochlear implant use, provided that they receive appropriate training. Improvements in both the accuracy of the production of individual speech sounds, as well as an increase in the number of different sounds produced, have been documented (Tobey, Geers, & Brenner, 1994; Dawson, Blamey, Dettman, Rowland, Parker et al., 1995; Robbins, Kirk, Osberger, & Ertmer, 1995). In one study (Osberger, Robbins, Todd, & Riley, 1994), the speech intelligibility of children in oral communication and total communication settings was compared. These children were matched on important variables, such as the age at which they lost their hearing, the age at implantation, and duration of implant use. Although there was a wide range of measured speech intelligibility across the children, the average intelligibility of children in oral settings was double that of the children using total communication. In fact, none of the children using total communication were as intelligible as the most intelligible children in the oral group.

Future Directions

Cochlear implantation is a relatively young field, and advances in the technologies will continue as more research is done and as computer technology improves. Past research has shown that as the signal processing improves, so does performance with cochlear implants. As more and more advanced speech coding strategies are developed, it is expected that performance with implants also will increase. For example, it is possible that the stimulation of a greater number of electrodes at faster rates will improve performance (Patrick & Evans, 1995). Speech processors will become smaller, so that they are more attractive cosmetically.

Recently Cochlear Corporation introduced, under clinical investigation in the United States, a new multichannel system, the Nucleus 24 Cochlear Implant System (Figure 6). This system consists of a new cochlear implant and two speech processors, one body-worn (SPrint) and the other an ear-level processor (ESPrit). The Nucleus 24 cochlear implant uses the same electrode array as the Nucleus 22, with the addition of two extracochlear reference electrodes. It includes a new integrated circuit that will allow programming of a variety of different

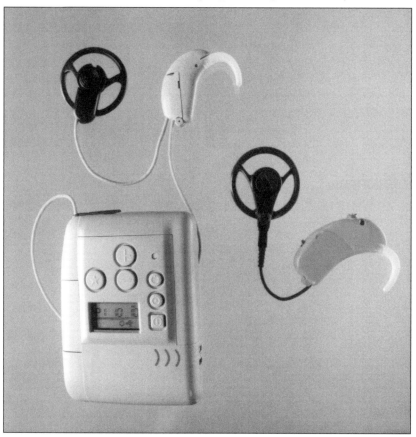

Figure 6   The Nucleus 24 cochlear implant system.

coding strategies, including Spectral Peak type strategies and continuous interleaved sampling strategies, as well as others.

The SPrint speech processor stores up to four different programs, as well as a number of features that can be programmed for the specific needs of the individual. Some of these, such as the ability to lock the user-operated controls, may prove to be particularly useful in children. Because of its flexibility, this processor is the platform for implementation of new coding strategies for the Nucleus 24 cochlear implant. The ear-level ESPrit stores two separate programs and is designed to be a cosmetic alternative to the body-worn processor (Cochlear Corporation, 1997; Lai, Dillier, Laszig, & Fisch, 1996).

In the future, selection criteria for children may be broadened to permit even younger children to receive a cochlear implant. Research with congenitally deafened young children who have implants suggests that the earlier sound experience is provided to children, the faster they progress in learning to use sound for meaningful communication (Dowell & Cowan, 1997; Robbins, Svirsky, & Kirk, 1997; Staller et al., 1994). Thus, it may be beneficial to give children a cochlear implant as early as feasible, after it has been determined that hearing aids are insufficient. In addition, as cochlear implant results continue to improve, children who gain minimal benefit from hearing aids may be considered as cochlear implant candidates.

References

Advanced Bionics Corporation. (1997a). *Strategies: Advanced Bionics information update: The power of Clarion.* Sylmar, CA: Author.

Advanced Bionics Corporation (1997b). *Clarion pediatric clinical study.* Sylmar, CA: Author

Beiter, A.L., & Estabrooks, W. (1996). The cochlear implant and auditory-verbal therapy. In W. Estabrooks (Ed.), *Auditory-verbal therapy for parents and professionals.* Washington, DC: A.G. Bell Association for the Deaf.

Beliaeff, M., Dubus, P., Leveau, J.M., Repetto, J.C., & Vincent, P. (1994). Sound signal processing and stimulation coding of the Digisonic DX10 15-Channel Cochlear Implant. In I.J. Hochmair & E.S. Hochmair (Eds.), *Advances in cochlear implants* (pp. 198–203). Vienna, Austria: Manz.

Brimacombe, J.A., & Beiter, A.L. (1996). Cochlear implants. In S.E. Gerber (Ed.), *The handbook of pediatric audiology.* Washington, DC: Gallaudet University Press.

Caleffe-Schenck, N. (1993). Pediatric cochlear implant candidacy: Educational, therapeutic and parental issues. *Auricle.* Auditory-Verbal International, Alexandria, VA.

Clark, G.M. (1997). Historical perspectives. In G.M. Clark, R.S.C. Cowan, & R.C. Dowell (Eds.), *Cochlear implantation for infants and children.* San Diego, CA: Singular Publishing.

Cochlear Corporation. (1997). *Nucleus CI24M Cochlear Implant System information.* Englewood, CO: Author.

Cowan, R.S.C., & Clark, G.M. (1997). The Melbourne Cochlear Implant Clinic Program. In G.M. Clark, R.S.C. Cowan, & R.C. Dowell (Eds.), *Cochlear implantation for infants and children.* San Diego, CA: Singular Publishing.

Dawson, P.W., Blamey, P.J., Dettman, S.J., Rowland, L.C., Parker, E.J., et al. (1995). A clinical report on speech production of cochlear implant users. *Ear & Hearing, 16,* 551–561.

Dorman, M.F., Hamsly, M.T., Dankowski, K., Smith, L., & McCandless, G. (1989). Word recognition by 50 patients fitted with the symbion multichannel cochlear implant. *Ear & Hearing, 10,* 44–49.

Dowell, R.C., & Cowan, R.S.C. (1997). Evaluation of benefit: Infants and children. In: G.M. Clark, R.S.C. Cowan, & R.C. Dowell (Eds.), *Cochlear implantation for infants and children.* San Diego, CA: Singular Publishing.

Durrant, J.D., & Lovrinic, J.H. (1977). *Bases of hearing science.* Baltimore: Williams & Wilkins.

Eddington, D.K. (1983). Speech recognition in deaf subjects with multi-channel intracochlear electrodes. *Annals of the New York Academy of Sciences, 405,* 241–258.

Geers, A.E. (1994). Techniques for assessing auditory speech perception and lipreading enhancement in young deaf children. In A.E. Geers & J.S. Moog (Eds.), Effectiveness of cochlear implants and tactile aids for deaf children: The sensory aids study at Central Institute for the Deaf. *Volta Review, 96* (5), 85–96.

Geers, A.E., & Brenner, C. (1994). Speech perception results: Audition and lipreading enhancement. In A.E. Geers & J.S. Moog (Eds.), Effectiveness of cochlear implants and tactile aids for deaf children: The sensory aids study at Central Institute for the Deaf. *Volta Review, 96* (5), 97–108.

Geers, A.E., & Moog, J.S. (1987). Predicting spoken language acquisition of profoundly hearing-impaired children. *Journal of Speech and Hearing Disorders, 52,* 84–94.

Hochmair-Desoyer, I.J., Steinwender, G., Klasek, O., Sürth, W., & Kerber, M. (1994). Results with the Med-El devices in ossified cochleas. In I.J. Hochmair-Desoyer & E.S. Hochmair (Eds.), *Advances in cochlear implants* (pp. 483–487). Vienna: Manz.

House, W.F. (1996). *The AllHear Cochlear Implant System: The AllHear devices, their manufacture, preliminary test results and the future.* Newport Beach, CA: AllHear.

House, W.F., & Berliner, K.I. (1991). Cochlear implants: from idea to practice. In H. Cooper (Ed.), *Cochlear implants: A practical guide.* London, UK: Whurr.

Kessler, D.K., & Schindler, R.A. (1994). Progress with a multistrategy cochlear implant system: The Clarion. In I.J. Hochmair-Desoyer & E.S. Hochmair (Eds.), *Advances in cochlear implants* (pp. 354–361). Vienna: Manz.

Lai, W.K., Dillier, N., Laszig, R., & Fisch, U. (1996). Results of a pilot study with the Nucleus CI24M/SP5 Cochlear Implant System. Paper presented at the Third European Symposium on Pediatric Cochlear Implantation, June 6–8, Hanover, Germany.

Luxford, W.M., & Brackman, D.E. (1985). The history of cochlear implants. In R.F. Gray (Ed.), *Cochlear implants*. San Diego, CA: College Hill Press.

Mecklenburg, D.J., & Lehnhardt, E. (1991). The development of cochlear implants in Europe, Asia and Australia. In H. Cooper (Ed.), *Cochlear implants: A practical guide*. London, UK: Whurr.

Med-El Corporation. (1997). *Information for candidates, COMBI 40+*. Innsbruck, Austria: Author.

National Institute of Health Consensus Statement. (1995, May 15–17). *Cochlear implants in adults and children, 13* (2), 1–30.

Osberger, M.J. (1997, May). Clarion Multistrategy Cochlear Implant Pediatric Clinical Trial update. Paper presented at the Auditory-Verbal International Conference, Ottawa, Canada.

Osberger, M.J., Robbins, A.M., Todd, S.L., & Riley, A.I. (1994). Speech intelligibility of children with cochlear implants. In A.E. Geers & J.S. Moog (Eds.), Effectiveness of cochlear implants and tactile aids for deaf children: The sensory aids study at Central Institute for the Deaf. *Volta Review, 96* (5), 169–180.

Patrick, J.F., & Clark, G.M. (1991). The Nucleus 22 Channel Cochlear Implant System. *Ear & Hearing, 12* (4), 3S–9S.

Patrick, J.F., & Evans, A.E. (1995). Implant design for future coding strategies. *Annals of Otology, Rhinology & Laryngology, 104* (9) (Suppl. 166), 137–138.

Rebscher, S.J. (1985). Cochlear implant design and construction. In R.F. Gray (Ed.), *Cochlear implants*. San Diego, CA: College Hill Press.

Robbins, A.M., Kirk, K.I., Osberger, M.J., & Ertmer, D. (1995). Speech intelligibility of implanted children. *Annals of Otology, Rhinology & Laryngology, 104* (9) (Suppl. 166), 399–401.

Robbins, A.M., Svirsky, M., & Kirk, K.I. (1997). Children with implants can speak but can they communicate? *Archives of Otolaryngology—Head & Neck Surgery, 117* (3, Pt. 1), 155, 160.

Schindler, R.A., & Kessler, D.K. (1993). Clarion Cochlear Implant: Phase 1 investigational results. *American Journal of Otology, 14,* 263–272.

Seligman, P., & McDermott, H. (1995). Architecture of the Spectra 22 speech processor. *Annals of Otology, Rhinology & Laryngology, 104* (9) (Suppl. 166), 139–141.

Simmons, F.B. (1966). Electrical stimulation of the auditory nerve in man. *Archives of Otolaryngology, 84,* 2–54.

Staller, S.J. (1985). Cochlear implant characteristics: A review of current technology. *Seminars in Hearing, 6,* 23–32.

Staller, S.J., Beiter, A.L., & Brimacombe, J.A. (1994). Use of the Nucleus 22 Channel Cochlear Implant System with children. In A.E. Geers & J.S. Moog (Eds.), Effectiveness of cochlear implants and tactile aids for deaf children: The sensory aids study at Central Institute for the Deaf. *Volta Review, 96* (5), 15–39.

Staller, S.J., Beiter, A.L., Brimacombe, J.A., Mecklenburg, D.J., & Arndt, P. (1991). Pediatric performance with the Nucleus 22 Channel Cochlear Implant System. *American Journal of Otology, 12* (Suppl.), 126–136.

Staller, S.J., Menapace, C., Domico, E., Mills, D., Dowell, R.C., Geers, A.E., et al. (1997). Speech perception abilities of adult and pediatric implant recipients using the Spectral Peak (SPEAK) coding strategy. *Archives of Otolaryngology—Head & Neck Surgery, 117* (3, Pt. 1) 236–242.

Tobey, E., Geers, A.E., & Brenner, C. (1994). Speech production results. In A.E. Geers & J.S. Moog (Eds.), Effectiveness of cochlear implants and tactile aids for deaf children: The sensory aids study at Central Institute for the Deaf. *Volta Review, 96* (5), 102–129.

Tyler, R.S., Fryauf-Bertschy, H., Kelsay, D.M.R., Gantz, B.J., Woodworth, G.P., & Parkinson, A. (1997). Speech perception by prelingually deaf children using cochlear implants. *Archives of Otolaryngology—Head and Neck Surgery, 117* (31, Pt. 1), 180–187.

Tyler, R.S., & Tye-Murray, N. (1991). Cochlear implant signal processing strategies and patient perception of speech and environmental sounds. In H. Cooper (Ed.), *Cochlear implants: A practical guide.* London, UK: Whurr.

Waltzman, S.B., Cohen, N.L., Gomolin, R.H., Shapiro, W.H., Ozdomar, S.R., & Hoffman, R.A. (1994). Long-term results of early cochlear implantation in congenitally and prelingually deafened children. *American Journal of Otology, 15* (Suppl. 2), 9–13.

Wilson, B.S. (1993). Signal processing. In R.S. Tyler (Ed.), *Cochlear implants: Audiological foundations.* San Diego, CA: Singular Publishing.

Wilson, B.S., Lawson, D.T., Finley, C.C., & Wolford, R.D. (1991). Coding strategies for multichannel cochlear prostheses. *American Journal of Otology, 112* (Suppl.), 56–61.

Wilson, B., Lawson, D., Zerbi, M., & Finley, C. (1994). Recent developments with CIS strategies. In I.J. Hochmair-Desoyer & E.S. Hochmair (Eds.), *Advances in cochlear implants* (pp. 103–112). Vienna: Manz.

Yost, W. , & Nielsen, D.W. (1977). *Fundamentals of hearing: An introduction.* New York: Holt, Rinehart & Winston.

Zierhofer, C., Peter, O., Brill, S., Czylok, T., Pohl, P., Hochmair-Desoyer, I.J., & Hochmair, E. (1994). A multichannel cochlear implant system for high-rate pulsatile stimulation strategies. In I.J. Hochmair-Desoyer & E.S. Hochmair (Eds.), *Advances in cochlear implants* (pp. 204–207). Vienna: Manz.

CHAPTER 2

Cochlear Implants for Young Children: Ethical Issues

Thomas Balkany, M.D.
Annelle V. Hodges, Ph.D.
Kenneth W. Goodman, Ph.D.

Ethics is the study of such concepts as goodness, duty, rightness, and obligation. In bioethics, these concepts are applied to practical problems raised in health care and biomedical research. Many of these problems arise along with the testing and adoption of new medical technologies. The second half of the 20th century has seen an extraordinary array of new and evolving technologies, ranging from organ transplantation and gene manipulation to life support systems and electronic medical records. This chapter considers ethical controversy surrounding another technological development: cochlear implants for children, and is based in part on the authors' previous work in this area (Balkany, Hodges, & Goodman, 1996).

Cochlear implants (CIs) represent an emerging technology that has the potential to change fundamentally the way people live. From the medical point of view, the CI is a safe and effective treatment for a severe disability — profound deafness. From the point of view of Deaf culture, however, it is unnecessary technology that is demeaning to deaf people's way of life (Lane, 1993). In the opinion of some Deaf activists, anything that prevents deafness or restores hearing to children who are deaf, threatens Deaf society (Lane, 1993; Pollard, 1987). As a result of this perceived threat, there have been organized attempts to suppress CIs throughout the 1990s (Balkany, 1993).

It is essential to appreciate that Deaf society is dependent for perpetuation of itself on children who are deaf whose parents have normal hearing. Since 90 percent of children who are deaf are born to two hearing parents and 97 percent to at least one hearing parent, it is widely thought that if parents were given a safe and effective option to provide hearing to their child, many would choose to do so. If a large number of children who are deaf did not enter Deaf society, that society could be essentially changed. And because medical technology affects society, conflicts of an ethical nature may occur.

Members of mainstream society, or even the blind (who share with the deaf the inability to utilize one of humankind's dominant senses, but may not otherwise be similar), may have difficulties understanding opposition to providing a child who is deaf with the ability to hear. However, many in the Deaf community see their way of life as emotionally fulfilling, promising, and independent without hearing (Balkany, 1993; Balkany & Hodges, 1995: Balkany, 1995). Some Deaf leaders also claim that the deaf are an oppressed linguistic minority and that any intervention to provide hearing to children who are deaf is inherently racist (Lane, 1993).

In the case of cochlear implants for children, the elements of conflict may be framed as issues that concern honesty, autonomy, beneficence, the best interests of the child, the needs of a linguistic minority to perpetuate itself, the cost of deafness to society, and acceptance of diversity.

Truthfulness

It is inherent that CI teams recommending implantation truthfully provide full information to parents as part of the process of obtaining informed consent. This includes not only describing the risks and benefits of the operation, but also ensuring that parents understand the limitations of the technology, the requirement for auditory (re)habilitation, as well as the options of joining Deaf society, communicating in American Sign Language (ASL), and avoiding "treatment" of deafness entirely.

Deaf culture is rich and diverse, and its members are bonded by ASL as well as by social and political organizations (Balkany, 1993; Lane, Hoffmeister, & Bahan, 1996). Deaf people attend parties, date, marry, have families, and raise children. In short, there are many positive aspects of life in the Deaf community, and they are best described to parents by a member of Deaf society.

Just as CI teams do with CIs, Deaf society proponents have an inherent responsibility to describe fully the positive as well as the negative aspects of life in Deaf society and to state their reasons for opposition to restoration of hearing. As in the informed-consent process for surgery, this discussion needs to be truthful and complete, allowing parents the autonomy to decide for themselves whether their child should receive a CI. Unfortunately, many members of Deaf society have been misinformed about CIs. One reason this has occurred is that the average graduate of a Deaf residential high school reads at a third- to fourth-grade level (Dolnick, 1993; Conrad, 1979) and is thus incapable of accessing moderately sophisticated published information in the lay media. Since there is no written form of ASL, many in the Deaf community rely on informal sources of information such as newsletters and storytellers at Deaf clubs. Deaf leaders and educators who, to a substantial degree, control this information, have misled the Deaf community in a highly successful effort to generate opposition to CIs (Balkany, 1995).

Examples of the misleading, pejorative picture of CIs painted by Deaf leaders include articles in Deaf culture newsletters:

"I would be remiss not to equate cochlear implants with genocide" (Silver, 1992).

"There is absolutely no question that our government has a hidden agenda for deaf children much akin to Nazi experiments on Holocaust victims" (Silver, 1992).

"Using deaf children as 'lab rats' and medical guinea pigs is profoundly disturbing" (Roots, 1994).

Much more distressing, however, are inventions by respected colleagues designed to sway public opinion. Dr. Yerker Andersson, Professor and Chairman, Department of Deaf Studies at Gallaudet University and Emeritus President of the World Federation of the Deaf, published an article in the *World Federation of the Deaf News* in which he reported (without supporting reference) a surgeon who was "eager to use his skills on 17 Deaf individuals." According to Prof. Andersson, "Three died due to complications and one became mentally ill. The rest were failures" (Andersson, 1994). In fact, no deaths or cases of mental illness have been caused by CIs, and after hundreds of scientific papers and years of study, the U.S. Federal Drug Administration, medical oversight organizations, and even insurance carriers have concluded that CIs are safe and effective (Balkany, 1993). To say simply that Andersson was incorrect is to underestimate his scholarly abilities.

It is generally considered unethical to mislead people purposefully in order to persuade them to a point of view. The ethical principle violated by Andersson and others is autonomy as it relates to self-determination. People are deprived of their right to decide for themselves when they have been purposefully misled.

It is not surprising that, as a result of widespread misinformation, there is widespread misunderstanding. Many people who are deaf fervently believe that CIs are often fatal or severely damaging to children and they are therefore opposed to them. The following are representative verbatim quotations from the future leaders of the Deaf community, college students at Gallaudet:

"I read few articles about how cochlear implant. For deaf people died from cochlear implant. It was explained about how cochlear implant affected to brain damage."

"I feel that cochlear implants are wrong because it makes the recipient a robot with wires sticking out of their head."

"I may not aware of cochlear implant much but I do have a strong against it" (letters to the William House Cochlear Implant Study Group, a committee of the American Academy of Otolaryngology — Head and Neck Surgery, 1993; author's files).

Internal Inconsistency and Conflict of Interest

Other examples of failure to respect the value of truthfulness are seen in Deaf leaders' advocacy of mutually contradictory positions. For example, it is claimed that deafness is not a disability and, at the same time, that people who are deaf are entitled to disability benefits amounting to billions of dollars per year. Another is that CIs do not work and also that they work so well as to eliminate deafness (genocide). Consciously supporting both sides of mutually exclusive arguments in order to influence public opinion is not considered ethical behavior. Deaf advocates must decide whether to tell parents that the deaf or hard of hearing are independent or that the majority require disability (and other entitlement) benefits. They must decide whether it is ethical to say to parents that CIs don't work and to politicians that CIs work so well that they are genocidal.

Deaf activists who believe that their way of life is threatened by CIs may find themselves in conflict of interest. Barbara White, writing as an Associate Professor at Gallaudet, succinctly reveals this conflict of interest: "... the future of the deaf community is at stake. An entire subculture of America will no longer exist" (letters to the William House Cochlear Implant Study Group, a committee of the American Academy of Otolaryngology — Head and Neck Surgery, 1993; author's files). (Ear surgeons may be at similar risk for conflict of interest. It is estimated that CI surgery, however, constitutes less than one-tenth of one percent of the operations performed by otologists. A CI program, rather than generating income, actually costs a great deal to sustain by cost shifting and philanthropy.)

This potential conflict of interest among members of the Deaf community may operate to the disadvantage of individual children who are deaf. Australian physician Henley Harrison wrote, "The motive in opposing cochlear implants in children is self-interest rather than the children's welfare... it is the welfare of the children that should be borne in mind, not some other group" (Harrison, 1991).

Ethical standards hold that Deaf advocates should reveal such conflicts of interest to parents who are considering the merits of life in Deaf society for their children. As a three-generation member of the Deaf community warns, "Parents should cast a cautious eye towards anyone wanting to sacrifice a deaf child towards preserving a culture" (Bertling, 1994).

In short, representatives of the Deaf community who wish to influence parents and the public must begin truthfully to reveal both the advantages and the disadvantages of life in Deaf society. Only in this way can parents make an informed decision regarding the best interests of their child.

Is Deafness a Disability?

Examination of the position that deafness constitutes neither a handicap nor a disability, but only an oppressed linguistic minority (Lane et al., 1996) is a central issue in the discourse about CIs for children. Deaf leaders surely understand that if deafness is not a disability, people who are deaf or hard of hearing must give up billions of dollars in public assistance that is intended for the disabled. In writing from the ethical perspective, Englehardt (1986) defines disability as the failure to achieve an expected state of function. Boorse (1975) more precisely defines disability as occurring (a) when a specific function is impaired, (b) there is reduced ability below typical efficiency, or (c) a limitation of functional ability occurs with reference to the patient's age or gender group.

It is clear that, in addition to its cultural definition, deafness fits the functional definition of a disability; but how does it compare with other disabilities? According to a California Department of Rehabilitation survey published in 1993, in which clients with all types of disabilities filled out self-assessment forms, deafness was associated with the lowest educational level, the lowest family income, the lowest percentage working, the lowest percentage in professional/technical jobs, and the poorest *self-assessment* of well-being (Harris, Anderson, & Novak, 1995). This study suggests that deafness is not only a disability, but that it may be among the most disabling of disabilities.

To deny that deafness is a disability, Deaf leaders must also deny its cost to society: $377,000 per child in K–12 residential Deaf school education (estimated $121.8 billion for educating all people who are deaf or hard of hearing at residential schools), $2.5 billion per year in lost workforce productivity, and more than $2 billion annually for the cost of equal access, Social Security Disability Income, Medicare, and other entitlements of the disabled (National Institutes of Health, 1992). As Tom Bertling, a third-generation member of Deaf culture, notes in his book, *A Child Sacrificed,* "Virtually every aspect of the deaf community is dependent on government support for the disabled" (Bertling, 1994).

Perhaps the greatest monetary cost to society of the disability of deafness is in education. It is estimated that the cost of kindergarten through 12th-grade education in Rhode Island is about $9,000 per hearing child. For children who are deaf who are mainstreamed in public schools, the cost jumps to $44,000 per child. If the same deaf students attend residential schools for the Deaf, the cost becomes $429,000 per child (Johnson, Mauk, Takeawa, Simon, et al., 1993).

At this high cost, what are the outcomes of current methods of, and approaches to, educating students who are deaf or hard of hearing? The average reading level of an adult who is deaf is at third or fourth grade (Conrad, 1979); further, when students who are deaf or hard of hearing finish high school, three of four cannot read a newspaper (Dolinick, 1993). In large part because of this low educational outcome, the deaf are too often unemployed or underemployed, resulting in a cost to society of $2.5 billion per year in lost wages (National Institutes of Health, 1992).

The Deaf community is well aware of the rights of the disabled under the Americans with Disabilities Act. As an example, a woman who was deaf sued a Maryland volunteer fire department because she was not selected to be a fire fighter (Strom, 1994). She was presumably unable to hear sirens, alarms, calls for help, or instructions for emergency action, and she could not express her own needs or instructions with sign language while holding a fire hose or climbing a ladder.

A controversial risk of deafness that is rarely discussed with parents is the prevalence of psychological disorders. Although this relationship has been confirmed by hundreds of independent investigators and scientific papers, the data on morbidity have been attributed by Deaf leaders both to poor parenting and to culturally/linguistically biased testing (Lane, 1993). Debate over the value of such data notwithstanding, ethical representatives of Deaf society must decide whether it is appropriate to discuss these studies with parents whom they are counseling about life in Deaf culture.

Another area that remains obscured from parents is much more difficult to approach delicately. Tom Bertling, in his second book, *No Dignity for Joshua* (1997), describes in painful detail the ongoing problem with the physical, emotional, and sexual abuse that occurs, especially to very young children, in residential Deaf schools. He feels that abuse is widespread, owing to a combination of low salaries paid to the nonprofessional members of the staff at state-run Deaf schools, a tendency among the Deaf community to conceal internal affairs, quasi-acceptance of such behavior within Deaf culture, and difficult communication between parents and their children who use ASL. Bertling's experiences are supported by scientific studies of over 480 abused children by Sullivan and colleagues (Sullivan, Brookhouser, Scanlan, Knutson, et al., 1991) showing a high incidence of sexual abuse in residential Deaf schools. On the basis of this awareness, several states are interceding to provide better supervision, especially for children who are deaf under the age of five years (Bertling, 1994). Although similar problems may also occur at any residential school where poorly trained staff are underpaid, Deaf advocates must decide whether the ethical principle of truthfulness requires that parents be made aware of possible problems of sexual and other abuse at residential Deaf schools.

Deaf Leaders vs. Parents

Deaf activists hold conferences on the unseemly topic, "Who Owns the Deaf Child?" (Barringer, 1993). Their answer is that children who are deaf or hard of hearing are de facto members of the Deaf community and that hearing parents are obliged to "give up the child" (a phrase used by the Deaf) to be acculturated by Deaf society (Dolnick, 1993).

By this, Deaf activists mean that the usual values taught in families, including morals, ethics, religion, love, security, self-esteem, as well as language, should be taught by culturally Deaf adults who are not part of the child's family (Lane, 1993). This process is termed *horizontal acculturation* (as opposed to *vertical acculturation,* in which these values are taught by parent to child, generation after generation). They claim that horizontal acculturation is best accomplished by removing the child from the home and placing him or her in a residential Deaf school (Lane, 1993).

Dr. Marina McIntire, director of ASL programs at Northeastern University, notes, "It has been argued that hearing parents have 'the right' to raise youngsters who are linguistically and culturally like themselves. We disagree" (letters to the William House Cochlear Implant Study Group, a committee of the American Academy of Otolaryngology – Head and Neck Surgery, 1993; author's files). Roz Rosen, president of the U.S. National Association of the Deaf in 1992, concurs: "Hearing parents are not qualified to decide about implants" (Coffey, 1992). In his book, *The Mask of Benevolence,* Dr. Harlan Lane states that parents cannot make decisions for their own child who is deaf because they don't "really know the patient" and are in a "conflict of interest with their own child." Lane has previously taken the position that a culturally Deaf adult who is not related to the child should be empowered to override the child's parents and make the decision as to whether a child should receive a CI (Lane, 1993).

This proposed intrusion into the American family is in direct conflict with Public Laws 94-142 and 99-4457, which ensure that children who are deaf are educated in the least restrictive environment (i.e., most like nonhandicapped children). These laws empower families of deaf children, and are directly opposed to horizontal acculturation (Gearhart, Wright, 1979; Katz, Marthis, & Merril, 1978).

Important Questions

Thus, two important questions arise regarding CIs for children: (1) Who should decide for the child? and (2) According to what standards should the decision be made?

The courts, as well as legal scholars and ethicists, concur that the rights and concerns of self-interest groups should be strictly excluded from decisions concerning the well-being of individual children (Buchanan & Brock, 1989). Interference from outside groups deprives families of their right to privacy. As Buchanan and Brock (1989) state in their book, *Deciding for Others: The Ethics of Surrogate Decision Making,* "the family must have great freedom from oversight, control and intrusion to make important decisions about the welfare of its children. Society should be reluctant to intercede in a family's decision."

Parents exercise free informed consent on behalf of their children. "Others do not have the right to intervene in their... actions" (Englehardt, 1986).

In addition, "There must be a clear locus of authority or decision making will lack coherence, continuity and accountability" (Buchanan & Brock, 1989). Only the child's parents, or in their absence, a legal guardian who has authority for all aspects of the child's life, can provide such continuity and accountability. The suggestion that a culturally Deaf individual be appointed to decide whether a child should or should not receive a CI (or, for that matter, any other medical treatment or procedure) would violate the principle of a clear locus of authority because that individual would not have authority or responsibility for any aspect of the child's life.

However, parental rights to make health care decisions for children, while broad, are not unlimited. For instance, a decision to forgo treatment for a disability or other treatable disorder might appropriately be regarded as neglect. Nonetheless, the exercise of a parent's judgment is rarely constrained, and only in extreme cases of neglect is parental judgment overridden.

Parents must bear the consequences and are financially responsible for decisions made about their children. Thus, only parents can decide for the child. But according to what principles should the choice be made?

Autonomy and Beneficence

Buchanan and Brock (1989) identify two underlying ethical values in making decisions for others: respect for self-determination (autonomy) and concern for well-being (beneficence).

In foreseeing the desire of special-interest groups such as Deaf society for influence, Engelhardt (1986) states, "This principle of autonomy provides moral grounding for public policies aimed at defending the innocent." In exercising autonomy for their children, parents act within the rights of their children, which include freedom of choice, respect for the individual, and free, informed consent to make decisions on behalf of their child. Engelhardt (1986) defines free choices as "being unrestrained by prior commitments or justified authority, and being free from coercion."

Associated with the right to self-determination is the right to privacy. When Deaf activists attempt to impose their wishes on parents of deaf children and suggest that parents are in conflict of interest with their own children, that they are not aware of their own children's best

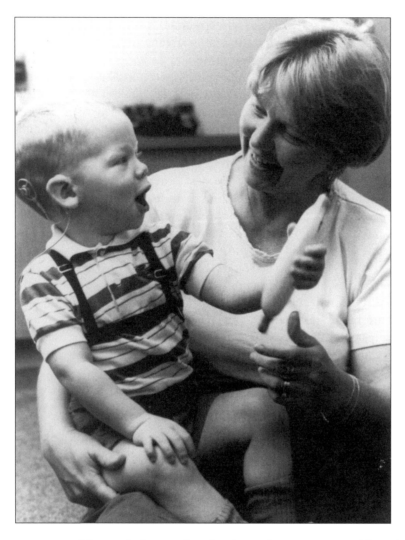

Figure 1   The underlying ethical values of autonomy and beneficence apply to the child as represented by his parents.

interests, and that only culturally Deaf adults should be allowed to act as proxy decision makers on behalf of the deaf child (Lane, 1993), they ignore the family's right to privacy and self-determination and, in doing so, trample the family's autonomy.

The ethical value of beneficence also guides parents. In simplest terms, it involves a prudent effort to do good and avoid evil

(Englehardt, 1986). Advocates of Deaf culture who claim that making CIs available to children who are deaf is tantamount to "genocide" for Deaf culture are more concerned with doing good and avoiding evil to their culture than honoring the value of beneficence as it applies to the child.

Beneficence also applies to the child's "right to an open future" (Buchanan & Brock, 1989). Children have clear interest in maintaining and developing functional abilities. The ability to hear not only has communicative value but also provides auditory enjoyment and is important to safety. Children who are deaf or hard of hearing also have an "opportunity interest" regarding preservation of opportunity for their future education, employment, and interpersonal relationships. Educational and employment expectations for culturally Deaf persons are unfortunately lower than those for hearing people (Balkany & Hodges, 1995; Dolnick, 1993). Since 99.8 percent of the population of the United States cannot communicate in ASL (Padden, 1987), opportunities for personal relationships (teachers, bus drivers, neighbors, friends) are highly restricted by primary or sole communication in ASL. Conversely, entering the hearing world may increase opportunity for education, employment, and personal relationships.

Standards for Making Surrogate Decisions

In addition to the two ethical values mentioned, there are three well-established standards for making surrogate decisions: advance directive, substituted judgment, and best interest. If an advance directive has been established by the patient, such as a living will or a specific nomination of surrogate, it should be meticulously followed. If none is available, a family member should make decisions on the basis of substituted judgment (using knowledge of the person, the surrogate does what he or she believes the person would do under the circumstances, if the person were competent). Neither of these first two standards applies to children. The third guiding standard, which does apply to children, is that of best interest. It is the parents' responsibility to make decisions according to their understanding of what is in the best interest of their child.

Diversity

A possible solution to the ethical conflict between the child's best interest and the needs of Deaf society to perpetuate itself lies in the well-established principle of social diversity. Efforts by Deaf leaders to keep the Deaf community pure, however, systematically exclude people who may be slightly different, for example, children who are deaf or hard of hearing and who have CIs. This demand for cultural purity, and the attendant exclusionary behavior, is generally not tolerated in advanced societies.

Diversity is a valued strength of modern society that requires open-mindedness and fairness. Whereas Deaf leaders rightfully insist that mainstream society accept Deaf persons, Deaf society itself systematically excludes children who are deaf or hard of hearing and who use CIs. As Bienvenue and Colonomos state, "... implanted children can never be fully accepted within the Deaf community" (letters to the William House Cochlear Implant Study Group, a committee of the American Academy of Otolaryngology — Head and Neck Surgery, 1993; author's files). Lane (1993) agrees that if CI patients "turn to the deaf community for support, they experience discrimination." Donnel Ashmore states that "if a child shows 'signs of hearism' this will result in a hostile, silent reprimand" (Lane, 1993).

CI recipients in elementary school have recently been taught a new sign for CIs by adult interpreters for the Deaf: the sign for "snake bite" made behind the ear. Such stigmatization is typical of societies that attempt to keep their ranks "pure" and avoid diversity.

Deaf advocates who oppose the diversity that children with CIs might bring seem to ignore the fact that the Deaf community is already diverse — socially, economically, educationally, and politically. Welcoming children who are deaf or hard of hearing and who are "different" (because they can use the CI to help them communicate) to be part of their community may enlarge and strengthen Deaf society.

Changing with the Times

Two recent strategic shifts in position have been notable in opposition to CIs: (a) in view of data showing remarkable hearing and language acquisition by children with CIs, some leaders have stopped emphasizing that CIs don't work and have begun to promote the notion that even if CIs restored hearing perfectly, they would be unacceptable (Lane, 1993); and (b) many Deaf leaders have retreated from their arguments that a representative of Deaf culture must decide whether a child receives a CI. They now agree that parents must be allowed that choice (Lane et al., 1996). It is hoped that others will follow this logic.

Another recent position adopted by some Deaf leaders is that cochlear implant professionals are in violation of United Nations conventions proscribing limitation of the growth of linguistic minorities. It would follow that since CIs work, they would limit the growth of the Deaf community (a linguistic minority): therefore, CIs are forbidden by the United Nations. This line of reasoning clearly establishes that these leaders are more concerned with the needs of their culture than with the best interests of deaf children.

In summary, the term deafness describes both an important, respected way of life and a disability. The ethical standard of truthfulness requires that representatives of Deaf society inform parents of both the positive and the negative qualities of life in Deaf society and that CI teams do the same regarding CIs.

The ethical values of autonomy and beneficence and the need for a single locus of authority in raising children determine that *parents* decide whether their child should receive a CI. The guiding standard for such a surrogate decision is best interest. Thus, parents must determine what is in the best interest of their child. The need of Deaf society to perpetuate itself has no bearing on that decision, although parents should consider the opinions and experiences of truthful Deaf adults.

The Deaf community should demand the same acceptance of diversity from itself that it does from mainstream society. There must be room for all who wish to join. Deaf society's goal of ethnic purity and its exercise of discriminatory exclusion of deaf children who have CIs countervail the norms of ethical behavior and weaken its moral position.

References

Andersson, Y. (1994). Do we want cochlear implants? *World Federation of the Deaf News, 1,* 3–4.

Balkany, T. (1993). A brief perspective on cochlear implants. *New England Journal of Medicine, 328,* 281–282.

Balkany, T. (1995). The rescuers, cochlear implants: Habilitation or genocide? *Advances in Otorhinolaryngology, 50,* 4–8.

Balkany, T., & Hodges, A.V. (1995). Misleading the deaf community about cochlear implantation in children. *Annals of Otolaryngology, 104* (Suppl. 116), 148–149.

Balkany, T., Hodges, A.V., & Goodman, K.W. (1996) Ethics of cochlear implantation in young children. *Archives of Otolaryngology—Head & Neck Surgery, 114,* 748–755.

Barringer, F. (1993, May 16). Pride in a soundless world. *New York Times* (pp. 1, 14).

Bertling, T. (1994). *A child sacrificed to the deaf culture.* Wilsonville, OR: Kodiak Media Group.

Bertling, T. (1997). *No dignity for Joshua*. Wilsonville, OR: Kodiak Media Group.

Boorse, C. (1975). On the distinction between disease and illnesses. *Philosophy and Public Affairs, 5,* 61.

Buchanan, A.E., & Brock, D.W. (1989). *Deciding for others. The ethics of surrogate decision making*. Cambridge, MA: Cambridge University Press.

Coffey, R. (1992). Caitlin's story on "60 Minutes." *The Bicultural Center News, 53,* 3.

Conrad, R. (1979). *The deaf school child: Language and cognitive function*. New York: Harper & Row.

Dolnick, E. (1993, September). Deafness as culture. *The Atlantic Monthly,* 37–53.

Englehardt, H.T. (1986). *The foundation of bioethics*. New York: Oxford University Press.

Gearhart, B.R., & Wright, W.S. (1979). *Organization and administration of educational programs for exceptional children*. Springfield, IL: Charles C. Thomas.

Harris, J.P., Anderson, J.P., & Novak R. (1995). An outcome study of cochlear implants in deaf patients. *Archives of Otolaryngology—Head & Neck Surgery, 121,* 398–404.

Harrison, H.C. (1991). Deafness in children. *Medical Journal of Australia, 154,* 11.

Johnson, J.L., Mauk, G.W., Takekawa, K.M., Simon, P.R., et al. (1993). Implementing a statewide system of services for infants with hearing disabilities. *Seminars in Hearing, 14,* 105–118.

Katz, L., Marthis, S.L., & Merril, E.C. (1978). *The deaf child in the public schools*. Danville, IL: Interstate Printers.

Lane, H. (1993). *The mask of benevolence*. New York: Vintage Books.

Lane, H., Hoffmeister, R., & Bahan, B. (1996). *A journey into the deaf world*. San Diego, CA: Dawn Sign Press.

National Institutes of Health Consensus Statement. (1992). *Early identification of hearing impairment in infants and young children, 11* (1), 1–12.

Padden, C.A. (1987). American Sign Language. In *Gallaudet encyclopedia of deaf people and deafness* (Vol. 3, pp. 43–53). Washington, DC: Gallaudet University Press.

Pollard, R.Q. (1987). Cross cultural ethics in the conduct of deafness research. *Rehabilitation Psychology, 37,* 87–99.

Roots, J. (1994). Deaf Canadian fighting back. *World Federation of the Deaf News,* 2–3.

Silver, A. (1992). Cochlear implant: Surefire prescription for long-term disaster. *TBC News, 53,* 4–5.

Strom, K.E. (1994, February). Disability regulations review. *Hearing Review,* 12–14.

Sullivan, P.M., Brookhouser, P.E., Scanlan, J.M., Knutson, J.F., et al. (1991). Patterns of physical and sexual abuse of communicatively handicapped children. *Annals of Otology, Rhinology & Laryngology, 100,* 188–194.

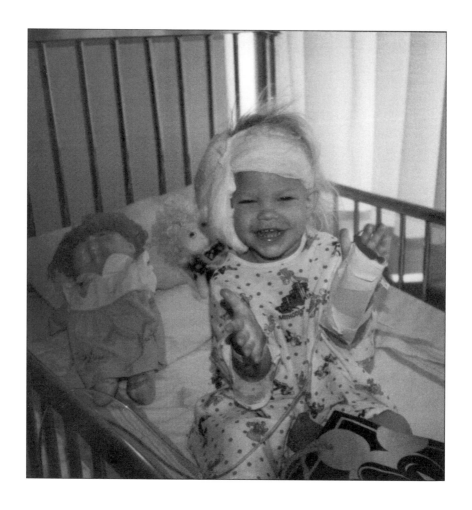

PART II

Surgery and Programming

Overleaf: Mandi Zbikowski, San Antonio, Texas, USA

CHAPTER 3

Cochlear Implant Surgery: What Parents Need to Know

Noel Cohen, M.D.

After the decision has been reached that your child is a candidate for receiving a cochlear implant, you will meet with the surgeon, who will explain to you and the child (if he or she is old enough) what is involved in the surgery. This chapter is written from the perspective of one surgeon and his team, and is not meant to contradict what you may hear from your surgeon. As with so many other things, there is more than one opinion on some aspects of cochlear implant surgery, and more than one possible technique. Wherever feasible, I have attempted to mention several approaches to a particular aspect.

The actual surgery occupies but a small percentage of the total time taken up by the testing, evaluation, stimulation, programming, and rehabilitation of your child who is hearing impaired, yet it is a period of anxiety, great tension, and potential risk. If the surgery is not correctly performed, the child may suffer complications or the implant may not function properly.

How to Prepare Your Child for the Surgery

For the very young child, there is no realistic way in which you can prepare him or her for the cochlear implant surgery. But for the older child, it may well be possible to explain that you both will be going to another place for a few days, and that he or she will go to sleep and wake up with a bandage and a "boo-boo" on the side of the head. The child can be told that you will go to another part of the doctor's office, where people will put things on the arm and finger, and there will be a mask with something to smell. You can tell the child that you will go with her or him until it is sleeping time, and that you will be there when it is time to wake up. You can also be reassuring that all the people will be very nice, and that there are lots of other kids who have had the same experience. There may even be a balloon to blow up! It is important for the child to understand that you will not leave, but will be there until you can go home, even though it may be the next day. The older child may want to know that there may be some discomfort, but you can say that it will go away with some medicine, and that there may also be some dizziness, which will also go away. All of this can be related to the fact that the visit to the hospital and the operation are to help him or her to hear better.

Where Will the Operation Take Place?

Cochlear implant surgery is usually an in-patient procedure, meaning that the patient spends the night of surgery in the hospital. Usually, the child is admitted early in the morning of surgery, goes to the recovery room following the operation, and then spends the rest of that day, as well as the night, in the pediatric unit of the hospital. You can count on being allowed to stay with your child in the hospital, except when the operation is actually going on. The operating room staff will help you to change into appropriate gowns to be able to take your child into the operating room, and will tell you where to wait until the surgery is finished. You will also be able to be in the recovery room, and will go to the pediatric unit with your child. The recovery room is often a rather intimidating place since there are so many other patients there, and your child may be disoriented, nauseated, and frightened. The nurses in the recovery room will periodically take the child's vital signs, record blood pressure, and check for bleeding.

Recently, some insurers and HMOs (health maintenance organizations) have insisted that cochlear implant surgery be performed as ambulatory surgery. This means that the child will be discharged to go home later on the day of surgery and will not be permitted to spend the night in the hospital. If there is any reason for concern, the surgeon can insist that the child be admitted and spend the night. Most often, this is done because of nausea or imbalance, which typically clear sufficiently the day following surgery for the child to be discharged. Regardless of whether the surgery is performed as an in-patient or ambulatory procedure, you will be given instructions about what to expect, what to give the child for pain (typically, nothing more than Tylenol), and when to see the surgeon next.

Going to the Hospital

In all probability, your child will be admitted to the hospital, or the ambulatory surgery unit, early on the day of the surgery, perhaps as early as 5:30 a.m. if it is the first surgery of the day. It is a good idea to bring a few favorite toys, a change of clothes for both of you, and perhaps a "security blanket" if the child has one.

It is important that the child not have *anything* to eat or drink after midnight in order to avoid vomiting during the induction of anesthesia. If the child is taking any oral medications, or is not feeling well in any way, check with the surgeon for specific instructions. You will go to an admitting area where you will be interviewed by several people, the child will be examined, and instructions will be given for the trip to the operating room. The child will be given an operating room gown, and you will either change into a scrub suit or be given a disposable overall to put on top of your clothes. If your child is old enough to comprehend, explain that you are both going to a very noisy place with lots of people who are going to help him or her. Also, try to explain about the operating table, anesthesia, and pulse monitor, which is a little band-aid with a red light that is put on the child's finger. The child may also be asked to blow up a "balloon" with gas in it to initiate the anesthesia process. All this is confusing, intimidating, and frightening, but you can reassure the child that you will be right there.

How Is the Operation Performed?

Cochlear implant surgery is performed under general anesthesia; that is, the child will be asleep throughout the procedure. Entering the operating room and beginning the anesthesia are the most difficult moments for the small child, and require the most tact and patience on the part of all the adults involved. The child usually cries as the anesthesia (most often a gas) is begun, but the associated deep breathing actually helps to speed the process since more of the gas is absorbed. After the child is asleep, you will usually be asked to wait outside during the rest of the procedure. Once the child is asleep, an intravenous drip is begun, a stethoscope and blood pressure cuff are placed, and a breathing tube is inserted through the mouth into the trachea (windpipe). This allows the anesthesiologist to administer the proper mixture of anesthetic agent and oxygen for the rest of the case. Some surgeons place facial-nerve monitoring electrodes next to the patient's mouth and eyes at this point. Antibiotics are usually given during the surgery and for a short time afterwards.

Hair is shaved behind and above the ear, the skin is washed and prepared with an antiseptic solution, and sterile drapes are placed around the ear as well as over the entire body. The position of the cochlear implant itself is then drawn on the scalp and the incision is marked, allowing sufficient space around the device.

A variety of incisions are used, depending on the surgeon's preference as well as the presence of any scars from prior surgery. The most commonly used incisions in North America are the inverted J and the C. Both offer good visualization of the operative field and are cosmetically acceptable, since the scar is hidden by the hair and the ear.

Many surgeons inject the incision with adrenaline in order to limit blood loss, and mark the site of the center of the well for the body of the implant with a drop of blue dye. The incision is then made using either a scalpel or the cutting current, which is a sort of electric knife. This has the advantage of sealing the blood vessels of the scalp as they are cut. The scalp is then separated from the bone above and behind the ear, exposing the bone.

An electric or air-driven drill is then used to create a recess or well in the bone behind the ear in order to accommodate the body of the implant. Small holes are then drilled above and below the well to allow sutures to be placed around the device. This combination of a well and tie-down sutures accomplishes several purposes: (a) it lowers the profile of the device so that it does not bulge under the scalp, (b) it renders the device less vulnerable to external trauma, and (c) it firmly secures the device to the side of the head so that it cannot move. This is particularly important, since movement of the implant may jostle the electrode out of the cochlea or cause erosion of the device through the scalp, or even failure of the implant itself. The mastoid bone, directly behind the ear, is then hollowed out with the drill, and a channel is created for the electrode between the well and the mastoid cavity.

Working through the mastoid cavity, with the assistance of an operating microscope, the surgeon then locates the facial nerve and creates an opening (the facial recess) just in front of it, into the middle-ear space. This then exposes the area of the round window, which is where the opening into the cochlea (the cochleostomy) will be made. Using a very fine drill bit, the surgeon creates an opening into the lower fluid-

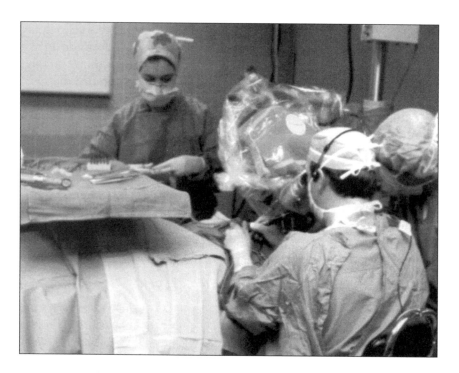

Figure 1   The surgeon inserts the internal components of the system, consisting of the electrode array and the implant electronics. The electronics are placed under the skin and behind the ear on the mastoid bone; the electrode array is inserted into the cochlea through the round window.

filled compartment of the cochlea (the scala tympani). At this point, depending on the device used, either the electrode is inserted and then the device placed and sutured into the well, or the device is fixed prior to inserting the electrode. Regardless of the order of steps, the electrode insertion is the most critical step in the operation and must be performed with great accuracy and delicacy. An attempt is made to insert all the electrodes, but force should never be used: it is much better to leave a few electrodes outside the cochlea than to take a chance of damaging the electrode array.

Once the electrode is inserted and the device is secured, the implant can be checked electronically to ensure that it is functioning, and that the patient is receiving the signal. At present these steps are somewhat complex, and not all centers are able to perform the full series of checks, but newer software is being developed to simplify these procedures. Tissue is then packed around the electrode in the cochleostomy to prevent any leakage of fluid out of the inner ear, and more tissue is placed in the facial recess in order to stabilize the electrode. A variety of techniques may be employed at this point to minimize the chance that the electrode might come out of the cochlea over time.

The incision is closed, using sutures and/or stainless steel staples, and a large dressing is placed over the ear. Sometimes the surgeon may place a drainage tube under the scalp for a day, but this is usually not necessary. We always take a single x-ray in the operating room to be absolutely sure of the electrode's position.

The child is then allowed to awaken and is taken to the recovery room, where you can also be present.

What Are the Risks of the Surgery?

There is always some slight risk that an accident will occur during the administration of general anesthesia. Since the large majority of children receiving cochlear implants are basically healthy, this risk is very, very small. In addition, there can always be excessive bleeding or infection following any surgical procedure, but these are, again, very rare in the case of cochlear implant surgery. The preoperative evaluation and work-up of your child will include questions and tests designed to minimize the chance of excessive bleeding, and the operation is always performed under an umbrella of prophylactic antibiotics.

There are several potential complications that are inherent in ear surgery: one is injury to the facial nerve, which would give rise to deformity of the face. The surgeon must work quite close to the facial nerve in opening the facial recess, but this is an approach used for many other ear operations, and facial-nerve injury is very uncommon. The risk is potentially greatest when dealing with a child with a congenital abnormality of the development of the inner ear (Mondini deformity); special care should be taken for these children. It is advisable for the surgeon to use a facial-nerve monitor when operating on patients with a congenital malformation of the inner ear, and some surgeons choose to use the monitor in all cases. The facial nerve is also vulnerable to thermal injury when the cochleostomy is being performed, but the techniques of avoiding this are well known.

Another potential complication of any surgery on the inner ear is postoperative dizziness. If there is any function remaining in the balance part of the ear that is chosen to receive the cochlear implant, opening into the inner ear in order to place the electrode may cause temporary imbalance. In fact, immediately after the operation it is not unusual for the child to vomit and have some imbalance for a day or two. This invariably subsides rapidly, leaving the child exactly as he or she was preoperatively in terms of balance. If the child has a Mondini deformity, there may be an abnormal communication between the inside of the head and the inner ear; this can give rise to a "gusher" during surgery, that is, a steady flow of spinal fluid coming through the cochleostomy. The surgeon can handle this by packing the cochleostomy to "cork" it against the flow of fluid. It may occasionally be necessary to place a drain in the child's spinal canal for a few days. It is very important that a gusher be stopped since it can cause headaches, imbalance, and a vulnerability toward meningitis. Fortunately, this is also extremely rare in the worldwide experience with cochlear implants in children.

The final potential risk with an implant is that of infection. Infections of the flap are very rare and are prevented by the appropriate use of antibiotics as well as a gentle surgical technique. At one time it was feared that children with cochlear implants might be more prone to middle-ear infections, or that these infections might be complicated by the presence of a cochlear implant. Fortunately, this has not turned out to be the case: children with implants have no more frequent ear infections than others, and there have been to date no serious complications of otitis media attributed to the presence of the cochlear implant. However, it is important that children with implants be appropriately and vigorously treated for middle-ear infection, and that the pediatrician work with the implant surgeon to coordinate their efforts.

The Postoperative Period

Immediately after the surgery, your child will be very sleepy and may complain of the tight bandage around the head. There may also be a drainage tube emerging from beneath that bandage. Fortunately, implant surgery is not particularly painful, and the child will not require any strong pain medications. Usually, the child sleeps through most of the remainder of the day of surgery. It is not unusual for the child to vomit later during the day of surgery.

The following day, your child will be allowed out of bed and may be a bit "wobbly" on taking the first few steps. There may also be further vomiting, the result of anesthesia and inner-ear imbalance. This

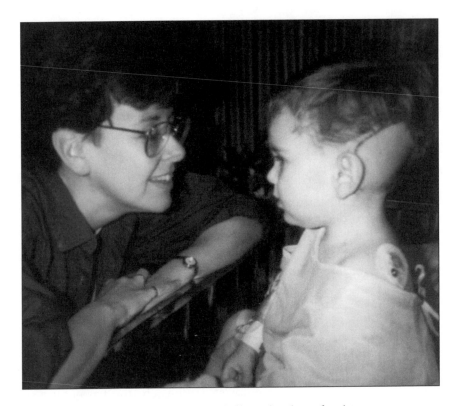

Figure 2   Mom visits with Eric Sieloff on the day after his surgery.

will subside during the course of the day. The large bandage will be removed by one of the doctors or nurses, and you can take the child home with no dressing over the wound. Again, typically pain medication is very mild; Tylenol usually suffices.

Taking the Child Home

Before you leave the hospital, you will be given instructions on how to take care of your child at home. In brief, you should avoid direct injury to the surgical site, but can bathe the child 24 hours after the operation. Use baby soap and shampoo, rinse the area well, and pat it dry. The stitches or staples can tolerate wetting but should not be soaked. The wound may appear slightly puffy but should not become more swollen or red after the child leaves the hospital. Typically, the child will not like to be touched in this area and will probably not want to sleep on that side. The swelling of the flap usually makes the ear appear more prominent, but this will go down over time. Continue to give the child Tylenol if necessary, and be careful if there is still some imbalance present. If there should be any progressive swelling or redness of the wound, or discharge from the ear, call your implant surgeon.

After a few days, the swelling will start to diminish and any imbalance should subside. The child should be able to attend school or a play group within a few days after surgery.

The Healing Period

The initial healing takes approximately 10 days, at which time stitches or staples will be removed by the surgeon or members of the team. Keep the ear dry for 24 hours after removal of the stitches or staples. After that, the child may bathe normally, but prolonged immersion of the incision should be avoided. During the next few weeks, the incision heals more strongly and can tolerate more direct manipulation of the area. At this time, it may seem that the implant has become more prominent. What actually is happening is that the swelling of the flap has gone down, making the outline of the implant seem more apparent. Any protrusion of the ear should also subside about this time.

Activity and Other Limitations

During the immediate postoperative period, vigorous physical activity that might expose the child to trauma over the implant should be avoided, but after approximately three or four weeks, even this limitation can be stopped. While it is impossible to prevent children from playing, siblings should be encouraged to avoid trauma to the surgical site.

After final healing has taken place, the child can resume normal activity, but should be firmly instructed on wearing protective headgear when engaging in sports such as baseball, football, soccer, horseback riding, and hockey, all of which may expose the child to the risk of trauma to the area. In addition, exposure to electrostatic discharge (ESD), such as that generated by plastic sliding ponds, should be avoided. This is best done by turning off the speech processor and actually removing it from the child's person. Although implants have become more resistant to ESD, an effort should be made to ground or spray computers and television sets in order to avoid the build-up of electrostatic charges. Aside from the above limitations, there is no reason why your child should not be able to participate fully in all the activities of growing up, using common sense and protective hardware. Considering the amount of uncontrolled activity in which children indulge, the problems with cochlear implants have been few and far between.

Long-Term Considerations

Cochlear implants are designed to last a lifetime, but the present generation of implants, of course, have only been used for less than 15 years. It may be that some of these devices will fail in the future and require replacement. On the other hand, the future may bring such a revolutionary change in implant technology that it will become desirable to replace the present cochlear implants with new devices, or to implant the second ear when possible. Only time will tell whether the emerging new generations of devices will prove to be substantially superior.

A significant long-term consideration is the fact that at the present moment cochlear implants should not be exposed to magnetic resonance imaging (MRI). Several possibilities for damage exist: the magnet may move because of the very powerful superconducting magnet in the MRI machine; the current in the MRI may cause damage to the implant itself; or, the current may be carried along the electrode array and damage the auditory nerve. For all these reasons, no current cochlear implant is considered MRI compatible. On the other hand, the multichannel auditory brainstem implant is MRI compatible, and there is a very significant likelihood that an MRI-compatible cochlear implant will be introduced in the near future.

What About Device Failures?

Cochlear implants are highly sophisticated, complex electronic devices. Although they are designed to last for decades, and undergo very rigorous quality-control testing, there is a certain small failure rate, as with all such electronic devices. Over the past few years, several failure modes have been identified by the manufacturers, and steps have been taken to minimize the chances of failure. These steps have included strengthening the attachment of the antenna, reinforcing the junction of the electrode with the body of the implant, changing the material of the implant case itself, and making changes to resist the effects of the electrostatic discharge.

Despite all these changes, some small failure rate is inevitable, and has actually occurred with all devices in use today. A device failure may manifest as a total sudden loss of hearing or as an intermittent malfunction. If you suspect that there has been a failure, make sure that the batteries are fresh and that the light on the speech processor goes on appropriately. Check also for breaks in the cable. Contact your cochlear implant center for an appointment to troubleshoot the entire system. There are tests that can be done at the center to ascertain whether the device has failed, but this may be very difficult in the case of an intermittent failure. Usually, an intermittent failure finally becomes total, and is then readily diagnosed.

If the device should fail, it will have to be replaced, requiring another operation. Fortunately, the second operation is usually less difficult than the first, and usually more successful. Typically, replacing the same device or even replacing one device with a different type gives rise to performance that is at least as good as that following the first operation. If your child has a device failure, be sure to inquire as to whether the implant is still under the manufacturer's warranty.

A Final Word

Cochlear implant surgery is technically challenging and absolutely critical for successful implantation. Nevertheless, it has been performed in over 15,000 cases by hundreds of surgeons in many countries. Although your young child cannot comprehend the experience, you, with the help of your surgeon and the hospital team, can prepare your child for the surgery and set the stage for successful implantation.

CHAPTER 4

Cochlear Implant Programming for Children: The Basics

William H. Shapiro, M.A.
Susan B. Waltzman, Ph.D.

P roviding a child with a cochlear implant requires decisions regarding candidacy, device, communication mode, rehabilitation strategy, and education. An effective team approach requires that all involved understand and appreciate the nature of the process, as well as the commitment of time required of family members. The purpose of this chapter is to provide basic information to parents, speech-language pathologists, educators of the deaf, and others who do not perform programming tasks.

Although the focus of this chapter is on programming the cochlear implant, it is important to have an overview of the process that leads up to postoperative care. The following sequence of events can be used as a guideline: questionnaire, evaluation, preparation for surgery, pre-programming, training, initial stimulation, programming techniques, and follow-up.

Questionnaire

Prior to initiating the formal evaluation, parents can be sent an intake questionnaire along with information about various implant devices. The questionnaire can include information regarding family, medical, educational, communication, and rehabilitation histories and general information regarding the implant program and process. When the family returns the questionnaire, they should include copies of the child's most recent audiometric and amplification data, as well as any relevant medical and rehabilitation information. The data obtained often serves to eliminate inappropriate referrals without subjecting the family to unnecessary and costly visits to the implant center. If the child is deemed a possible implant candidate, the next step in the process is the evaluation.

Evaluation

The evaluation requires the input and expertise of many professionals: audiologist, pediatrician, otolaryngologist (surgeon), radiologist, speech-language pathologist, psychologist, educational advisor, and social worker. In larger programs a team coordinator can facilitate the scheduling of appointments and the communication between the various professionals and the family.

In addition to beginning the assessment of the child's auditory function, the initial visit to the implant center should provide the parents with the information and guidance that they need regarding both the process and the cochlear implants available. The number of appointments necessary to complete the audiological and perception test battery is determined by the age and abilities of the child. Following the completion of these initial tests, the child may or may not be deemed a candidate based on either pure-tone audiometric data and/or the level of aided speech perception attained. If the child meets the audiologic criteria for implantation, the evaluation can proceed to include appointments with the surgeon, radiologist, and speech-language pathologist, among others. The age, mode of communication, amplification history, and related medical and social issues of both the proposed candidate and the family will often determine which of the team members need to be involved in the initial evaluation.

Young children are often referred for cochlear implants without having had the benefit of appropriate amplification and aural rehabilitation. Prior to the final decision regarding implantation, a trial period with hearing aids and habilitation/rehabilitation should take place. The length of the trial depends upon the skills of the child and the philosophy of the implant center. Upon completion, a second evaluation is performed to assess perceptual and linguistic progress. Considerations such as lack of growth of linguistic competence should be included in making the final decision. A formal evaluation can include standard audiometric procedures, measures to assess speech perception, language development, speech production, academic and psychological development (when appropriate), CT scans and MRI, if necessary, and other required medical tests. Then a decision regarding implantation can be made and surgery scheduled.

Preparation for Surgery

It is imperative to prepare the child for the surgery in order to minimize the trauma of the experience. The type and amount of orientation required depend on the age and needs of the child. The parents can best determine the extent to which the child needs to be exposed to the hospital environment prior to surgery. Often a booklet and a brief explanation suffice; some children are, however, more curious and require more detailed descriptions, or even a tour of the hospital.

A second part of the preparation is the postsurgical preprogramming training and adjustment to the device. During the one-month postoperative period, children who require additional orientation to auditory concepts can be trained to respond appropriately in preparation for the initial stimulation. The techniques used depend upon the age and developmental stage of the child and the methods preferred by the clinician. Continued use of conventional amplification on the nonimplanted ear during the one-month period between the surgery and initial stimulation is critical. If a child is extremely fearful or reticent or highly anxious, familiarizing him or her with the physical area where the programming will take place can be helpful.

Programming

The physical environment in which the programming takes place is critical in establishing a comfortable situation for the child and the parents, and should promote compliance and cooperation. The room should be equipped with child-sized chairs and table. The computer equipment necessary for programming should be placed facing away from the child. It can be comforting for the child if the walls are decorated with pictures, wall hangings, and drawings made by other children. Bright, but not overwhelming, colors on the walls and an adjacent observation room with a one-way mirror are desirable. It is imperative to have a variety of toys such as sponge blocks, pegboards, and wooden rings, which can be used to help condition the child to the electrical stimulus. Parents are encouraged to bring the child's favorite toy, especially for the initial stimulation.

Initial Stimulation

The day of the initial stimulation is clearly a time of great anticipation for parents. It can also generate much excitement and nervousness, which can be transmitted to the child and affect the child's behavior. Although it is impossible to eliminate or even reduce these emotions,

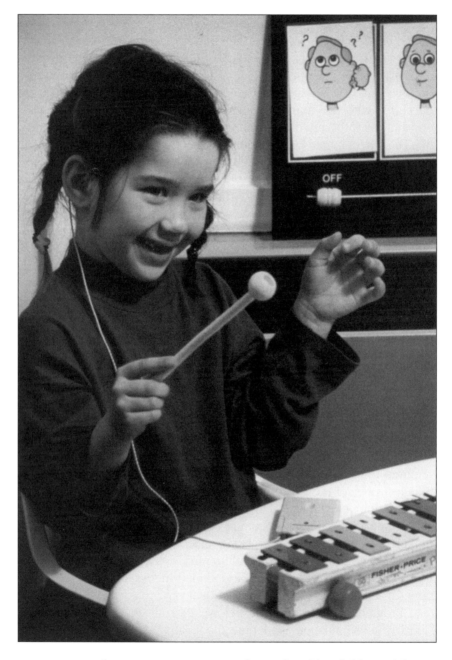

Figure 1 A pleasant environment with comfortable, child-sized furniture, interesting toys, and bright decorations will be more conducive to successful programming of the cochlear implant.

parents need encouragement to remain calm, particularly when very young children are involved. If the child is older or can separate easily from the parents, it is preferable that the only people in the room be the audiologists who are working with the child so that the parents do not inadvertently transmit their anxieties to the child. If the parents do not agree with this approach, they can stay in the room but must be encouraged to be unobtrusive so as not to interfere with the process.

The videotaping of programming sessions is very advantageous and serves a dual purpose: first, it helps the clinicians to document progress and secondly, it enables them to assess the methods used and the responses obtained. It is often difficult, however, to make judgments and adaptations during sessions. Videotaping allows for an objective review of the programming sessions so that modifications in methodology can be implemented when necessary.

Ideally two audiologists will participate in the programming: one will work with the child and one will program the device using a computer. Familiarity with all basic programming methods and options is essential prior to instituting a children's cochlear implant program. Although experience in programming adult implantees is helpful, the clinical acumen acquired by programming large numbers of children is irreplaceable. A broad range of professional training workshops and conferences offer clinicians the opportunity to share ideas and to discuss methods that can be adapted to the clinical environment.

The initial stimulation should be scheduled over a three-day period consisting of approximately three hours each day. The time is spent primarily in obtaining psychophysical measures, although the time required to program the electrodes is device related. For example, half the electrodes of the Nucleus device might be programmed on the first day and the remaining electrodes on the second day. The third day could then be used for fine-tuning (Cochlear Corporation, 1996). The Clarion device, however, has fewer electrodes but has the ability to store multiple programs so that, although the psychophysical measures for individual electrodes might be obtained in less time, the remaining time can be used for developing optional programs, when appropriate (see Programming Techniques, below). Not all children will respond similarly to stimulation, and thus the process could potentially take longer than three days. Thresholds (defined as the lowest level of response to electrical stimulation for a given electrode) and comfort levels (defined as the loudest level one can comfortably listen to for an extended period of time) that are established during the first or second day will most likely not be ideal. First, the children need time to adjust to the new signal. Tolerance for the loudness of the signal does increase over time. Secondly, physiologic changes occur which are reflected in the changes in thresholds over a period of months. Since accurate thresholds are basic to the access to sound and, therefore, to postoperative performance, it is advisable to schedule programming sessions at frequent intervals to reestablish both thresholds and comfort levels.

Programming Techniques

Encoding strategies can be defined as the method by which a given implant translates the incoming acoustic signal into patterns of electrical pulses, which stimulate the existing auditory nerve fibers. Despite the different strategies used by various devices, the basic elements of programming are not device dependent. That is, the audiologist needs to obtain thresholds and comfort levels on all electrodes for each device. The techniques, however, can differ. One of the most important parameters in effecting threshold and comfort levels is the stimulation mode. The Nucleus 22 device can be programmed in a bipolar mode (current flows between an active electrode and a ground electrode) or a common-ground mode (one electrode is stimulated while all others act as a ground), while the Clarion implant most frequently utilizes monopolar stimulation with children. The ground electrode in monopolar stimulation is outside the cochlea, while in common-ground and bipolar stimulation both the active and ground electrodes are within the cochlea. The wider area of stimulation provided by the monopolar configuration can serve to reduce threshold values. At this writing the Nucleus CI24M, which can also utilize monopolar stimulation, is undergoing clinical trials on adults and children in the United States. The Med-El COMBI 40 multichannel cochlear implant, which can also utilize various strategies, manufactured in Austria, is currently involved in clinical trials on adults in the United States.

On the initial day of programming the Nucleus device, the stimulus control knob can be used as a first pass at setting the thresholds. After the thresholds are established for half the electrode array, the audiologist can revert to keyboard control to obtain more accurate thresholds. A threshold is set at the lowest level at which the child responds 100 percent of the time. While the child is engaged in some activity, comfort levels for the same electrodes can be established. If the child is old enough, he or she can tell the audiologist when the sound is comfortable. With a young child, 25 to 50 units between the threshold and

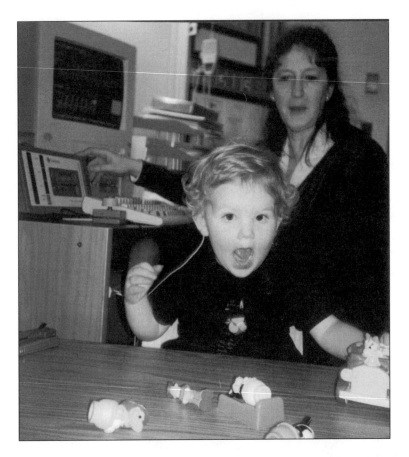

Figure 2   After thresholds and comfort levels are established for half the electrode array, the audiologist can work from the computer keyboard to obtain a more accurate threshold for each electrode.

comfort level is acceptable for the initial stimulation. Underestimating comfort levels can allow for a more rapid and fluid adjustment to the implant by reducing the possibility of frightening the child with a new and loud auditory sensation. The audiologist rotates the stimulus control knob slowly upward in order to note any adverse effects. All comfort levels are then checked to ensure that no adverse reactions occur. The same procedure is performed for the remaining electrodes on the second day of stimulation.

After the thresholds and comfort levels are obtained for all electrodes, the computer assimilates this information and translates it into an operating program that is placed into the child's speech processor. Live voice stimulation can then be initiated. Although many parameters — including global increases in thresholds and comfort levels and the determination of which sounds are directed to individual electrodes — can be manipulated, it is advisable with most children to remain as close as possible to the values suggested by the manufacturer until there is greater certainty regarding the accuracy of the child's responses.

In principle, establishing thresholds and comfort levels is the same with the Clarion device (Advanced Bionics Corporation, 1995). As with the Nucleus device, many parameters can be manipulated in an attempt to achieve optimum performance. The Clarion device currently has the capability of storing three different programs, which ultimately can be used in different listening environments. Switching between multiple programs, however, with young children recently stimulated is often confusing and counterproductive, and should be used with caution. A viable option is to store the same basic program in the three slots, with the only change being the loudness of each program.

Electrophysiologic (objective) measures have been proposed as an alternative to standard device programming. Although electrical auditory brainstem responses and electrical stapedius reflex (contraction of the muscle in the middle ear) measurements can be used to provide limited information on thresholds and comfort levels for initial stimulation, they cannot replace the accuracy of behavioral device-setting procedures, as described above, particularly at follow-up programming sessions.

Initial Responses

The initial response to hearing with the implant varies greatly. Many children show little or no response, while others may react fearfully. Very few young children exhibit positive initial reactions when first hearing an electrical signal. The audiologist must be able to differentiate between a device problem and a behavioral issue. Depending upon the age and emotional state of the child, informal responses to speech can be explored.

One of the most important aspects of the initial programming sessions is the parent's orientation. Although expectations are addressed during the evaluation period as well as prior to stimulation, it is imperative to repeat what can and cannot be expected of the child during the initial stages of using a cochlear implant. Excitement over the presence of heretofore-unseen auditory responses by the child often leads to unrealistic short-term goals that can be detrimental to the child's over-all progress. Parents must also learn the intricacies related to the daily care and troubleshooting of the device.

Daily Care and Troubleshooting

External equipment — including the speech processor, headset, and cables — is built to withstand activities of daily living. There are times, however, when malfunctions occur with or without provocation. Spare parts (including extra batteries, cables, and possibly, an additional headset) can be kept in inventory by the parents and the school to solve a simple problem. If replacing cords, batteries, or a headset does not help, then a phone call and, most likely, a visit to the implant center are necessary. There are daily-care recommendations outlined by each manufacturer that will assist in minimizing breakdowns. Parent kits, which accompany each implant unit, provide guidelines for troubleshooting to determine the nature of the problem, and the audiologist will review these with the parents during the initial stimulation period. It is important to remember, however, that electronic devices of any type can fail. The failure rate of the internal portion of cochlear implants in general is low; however, should a failure occur, reimplantation is necessary. To date, there have been no reports of complications or decreased performance following reimplantation.

Electrostatic discharge (ESD) is an ongoing problem for children using cochlear implants. This transfer of static electricity to the implant system can cause a breakdown in the electronics package or a corruption or elimination of the program stored in the processor. If this occurs numerous times, the processor may need to be repaired or replaced. Manufacturers provide suggestions to help prevent or reduce the likelihood of this happening, but the best suggestion is to remove the processor and headset before exposure to high levels of static electricity, as when playing on plastic slides.

Follow-up Programming

Accurate electrical thresholds contribute to postoperative performance. Research has shown that a majority of young children have significant fluctuations in thresholds during at least the first year following initial stimulation. A programming schedule such as the following is advisable poststimulation: 2 weeks, 4–5 weeks, 3 months, 4.5 months, 6 months, twice between 6 months and 12 months, and again at 12 months (Shapiro & Waltzman, 1995). Additional visits should be initiated if changes indicate decrements in auditory behavior or speech production. These may include a decrease in auditory responsiveness, changes in auditory discrimination or identification, increased requests for repetition, addition and/or omission of syllables, prolongation of vowels, and change in voice quality. The need for a program adjustment should not be confused with the fact that modified programs sometimes result in a temporary decrement in auditory and/or speech production skills. The length of time necessary to adjust to a newly tuned processor varies greatly among children. Familiarity with the auditory adjustment patterns of each child is central to the programming schedule. Reports and feedback from parents, teachers, and therapists are essential to this process. Input from these team members can alert the audiologist to both the specific nature of the problem and the need for reprogramming.

Despite the need for adjustments, there are times when changes in auditory behavior are not related to a given program. When a child is not performing a specific skill, parents and therapists often focus on the program and attempt to dictate the modification of specific parameters. This can be counterproductive since ultimately, the most effective program is usually one that is accurate rather than overly creative. Although input from members of the team is always valuable, it is in the best interest of the child for the audiologist to determine which type of program changes, if any, are required.

Programming, however important, is just one of the variables that contribute to postoperative performance. Despite the most diligent efforts of the programmer, the progress of development of auditory and linguistic skills will vary greatly among children based on such factors as age at time of implantation, duration of deafness, communication approach, type and frequency of therapy or auditory skills training, educational placement, neurological involvements, and cognitive development.

Evaluations

Yearly formal evaluations are necessary to validate performance and progress. These evaluations are often the basis for determining the future directions of research involving processing strategies. Documentation of specific strengths and deficits can lead to changes in processor design that will ultimately provide greater benefit to a larger population of children. Since outcome measures are the basis of reimbursement in the current medical environment, it is mandatory that all professionals document and substantiate all claims of significant improvement. Parents must therefore be convinced of the importance of regular formal assessments encompassing both auditory and linguistic skills.

The field of cochlear implants has attained scientific and clinical gains that could not have been predicted 20 years ago. The collaboration and cooperation of children, family members, and professionals from many disciplines will ensure continued progress towards the goal of improved quality of life for children who are hearing impaired.

References

Advanced Bionics Corporation. (1995). *Clarion device fitting manual.* Sylmar, CA: Author.

Cochlear Corporation. (1996). *Technical reference manual.* Englewood, CO: Author.

Shapiro, W.H., & Waltzman, S.B. (1995). Changes in electrical thresholds over time in young children implanted with the Nucleus cochlear prosthesis. In G.M. Clark & R.S.C. Cowan (Eds.), International Cochlear Implant, Speech and Hearing Symposium, Melbourne, 1994. *Annals of Otology, Rhinology & Laryngology, 104* (9) (Suppl. 166), 177–178.

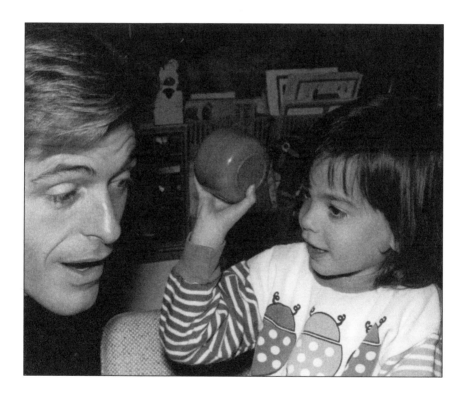

Habilitation

Overleaf: Warren Estabrooks with Dara Keller

Introduction

Warren Estabrooks, M.Ed., Cert. AVT

*P*art III consists of two chapters. In chapter 5, I have suggested a model that can be followed when helping a young child to learn to listen after he or she receives a cochlear implant.

In chapter 6, several of my professional colleagues from around the world have contributed detailed analytical therapy (lesson) plans for children with cochlear implants. It is an honor to present these works for the professional community at large and especially for parents.

The therapists were asked to present a detailed plan, complete with analysis, of a therapy session for a young child who has just received a cochlear implant, or who has had an implant for one to four years. The lessons are presented in that order, i.e., the lessons for children who have recently received their implant are given first.

Each plan provides the historical and audiological background of a particular child, as well as goals in audition, speech, language, cognition, and communication development. Each section of the lesson is explained in detail, with implications and ideas for effective target carryover from the therapy session to typical childhood activities.

It is hoped that the insights gained through these therapy plans, analyses, and carryover activities will provide guidance, and stimulate discussion among professionals and parents.

CHAPTER 5

Learning to Listen with a Cochlear Implant: A Model for Children

Warren Estabrooks, M.Ed., Cert. AVT

Never before in the history of the education of children who are deaf has there been such potential for *listening*. For many children who are unable to learn to hear and listen with hearing aids, cochlear implants can provide access to a world rich in sound and spoken language. Through consistent cochlear implant management and systematic auditory (re)habilitation (listening therapy) with maximum parental involvement, these children learn to listen to their own voices, the voices of others, and the sounds of the environment in order to communicate using speech.

As we approach the new millennium, children with cochlear implants will be using a variety of communication options: bilingual-bicultural, total communication (TC), cued speech, oral, auditory-oral, and auditory-verbal (Schwartz, 1996). Unfortunately, all of these options are not always available for all families. Regardless of the communication approach, the primary function of the cochlear implant is *to provide spoken language information through hearing sensation and active listening*. The exciting responsibility of helping children to maximize the use of this technology rests with the therapists, teachers, audiologists, parents, and caregivers.

This chapter provides a model for the development of spoken language through listening and can be used as a guideline when working and playing with any child who has a cochlear implant.

Getting Started

All children with cochlear implants need the same listening, language, communication, and learning foundations as children with typical hearing and those who wear hearing aids. Each child will need to pass through a number of stages of listening and talking (Table 1), but the

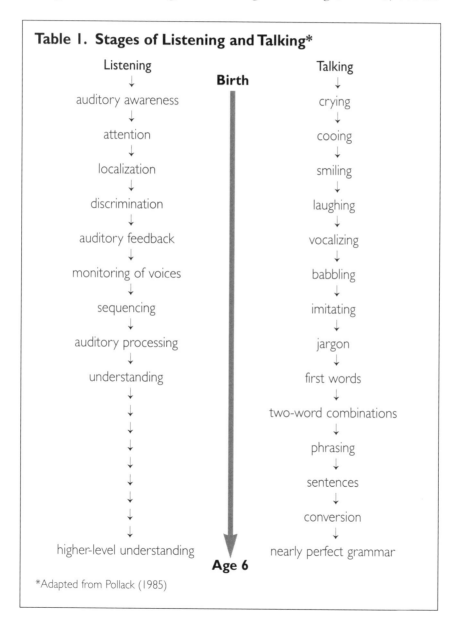

Table 1. Stages of Listening and Talking*

Listening	Birth	Talking
↓		↓
auditory awareness		crying
↓		↓
attention		cooing
↓		↓
localization		smiling
↓		↓
discrimination		laughing
↓		↓
auditory feedback		vocalizing
↓		↓
monitoring of voices		babbling
↓		↓
sequencing		imitating
↓		↓
auditory processing		jargon
↓		↓
understanding		first words
↓		↓
↓		two-word combinations
↓		↓
↓		phrasing
↓		↓
↓		sentences
↓		↓
↓		conversion
↓		↓
higher-level understanding	Age 6	nearly perfect grammar

*Adapted from Pollack (1985)

starting point may be steered by auditory experience, chronological age, linguistic abilities, and attitude. It is critical for the cochlear implant team to obtain accurate diagnostic information about auditory and cognitive-linguistic development at the beginning and throughout the habilitative process. The philosophy of *starting from scratch* is followed by many therapists who work with children immediately after the initial stimulation of the cochlear implant.

Since learning to listen and talk consists of a plethora of auditory-cognitive-linguistic tasks, professionals and parents need to record developmental behaviors. A variety of scales and measures are available that chart growth based on hearing age (time of full use of hearing aids and/or cochlear implant use to the present). The *Meaningful Auditory Integration Scale (MAIS)* (Appendix A at the end of this book) and its companion, the *Infant-Toddler: Meaningful Auditory Integration Scale (IT- MAIS)* (Appendix B), are particularly useful guidelines to help chart effective use of the cochlear implant by children immediately following stimulation of the cochlear implant. In addition, The *Auditory-Verbal Ages & Stages of Development (AVASD)* (Appendix C) may help to record progress in listening, receptive and expressive speech and language, and cognitive skills of the very young child who has a cochlear implant.

The Listening Environment

To maximize the use of hearing in learning spoken language through *listening* rather than *watching,* auditory skills programming needs to be carried out in the best possible listening conditions. This will ensure that information is easy to hear and to learn. The listening environment is enhanced by:

- parents and/or therapists sitting next to the child, on the side of the cochlear implant microphone ear.
- speaking close to the child's cochlear implant microphone.
- speaking at regular volume.
- minimizing background noise.
- using speech that is repetitive and rich in melody, expression, and rhythm.
- using *acoustic highlighting* (Table 2) to enhance the audibility of spoken language.

Some therapists and teachers choose to sit directly across from older children when they first receive their cochlear implant. These chil-

Table 2. Acoustic Highlighting

Acoustic highlighting encompasses a variety of techniques used to enhance the audibility of a spoken message. These may include: rewording, rephrasing, pausing, waiting, whispering, singing, and emphasizing specific suprasegmentals and/or segmental features.

Variable	Most Audible ⟶	Least Audible
Background noise	Absence	Presence (type and/or intensity)
Distance/Location	Close proximity to microphone of hearing aid or cochlear implant	Increased speaker distance
Repetition	Repetition(s) required	Spoken message presented only once
Length	Short utterance	Long utterance
Complexity	Simple utterance	Complex utterance
Rate	Slow rate of utterance	Individual rates of utterance
Suprasegmentals	Speech with emphasis on specific pitch, intensity, and/or duration cues	Little or no specific acoustic emphasis provided
Segmentals	Specific contrasting of acoustic features (place, manner, and/or voicing)	Little or no specific acoustic emphasis provided
Target position	End of word, [Middle] phrase, sentence, or whole message	Beginning of word, phrase, sentence, or whole message
Set	Closed	Open
Speaker familiarity	Familiar voice	Unfamiliar voice

dren may be highly visual and have little or no confidence in their newly acquired listening potential. The therapist may use an acoustic screen (such as an embroidery hoop covered with gauze) or the auditory-verbal technique known as the *hand cue* to encourage listening rather

---

The Hand Cue

The *hand cue* may consist of:

- the therapist, parent, or caregiver covering his or her mouth briefly, from time to time, when the child is looking directly at the adult's face. This encourages *listening* rather than *lipreading*. When the child is playfully engaged and not looking, this is unnecessary. The adult, however, must be close to the microphone of the child's cochlear implant (within earshot).

- the adult moving his or her hand towards the child, in a nurturing way, as a prompt for vocal imitation or as a signal for verbal turn taking.

- the adult talking through a stuffed animal, toy, picture, or book, placed in front of the speaker's mouth.

The hand cue signals the child to listen intently. The hand cue needs to be used only when necessary because its use may distort, smear, or eliminate the sound arriving at the microphone. As children come to rely on hearing, the use of the hand cue is reduced (Estabrooks, 1994). Once the child has "integrated hearing into his or her personality" (Pollack, 1985), the hand cue is rarely used.

---

than watching. During the process of learning to listen, many children become highly reliant upon listening and will require only ear contact, as opposed to eye contact, during formal listening sessions.

Speech Reception and Production

Accurate audiometric results, as plotted on the audiogram, remain one of the best predictors of speech reception. Most cochlear audiograms indicate that most children with cochlear implants have access to most speech information lying within the speech range from 250 Hz to 4000 Hz (Table 3). This auditory potential is a major variable in listening skills development and speech production among children who have a cochlear implant. Outcome results are also variable.

Table 3. Speech Information*

Availability at 250–4000 Hz (+ or – $^1/_2$ octave)

250 Hz	500 Hz	1000 Hz	2000 Hz	4000 Hz
• 1st formant of vowels /u/ and /I/	• 1st formants of most vowels	• Important acoustic cues for manner	• Important acoustic cues for place of articulation	• Key frequency for /s/ and /z/ morpheme audibility (critical for language learning)
• Fundamental frequency of females' and children's voices	• Harmonics of all voices (male, female, child)	• 2nd formants of back and central vowels	• 2nd and 3rd formant information for front vowels	– plurals
• Nasal murmur associated with the phonemes /m/, /n/, and /ng/	• Voicing cues	• Important consonant-vowel and vowel-consonant transition information	• Consonant-vowel and vowel-consonant transition information	– idioms – possessives – auxiliaries – 3rd person – questions – copulas – past perfect
• Male voice harmonics	• Nasality cues • Suprasegmentals	• Nasality cues	• Acoustic information for the liquids /r/ and /I/	• Consonant quality
• Voicing cues	• Some plosive bursts associated with /b/ and /d/	• Some plosive bursts	• Plosive bursts	
• Prosody		• Voicing cues	• Affricate bursts	
• Suprasegmentals patterns (stress, rate, inflection, intonation)		• Suprasegmentals	• Fricative turbulence	
		• Unstressed morphemes		

*Adapted from Ling (1996)

Speech Through Listening

Speech production is critical for the development of conversational competence. Listeners who have little or no experience communicating with children who are deaf or hard of hearing may find their speech difficult to understand. Intelligible speech and pleasant voice quality have a major impact on the successful inclusion of children who have cochlear implants in mainstream school programs. More importantly, these characteristics directly affect the self-esteem of these young children.

Systematic reception and production of the sounds of speech (Appendix E) have been extensively discussed by Ling (1976) in *Speech and the Hearing Impaired Child: Theory and Practice*. I have found that the skills and subskills for the production of the suprasegmentals and segmentals of speech as described in detail in Ling's classic work are particularly effective for use with children who have cochlear implants.

Some children will require specific teaching strategies to acquire sounds of speech, but all sounds at the phonemic, word, phrase, and/or sentence level need to be incorporated into meaningful conversation in typical childhood experiences.

Parent Participation

Like other children, kids who have cochlear implants learn language most easily when they are actively engaged in relaxed, meaningful activities with supportive, loving parents and caregivers (Kretschmer & Kretschmer, 1978; Ling, 1989; Ross, 1990; Estabrooks 1994, 1996).

Active parent participation is the cornerstone of the process and is critical for successful carryover of goals in listening and language learning for the child who has a cochlear implant. If parents receive adequate guidance, counseling, coaching, and support, they can acquire the confidence to implement techniques and strategies that will maximize the listening, speech, language, cognitive, and communicative development of their child. Parents need to be encouraged to observe, participate and practice, in order to learn to:

- model techniques for stimulating speech, language, and communication activities at home.
- plan strategies to integrate listening, speech, language, and communication into daily routines and experiences.
- communicate as partners in the therapy process.
- inform the therapist of the child's interests and abilities.
- interpret the meaning of the child's early communication.
- develop appropriate behavior management techniques.
- record and discuss progress.
- interpret short-term and long-term goals.
- develop confidence in parent-child interaction.
- make informed decisions.
- advocate on behalf of the child. (Estabrooks, 1994)

Variables Affecting Progress

Listening, communication development, and communication style vary from child to child and from family to family. As with children who wear hearing aids, auditory performance (detection, discrimination, identification, and comprehension of acoustic signals, including speech and environmental sounds) and spoken communication of children who have cochlear implants are variable and depend on:

- age at diagnosis.
- cause and degree of hearing impairment.
- effectiveness of audiological management.
- effectiveness of the cochlear implant.
- hearing and listening potential.
- health of the child.
- emotional state of the family.
- active participation of the family.
- skills of the professionals.
- child's learning style.
- child's intelligence.

Charting Auditory Development

Most children who have cochlear implants will require systematic, step-by-step habilitation, following such a model, enhanced by effective carryover in meaningful daily activities.

Even older children who have been deaf a short time before receiving a cochlear implant will benefit enormously from systematic, successful listening activities. The rationale for such structure is that under less redundant auditory conditions in the everyday environment of the real world, where the expected mode of linguistic input is speech in noisy environments, and at various distances, the child will optimally be able to use auditory cues in combination with all other visual, kinesthetic, and tactile cues to maximize spoken communication development (Estabrooks, 1994).

Development of auditory skills alone can be charted on the *Listening Skills Scale for Kids with Cochlear Implants* (Appendix D).

A Model for Listening

Children who have cochlear implants are, foremost, *children*. They require the same opportunities for play and frolic as other children. Parents and professionals are aware of the challenges in teaching and living with children who have cochlear implants, but sometimes forget the difficulties met by the children themselves, who face the greatest challenges in life. Professionals who have chosen a career working with children who are deaf or hard of hearing are responsible for providing support, guidance, and encouragement. It is hoped that this Model for Listening will help children who have cochlear implants to become active listeners, effective spoken language communicators, and exciting conversational partners.

A single, well-defined hierarchy of listening skills and speech-language development will not fit every child. It is critical, however, to establish specific short-term and long-term goals. The professional and parent can manipulate and adapt materials and reinforcers to meet the needs and interests of the child—but each stage in the model of listening skills must be covered. As stated earlier, the best guidance is to *start from scratch*.

The exemplary hierarchy of auditory skill development created by Erber (1982), which consists of four sequential, yet overlapping, levels, has been adapted in the formulation of the model. In chapter 6, the reader will find detailed therapy treatment plans (lesson plans) for children who have just received the initial stimulation of the cochlear implant and for children who have had cochlear implants for one to four years.

The Model*

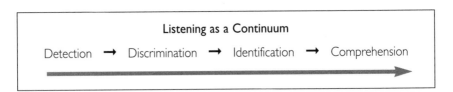

Listening as a Continuum

Detection → Discrimination → Identification → Comprehension

Detection
The ability to respond to the presence or absence of sound. Thus, the child learns to respond to sound, to pay attention to sound, and not to respond when there is no sound.

○ Spontaneous awareness of sound

- Child searches for sound by eye glancing or head turning, stopping his/her activity, becoming quiet, startling and/or vocalizing.

*Adapted from Erber (1982) and Estabrooks (1994)

○ Selective attention to sound

○ Detect and identify a variety of noisemakers and environmental sounds

○ Detect and identify *Learning to Listen Sounds* (Appendix F)

○ Detect and identify sounds (m, ah, oo, ee, sh, s) of *Six-Sound Test* (Ling)

○ Conditioned response to sound

• Child is required to perform an action when sound is heard (e.g., stack a ring on a pole, put a block in a bucket, put a marble in water).

• Six-Sound Test: these sounds are presented at random intervals for training and monitoring detection skills and for troubleshooting the cochlear implant; the sounds f, th, h, p, t etc. can be added to this test, and are especially important for children with cochlear implants since these sounds are generally detected more quickly than with hearing aids.

○ Searches for or localizes sound

Discrimination

The ability to perceive similarities and differences between two or more speech stimuli. The child learns to attend to differences between and among sounds, and to respond differently to different sounds.

• Same/different tasks are primarily used for clarification of identification and comprehension errors.

• Specific discrimination activities are generally used for remediation, such as confusion of singular and plural (flower, flowers) and/or place, manner, and voicing errors (see page 85).

Identification

The ability to label by repeating, pointing to, or writing the speech stimulus heard.

Suprasegmentals*

○ Prosodic features of speech (duration, rate, pitch, intensity, stress, intonation)

*Systematic speech teaching strategies for the development of suprasegmentals and segmentals are outlined by Ling (1976, 1989).

Duration
- awareness of changes in duration.
- long versus short sounds (speech and environmental).
- various combinations of duration.
- self-monitoring of changes in duration in conversation.

Rate
- awareness of changes in rate.
- fast and slow sounds in a closed-set task (speech and/or environmental).
- phrases spoken at fast, slow, or medium rates.
- recognition of sentences spoken at fast, slow, or medium rates in a closed-set task.
- self-monitoring of changes in rate in conversation.

Pitch
- awareness of changes in pitch.
- high and low pitch in a closed-set task.
- high, low, and moderate pitches.
- recognition of rising pitch and falling pitch.
- recognition of rising pitch, falling pitch, and monotone in a closed-set task.
- self-monitoring of pitch in conversation.

Intensity
- awareness of changes in intensity.
- high (loud) and low (quiet) intensity.
- recognition of high, moderate (conversational), and low intensity.
- self-monitoring of intensity in conversation.

Stress
- awareness of changes in stress patterns.
- stress patterns in a closed set.
- recognition of stress patterns in phrases.
- recognition of stress patterns in simple and complex sentences.
- self-monitoring of stress patterns in conversation.

○ Recognition of male, female, and child voices

- Fundamental frequency of male voice (125 Hz), female voice (250 Hz), and child's voice (325 Hz). Many children will do this with or without specific training.

○   Angry, sad, and happy voices

- The child learns to label the emotional content of a person's voice.

○   Respond to own name and names of other people

○   More *Learning to Listen Sounds* and word approximations

Segmentals

○   Phonemes by manner: b vs. m vs. h

○   Imitate a variety of phonemes (b, m, d, t, h, sh, s, f, th, etc.)

○   Words varying in number of syllables

- Child is required to identify spoken words from a small → large set of objects or pictures based on syllable length (ball, apple, dinosaur, rhinoceros, hippopotamus).

○   One-syllable words varying in vowel and consonant content

- Child is required to identify single-syllable words that are known (cup, shoe, boat, fish, house, tree, dog, cat). This is more difficult than the previous task.

○   Develop memory and expressive production for one word

- In phrase containing repetition of sound-word association:
  The airplane goes up, up, up.
  The ball can bounce, bounce, bounce.
  The top spins around and around and around.

- In single repetition of *Learning to Listen Sound:*
  The cow says moo.
  The sheep says baa.

- In phrases containing a range of suprasegmental features with a variety of nouns, verbs and adjectives (*Mmm, that's good* vs. *Pick up the flower* vs. *Brush, brush, brush your hair*).

- In simple sentences:

  – With varying vowel content and number of syllables:
    Can you see the fish? (apple, ice cream cone, pomegranate)

– Where key word is located at end of sentence:
Where are the *elephants?*

– Where word is located in the middle of a sentence:
Can you put the *flowers* on the table?

– Where word is located at the beginning of the sentence:
Dinosaurs are extinct.

○ Stereotypic messages (familiar expressions and directions)

- Recognition of typical phrases (brush your hair, tie your shoe, give it to me, put your coat on, don't touch it, it's hot, let's go home).

○ Words in which the consonants are identical and the vowels differ

- E.g., *boat, ball, bus, big, bat, bite, bean, key, car, cat, cow, coat.*

○ Words in which the vowels are identical and the consonants differ in manner and place of articulation, and in voicing

Manner: the way a sound is produced in the vocal tract. Different manner features include plosives (p, b, t, d, k, g); nasals (m, n, ng); fricatives (sh, s, f, th); affricates (ch, j); liquids (l, r); semivowels (y, w).

Place: the point of greatest constriction in the vocal tract during articulation; bilabial (b, p); labiodental (f, v); linguadental (th); alveolar (t, d); palatal (sh); velar (k, g); glottal (h).

Voicing: presence or absence of vocal fold vibration during articulation. Voiced/unvoiced pairs include: b/p, d/t, g/k, v/f, j/ch, z/s.

○ Words in which the vowels are identical and the consonants differ only in manner of articulation

- E.g., *bat, mat, fat, rat, sat, cat, house, mouse.*

○ Words in which the vowels are identical and the consonants differ only in voicing

- E.g., *fan, van; bat, pat; coat, goat.*

Comprehension

The ability to understand the meaning of speech by answering questions, following an instruction, paraphrasing, or participating in a conversation. The child's response must be qualitatively different than the stimuli presented.

Auditory Memory and Sequencing

○ Familiar expressions

- E.g., *Be careful, All gone, Wait a minute, All better, Peek-a-boo, It's stuck, Don't touch it, Shh baby's sleeping, That's yummy.*

○ Follow single directions

- E.g., *Give it to me, Take your coat off, Put your shoes on.*

○ Follow two directions

- E.g., *Close the door and sit down over there, Put the toast on the table and pour me some coffee.*

○ Sequence two → three → four critical elements

- Two critical elements: *On the table, In your pocket, Under the pillow, Purple hat, Big elephant, Tall giraffe.*

  – Develop two-item memory in phrases and simple sentences:
    noun + noun (get your hat and mittens)
    noun + verb (the girl is drinking)
    verb + object (wash the car)
    verb + verb (get up and dance)
    adjective + noun (find the purple ball)
    number + noun (I want three popsicles).

- Three critical elements: *On the big table, In daddy's pocket, Under mommy's pillow, Big purple hat, Big gray elephant, Tall yellow giraffe.*

- Four critical elements: *On the big brown table, In daddy's coat pocket, Under mommy's feather pillow, Big purple straw hat, Behind the big gray elephant, Beside the tall yellow giraffe, Daddy walks to the store, Mommy decorated the giant Christmas tree.*

○ Sequence three directions

- Auditory memory store is critical for language learning; the ability to process spoken conversation and participate at the discourse level is highly dependent on auditory memory.

- At the early levels, sequencing three directions may include such items as *Give the baby a drink, put her over your shoulder and burp her* or *Put the baby in the bed, kiss her good night and pull up the cover* or *Put your pajamas on, give mommy a kiss and get your teddy bear.*

- At the later levels, especially in school, the teacher may say *Draw a line under the last word, circle the word in the middle, and put a triangle around something you eat* (the school-age child is expected to follow many types of instructions in the classroom).

○ Sequence multielement directions

- There are many levels of difficulty within multielement directions in addition to the auditory capability to detect phonemes, identify language, and retain auditory information. Successful mastery requires a high level of linguistic competence at the semantic, syntactic, and pragmatic levels. (Estabrooks & Edwards, 1994)

- An early level may include: *Make the cow jump over the fence and move on to make the animal that gives us milk walk around a building used for storing corn.*

- At a higher level, the child will need to demonstrate the ability to extract salient auditory cues to identify objects in games such as I Spy, which contain a variety of embedded directions (*I spy something that is gray, has fins, swims in the ocean, and is very dangerous*).

○ Follow classroom directions

- E.g., *Close your books, Put your pencils away now, Draw a line under the last word, Circle the word in the middle, Draw a line under something you eat.*

- At a higher level (*Before you get your reading book out, remember that tomorrow is pizza day and you will need to bring money and a signed letter from your parents if you are planning to participate*).

Auditory/Cognitive Skills in a Structured Listening Set

○ Sequence series of multielement directions

○ Make identification based on several related descriptors

○ Sequence three → four → five events

○ Recall five details of an event, story, or lesson

○ Understand main idea of a lesson or complex story

Auditory/Cognitive Skills in Conversation

○ Answer questions requiring comprehension of the main idea of a short conversation

○ Paraphrase remarks of another

○ Offer spontaneous relevant remarks

Figure Ground

This is a hierarchy of figure ground activities for all levels of listening skills:

The presence of background noise interferes with the comprehension of speech for all children with a cochlear implant. Comprehension activities in the presence of noise distractions is a difficult but necessary part of listening. In listening therapy programs, it is essential to begin with the least interfering background noise and progress slowly to the most interfering noise condition. Successful listening experiences are paramount so that the child's attitude towards noise becomes positive over time.

The least interfering noise conditions are steady-state environmental noises, such as that from fans, overhead projectors, or the steam from a kettle. Moderately interfering noises include random environmental noises that are less predictable, such as cafeteria noise or traffic noise. The most interfering noise is speech from other talkers on topics of relevance or interest to the listener (for example, someone reading a familiar story is more interfering than the news report on the radio). Finally, the background noise from the speech of one to four speakers is more interfering than the noise created by 12 or more speakers. This latter condition resembles the less interfering random environmental noise.

○   Quiet environment → Regular noise → Noisy environment

At Varying Distances

○   Next to sound source → Five to six feet from the sound source → Across the room from sound source

Add the Presence of Distractions

○   Fan-type noise → Cafeteria noise → Four-speaker babble → Distance → Various background noises

References

Erber, N. (1982). *Auditory training.* Washington, DC: A.G. Bell Association for the Deaf.

Estabrooks, W. (Ed.). (1994). *Auditory-verbal therapy for parents and professionals.* Washington, DC: A.G. Bell Association for the Deaf.

Kretschmer, R.R., & Kretschmer, L. (1978). *Language development and intervention with the hearing impaired.* Baltimore: University Park.

Ling, D. (1976). *Speech and the hearing impaired child: Theory and practice.* Washington, DC: A.G. Bell Association for the Deaf.

Ling, D. (1989). *Foundations of spoken language for hearing impaired children.* Washington, DC: A.G. Bell Association for the Deaf.

Ling, D. (1996). *Acoustics, audition and speech reception.* AVI Video. Alexandria, VA. Auditory-Verbal International.

Pollack, D. (1985). *Educational audiology for the limited hearing infant and preschooler.* Springfield, IL: Charles C. Thomas.

Robbins, A.M. (1991). *Meaningful auditory integration scale (MAIS).* Bloomington, IN: Indiana University School of Medicine Publication.

Ross, M. (Ed.). (1990). *Hearing impaired children in the mainstream.* Parkton, MD: York Press.

Schwartz, S. (1996). *Choices in deafness* (2nd ed.). Bethesda, MD: Woodbine House.

Zimmerman-Phillips, S., Osberger, M.J., & Robbins, A.M. (1997). *Infant-Toddler meaningful auditory integration scale (IT-MAIS).* Sylmer, CA: Advanced Bionics Corporation.

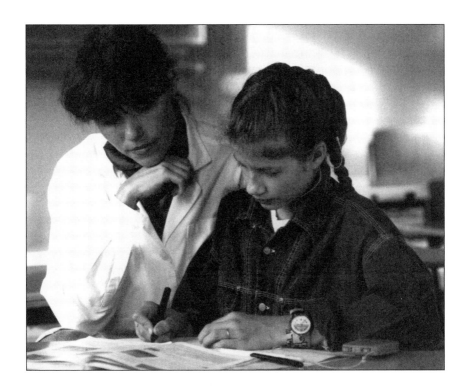

CHAPTER 6

Analytical Therapy Plans

Lesson Plan for Jonathan

Carol Zara, M.A., CCC-SLP

Your child has just received a cochlear implant! For many parents, this is both an exciting and a frustrating time. After the complicated decision to undergo an implant, followed by surgery and recovery, families eagerly await the initial activation of the device.

Since the majority of children who receive implants at around the age of two have congenital hearing losses, most have not had enough experience with sound to know what to do with the new information available to them. Despite careful counseling by the implant team, most families are disappointed when their children do not immediately respond to environmental sounds or turn to their names. The focus of the following lesson is to help establish improved responses to speech and help the child recognize his or her name and respond in an appropriate manner.

The Parents' Role in Therapy

The parents' role in the therapy process is critical to the child's attainment of speech, language, and auditory goals! Learning occurs not only in the formal therapy sessions, but in everyday shared experiences. All members of the family are encouraged to be active participants in the therapy process, both before and after the implant surgery.

The child who has recently received an implant, especially if he or she has also received intensive preimplant training, may demonstrate immediate detection of sound within a *set-to-listen* task. Parents and rehabilitation professionals, however, are often frustrated when this success is not repeated outside the structured setting of the therapy room or test booth. The child who has recently received a cochlear implant needs to learn *what* to listen for and *how* to respond. The therapist and family need to provide multiple opportunities for the child to hear sound and put meaning to it without falling into the habit of repeating or parroting the stimulus. A common behavior of such children may be referred to as *ear-to-mouth syndrome* (clinician or parent presents a sound or word and the child simply repeats it with no evidence that he or she has comprehended). When the child's name is called, however, there are a set number of responses that can be made, but imitation of that stimulus would be inappropriate.

One of the most gratifying experiences for parents occurs when the

Parents

While developing functional use of auditory skills with the child, bear in mind the acronym PARENTS:

- **P**atience. The child needs to learn how to *use* the sound that is now available. The implant team needs time to work with the child and arrive at the optimal program in the speech processor. Ongoing MAPping at regular and frequent intervals will assist in this process. Parental feedback to the implant team is essential. Be patient.

- **A**ccess. The cochlear implant gives the child access to the speech signal at audible levels, possibly for the first time. However, only through consistent use of the device and ongoing therapy does this new hearing potential become functional.

- **R**elevance. Targets and activities must be selected that are relevant and interesting to the child. As the processor is designed to code speech, use spoken language as the stimulus whenever possible. When using environmental sounds, select those that occur as a natural consequence of an activity.

- **E**xpectations. High, but realistic expectations for your child are critical. We assume the child can now hear! We must provide many opportunities for the child to hear and respond to speech. Naturally occurring situations are the best means of stimulating listening and language learning. To develop these skills, we like to make the most of activities such as getting dressed, cooking, and cleaning the house.

- **N**urture. Provide an abundance of affection, remembering that this little person is a child first and a recipient of a cochlear implant second.

- **T**ime. Learning to listen does not happen overnight. Learning speech and language through listening is an ongoing process. We need to be consistent.

- **S**uccess. With the energy and love parents put into this process, successful listening experiences will become an integral part of daily life.

child begins responding consistently to his or her name. In the following lesson, I will discuss the hierarchy of skills for name detection, discrimination, and identification with the child who has had an implant for a relatively brief period of time.

Background

Jonathan is a two-year, four-month-old boy who received his cochlear implant a week after his second birthday. He has a profound, bilateral sensorineural hearing loss of unknown etiology that was diagnosed when he was nine months of age, and he was aided shortly thereafter with a body-worn FM system.

At 11 months of age, Jonathan and his family began attending parent-centered, auditory-oral therapy two times per week, with each parent attending one session per week. Despite their intensive efforts, Jonathan's progress in developing auditory skills was minimal. His conventional amplification provided limited access to speech. Responses with the FM microphone activated were at 40 dB HL at 250 Hz and 500 Hz, 50 dB HL at 1000 Hz, 65 dB HL at 2000 Hz, and no responses above 2000 Hz.

After nine months of therapy, he inconsistently alerted to speech and nonspeech sounds and relied on lipreading to understand language. Jonathan was able to demonstrate some discrimination and identification of word associations and words through speechreading and listening. His speech sounds consisted of the vowels /a/, /o/, /au/, /uh/ and visible consonants /b/, /m/, /l/, and /w/. He was acquiring language, but frequently did not use his voice. At 18 months of age, his family, with the support of his therapist, began to investigate cochlear implantation. They met with other parents of children with cochlear implants and observed therapy sessions with children at a variety of stages post implant. After extensive testing by the implant team, Jonathan's candidacy for implantation was approved.

Surgery was uncomplicated, and a full insertion of the electrode array was obtained. All available electrodes were activated in a bipolar plus one (BP+1) stimulation mode. Jonathan wears his cochlear implant during all waking hours.

Introduction to the Lesson

This lesson takes place approximately 12 weeks after the initial stimulation. Jonathan has been back for three programming sessions since the activation of his cochlear implant. Prior to his receiving the implant, Jonathan's family had worked hard to develop a conditioned listening response. This involved waiting for a sound to be presented and performing a corresponding action (dropping a block in a bucket, throwing a ball across the room). As a result of pretraining, Jonathan is fairly consistent in responding during MAPping sessions. Within individual therapy sessions, he detects the six Ling sounds when he is *set to listen*. His parents report an increase in vocalizations when he is wearing the cochlear implant, but they are frustrated because he does not yet turn to his name nor respond consistently to sounds such as the doorbell or the telephone ringing.

Name recognition is a multifaceted task that requires the child to recognize his name and respond appropriately when called. An appropriate response when Jonathan hears his name may be any or all of the following:

- stopping the action in which he is engaged and looking up in search of the sound.
- pointing to himself.
- pointing to a picture of himself.
- holding out his hand in expectation of getting the object.
- attending to the speaker for the remainder of the comment, question, or command.

These behaviors and/or responses may need to be modeled and trained through auditory, visual, and even gestural means. It is helpful to have a third person present to model the expected response. In therapy the parent or therapist can perform this role. At home, a variety of people can help. In all activities, Jonathan should be given opportunities to act both as listener and speaker or director of the action. This reinforces use of his voice and spoken language to interact with those around him.

GOALS

Audition:
- to demonstrate detection of his name by looking up when his name is said by his mother or the therapist.
- to demonstrate discrimination of one versus three syllables (e.g., *Mom* vs. *Jonathan*) by selecting the correct picture or pointing to himself or his mother.

Language:
- to begin to understand and use two-word combinations to code possession (*Jonathan's shoe*) and action (*Jonathan sleeping*).
- to use his own name to label a picture of himself and use the words *Mom* and *Dad* to refer to his parents.

Speech:
- to attempt to produce three syllables for his own name.
- to demonstrate improved vowel production.

Pragmatics:
- to demonstrate turn-taking skills.
- to attend to the speaker for the duration of the message.

Where's Jonathan?

The theme of this lesson will be "Where's Jonathan?" Prior to starting the session, I collected all the necessary materials: photographs of Jonathan and his parents, a multicolored cloth bag, a shoebox with a slot in the top, a disposable camera, and assorted stickers.

I greet Jonathan in the waiting room, where I check his implant with the signal wand and find it to be in working order. As I check his device, the magnet falls from his head. His mother gets his attention and indicates through speech and gesture that he put it back on. He tries to lift the magnet to his head, and his mother helps him find the right position. She praises him for his attempt and informs me that, on occasion, he has begun to try to replace the magnet at home. I reply that this is a good sign, indicating he knows when the device is off and he is not hearing.

Ling Six-Sound Test

Each time Jonathan hears a sound he is expected to try to imitate it. He correctly imitates /a/ and /u/, but his production of /i/ is still imprecise. Jonathan produces a harsh, breathy sound for the fricative /sh/ and blows for /s/.

I introduce the next activity by picking up the pile of photographs that his mother has brought from home.

Shake, Shake, Shake

"Look what I have for you today. Do you want to see the pictures? Let's look at them together."

I show Jonathan the pile of photographs. Since he loves hiding and finding things, we place the photographs in the cloth bag. For added interest and language practice we make a production out of shaking the bag and taking turns saying, "Shake, shake, shake." This is a good opportunity for Jonathan to practice saying three syllables.

I take the first picture out of the bag and say, "Look. It's Mom." I point to his mother and place the photograph down in front of her. "Who wants a turn?" I ask.

His mom is familiar with this turn-taking game and replies: "Me. I want a turn." She takes the bag from me and shakes it up. "Shake, shake, shake. Ohhh. It's Jonathan! Hi, Jonathan. Look." She shows him the picture, which he takes from her and studies for a moment. "Do you want a turn?" He nods yes and takes out a picture, then points to his mother. We wait a moment to see if he uses her name, but Jonathan is silent.

"Is that Mom?" I ask.

"Ma." Jonathan imitates.

"That's right. Good!" Jonathan's mother tells him. "That's Mom. That's me."

Jonathan gets another turn and picks a picture of himself.

"Who is that?" I ask.

"A na," He attempts to produce his own name.

"Good try. That's Jonathan. Jo-na-than." I try to stress the three syllables, which are difficult for him to imitate at this point.

"Da na." he again tries to imitate.

"It's Mom's turn," I say, pointing to his mother. She turns over a picture but doesn't let him see. Mom uses the picture to cover her lips and says, "It's Jonathan." She waits to see if he will identify his own name, but Jonathan is frustrated and reaches out to grab the picture. Mom gives him the photograph and repeats, "See, it's Jonathan." Jonathan appears to be tiring of this activity, so we each take one more turn before moving on to the next phase of the lesson.

Shoebox

I reach under the table to retrieve the shoebox with a slit cut in the top. While I am doing this Jonathan becomes distracted and gets up to investigate some of the other toys in the room.

"Jonathan," I call, in an attempt to get his attention. No response. *"Jonathan,"* I repeat a little louder. "JONATHAN," I repeat again and knock loudly on the table at the same time. He looks around and, once I catch his attention, I hold out the box to show him. "Look what I have. Come sit down and let's play."

Jonathan is familiar with this shoebox, as we spent a previous session decorating it with stickers. We spend a minute looking at the animal stickers and practicing the animal sounds. Jonathan points to a cow and spontaneously says, "moo." We name a few more animals such as the duck (*quack quack quack*) and the pig (*oink oink oink*), practicing repeating three syllables.

For the next part of the task, I separate the pictures and take out only the ones of Jonathan. I give one to his mother.

"Listen," I instruct. His mom holds the picture up to her ear and waits. Using a mesh screen, I cover my mouth and after a moment, I say, "Jonathan."

"I heard that," his mom nods and points to her ear. Then she puts the picture in the slot. "In the box."

"Jonathan's turn." He holds his hand out for the picture, takes it, and holds it to his ear.

"Jonathan," I say. He smiles and moves to put the picture in the box. This is just a warm-up, since Jonathan demonstrates consistent detection of sounds. Next, I encourage Jonathan to respond only when he hears his name and not any other sound. We begin by having his mom model the targeted behavior. I hand her a picture of Jonathan.

"Listen. Listen for Jonathan. Ready?"

"I'm ready. Are you listening, Jonathan? Help Mommy listen," his mother says.

"Moo," I say. His mom wrinkles her brow and looks puzzled.

"No," she says as she shakes her head.

After a few seconds pass, I say, "Jonathan."

"Jonathan," she repeats, and smiles.

"Yes. That's right," I confirm. "Good job, Mom. Jonathan's turn." I hand him a picture which he attempts to put in the box. "No. You have to wait. Listen." I point to my ear, which cues Jonathan to hold the picture to his ear.

"Jonathan," I say. He puts the picture in the slot. "Good job. Here's another one. Listen. Woof, woof." Jonathan again moves to put the picture in the box. "No," I place my hand over the slot. "Woof, woof," I say again, and point to his picture with a puzzled look. "No. That's not a dog. That's Jonathan. Listen for Jonathan. Ready." He puts the picture back to his ear. "Jonathan," I say. He seems unsure. I repeat, "Jonathan" and nod my head slightly as a cue. He puts the picture in the box. Mom takes another turn, but it is clear that he is growing frustrated by the task. We say "goodbye" to the pictures and shoebox, and Jonathan puts them away on the shelf.

Play Dough

Because Jonathan has been quite cooperative with these challenging tasks, as a treat I take some play dough, one of his favorite activities, and offer him a choice.

"Do you want yellow or red?" I ask, showing him two containers.

"Eh," Jonathan attempts.

"Yellow? Try again. Ye-llow," I prompt.

"El-o." Jonathan improves his production, and I hand him the yellow play dough. He struggles to open it and hands it to his mother. She waits a moment, looking from Jonathan to the play dough. He points to the top of the container.

"What do you want me to do?" She asks.

"Opuh," he directs.

"Oh, open. Open the play dough. Okay. I'll take the top off." His mom takes the top off and looks into the can. "Oh. It's yellow. Nice, yellow play dough. Here you go."

Jonathan takes it, turns it over, and tries to get the play dough out. "Ay, ay, ay," he says, shaking the can.

"Great. You're shaking it," I reinforce. "Can I help you take some out?" He hands it to me and I take the play dough out for him. "Some for Mom?" I ask.

"Me. I want some," his mother responds. I hand her a piece. Jonathan vocalizes to get some of his own.

"Who wants some?" I ask, turning to him. He hold out his hand.

"Tell Carol... 'me,'" his mother says, while taking Jonathan's hand and putting it to his chest. "Me."

"Me," he tells us.

"Okay. Here's some for Jonathan." I put the extra play dough down beside him.

"Hey. How about me?" I ask, getting his attention. "I want some for me," I say, holding out my hand. Jonathan picks up a piece and hands it to me.

"Thank you," I reply. "Maybe we can *roll, roll, roll* the play dough." Mom imitates the three syllables of *roll, roll, roll.*

"You roll," his mom directs, taking his play dough and getting it started. He then attempts to imitate our actions.

"Look. I made a snake. Jonathan. *Jonathan.* JONATHAN." I attempt to get his attention, but he is much too interested in the play dough.

"Jonathan," his mother taps him and points to me, "Carol is talking to you." He looks up.

I repeat, "Look, a snake. *Sssssss.* He's coming to get you. *Ssss.*" Jonathan squeals and pretends to be afraid. "Go away, snake," I prompt him to say.

"Away," he indicates with a wave of his hand. Then, Jonathan pretends to attack me with his snake. He approximates the /s/ sound.

I comment to his mother that this is nice progress for him, as he has never been able to approximate a voiceless sound before. She reports that she is pleased with his progress and that the family sees changes from day to day. She says that she has some questions about his speech production and behavior that she would like to discuss. Jonathan plays with the play dough independently as we wrap up the remainder of the session. Jonathan's mother asks if I think he is making good progress, and I respond that I think his rate of improvement is well within what I expect after three months of implant use. She reports that there is pressure from Jonathan's grandparents that he is not *hearing* yet. I attempt to reassure her that Jonathan is, in fact, hearing quite well compared to his preimplant performance. We discuss some of the changes she has seen. I suggest that the grandparents be invited to attend a therapy session, and she agrees that this might prove helpful.

We terminate the session by saying, "Bye-bye," to the play dough and to Jonathan. Jonathan helps to clean up and opens the door independently to go back to the waiting/play area.

ANALYSIS
During this lesson, Jonathan has demonstrated the ability to sort pictures of himself and his mother and to approximate the names verbally. In a simple detection task he clearly demonstrates the fact that he hears his name. He continues to be inconsistent in discriminating his name from another sound. He also doesn't always demonstrate that he understands that his name *Jonathan* refers only to him and is a signal that he is supposed to stop what he is doing and attend to the person calling him. It may take several more weeks or even months for this knowledge to become fully established.

In a familiar play routine (play dough), Jonathan is improving his turn-taking skills and is using his known word associations and words more consistently. He is also more responsive to a speech model and willing to attempt to improve his productions. Jonathan's attempts to produce the voiceless /s/ are a clear indication that he is hearing this high-frequency sound.

Conclusion
Jonathan is making good progress with the information available to him through his cochlear implant. In familiar *set-to-listen* tasks, he is increasingly more confident and successful in detecting sounds. His imitation

Parent Guidance

✔ Continue to give Jonathan opportunities to hear his name in meaningful contexts. When you enter a room and he is engaged in an activity, call his name and observe whether he stops what he is doing and looks up. If there is another adult in the room, he or she may want to cue Jonathan by getting his visual attention and saying, "Listen. I hear someone." Then call his name again. If he doesn't respond, the other adult may point to you and tell him, "Mom was calling." Remember always to have a message to give him and not to call his name simply to get him to look. This establishes a *reason* for listening.

✔ Continue to have Jonathan practice saying his name and names of Mom, Dad, and siblings. Go through your family photo album and look at other pictures of Jonathan. Talk about who is in the picture and what they are doing. This activity helps to stimulate his vocabulary of both nouns and verbs.

✔ You might want to use your camera (a Polaroid for instant results) to take a series of pictures. This will be fascinating to Jonathan and provides many opportunities to develop such language as *wait, smile, push (the button),* and *pull (out the picture).* Take pictures of Jonathan doing a variety of actions (e.g., sleeping, eating, in the bath, on the swings). We will be able to use the same photographs to develop a variety of other language goals, including understanding of simple verbs.

✔ Bring some photos to the next therapy session. Jonathan can share them by telling me *who* is in the picture and *what* they are doing.

✔ In the next session, I would like to introduce possession (*Mommy's sock, Jonathan's sock*). Bring a pair of socks from each person in the family for this activity.

of speech presented to him indicates that he has access to both high-frequency and low-frequency sounds. The recent improvement in his productions of /sh/ and /s/ indicate that he is ready to have these used as more meaningful stimuli within therapy sessions.

Jonathan will continue to learn *how* to respond when his name is called. This will be achieved through ongoing practice, both in therapy and at home.

Lesson Plan for Sara

Pamela Steacie, M.Sc., Cert. AVT

Born to talk! Sara is the most gregarious person I have ever met. Now six, Sara has undoubtedly been outgoing since birth, but she has not been a verbal child for very long. Born in Lebanon, she was diagnosed at three months of age with a profound hearing loss but did not have access to hearing aids until she came to Canada at age two. Her older brother also has a profound hearing loss. Initially in a total communication (TC) program, Sara appeared, at that time, to have no useable hearing, and use of amplification was suspended. At age three, in the fall of 1993, she and her family joined our auditory-verbal program. She was using several signs, understood fewer than 20 spoken words, and used fewer than 10. She did not use her voice when she spoke.

One of our first challenges was to get earmolds to fit Sara's tiny ears. This took a couple of months and several remakes. Soon thereafter, she started to use her voice more consistently and to develop a few *learning to listen* sounds, containing relatively easy-to-hear, low-frequency vowel sounds and simple rhythm patterns. Lessons were a bit of a struggle, as Sara was extremely visual and very distractible. Her mother has always worked with admirable consistency, effectiveness, and determination to develop Sara's speech, language, and listening skills, as well as those of Sara's brother. As English was her mother's third and not very fluent language, she took English classes and volunteered at her son's school to increase her language competency.

Sara was given an FM system for home use to enhance listening further. Even so, she was still unable to process high-frequency sounds and found listening difficult all the time. Sara's audiologist and I met with her parents in the spring of 1994 to discuss the cochlear implant. They were reluctant to pursue investigation of it at that time. In December 1994, we gave Sara a frequency-transposition hearing aid to help her process high-frequency information. Soon, she began to detect /s/ and /f/, although she could not discriminate between them. She still was not able to hear place differences among front-plosive consonant /p/, mid-plosive /t/, and back-plosive /k/. She seemed to have more difficulty identifying low-frequency vowels /oo/ and /ah/ than she had with her ear-level hearing aids. Distance listening improved in that she could hear her name being called from up to eight feet away.

During 1995, Sara's speech and language progressed more quickly, but it was clear that her limited residual hearing made spoken communication laborious. After much soul searching, her parents chose a cochlear implant for Sara which she received in August 1996. It was switched on the following October. Prior to her implant surgery, vocabulary comprehension, as measured by the *Peabody Picture Vocabulary Test,* was at the two-year, five-month level. Understanding and use of language as measured by the *Zimmerman Preschool Language Scale-3* were at the levels of three years, one month and three years, two months, respectively. Sara expressed herself using short phrases of four to five words. By concentrating very hard, using listening alone, she could decode three-word phrases containing very familiar words when the context was known and limited. She needed to lipread to understand conversational speech.

Introduction to the Lesson

One week after being switched on, the cochlear implant gave Sara excellent listening potential. In order to exploit that potential fully, we needed, again, to find baseline diagnostic information, and then to reinforce skills at that level. This first lesson is heavily weighted with listening goals. Previously mastered speech and language goals are reinforced here through listening, and thinking skills are reinforced incidentally.

GOALS

Audition:
- phoneme detection; the Ling Six-Sound Test.
- phoneme identification of /bababa/, /ah/, /sh/, brbrbr (car sound), and /m/.
- responding to her name, i.e., turning toward the person calling her name.
- identification of familiar phrases: *Shut the door!; Ow, that hurts!; Sit down; Put it in the garbage.*
- identification of familiar verbs *Sit down, Sh! Go to sleep, Go up, up, up the stairs, Wash, wash, wash, wash (your hands, the car, the floor).*
- identification of familiar nouns *baby, hat, shoe, flower.*

Phoneme Detection

This is usually checked as soon as the first complete MAP is established, while the implant is still plugged into the MAPping computer. The six Ling sounds (/m/, /oo/, /ah/, /ee/, /sh/, and /s/) are used because they cover the full frequency range of spoken language. The same toys and the same procedure are used for this task as for conditioned play audiometry during audiological testing and cochlear implant MAPping:

- Sara holds a stacking ring or puzzle piece or block up to her ear.
- She listens for a sound stimulus (one of the Ling Six Sounds).
- If Sara hears the stimulus, she places the stacking ring on the stick or the puzzle piece in the puzzle or the block in the box.

Note: Depending on age and whether the child has developed residual hearing prior to receiving a cochlear implant and is proficient at conditioned play audiometry, he or she may be able to detect all six sounds even at this early stage. Sara was able to do so.

Parent Guidance

✔ Point out a variety of environmental sounds to Sara. Point often to your ear and cue her to *Listen!* Keep a daily note of the environmental sounds to which she does and does not respond.

✔ Perform the Ling Six-Sound Test with Sara daily. If she is unable to hear a sound, cue her to listen. Repeat the sound, closer to her and/or more loudly and/or more prolonged (e.g., /m→ / rather than /m/). Again, keep a daily record of the speech sounds detected or not. This information will be useful in refining Sara's cochlear implant MAP.

Phoneme Identification

Phoneme detection, as described above, is a simple task compared to the more complex tasks of discrimination (differentiating between *two* sounds, syllables, words or phrases, e.g., /f/ vs. /s/) and identification (telling which one of *several* possible sounds, syllables, words, or phrases has been said). Through phoneme identification tasks, I determine which sounds Sara can identify. As she can read a bit, I use a small number of printed letters and a happy face stamp for this activity. I use the staccato /bababa/; /a/ for the /ah/ sound with a long, slowly rising, then falling, intonation; /sh/ for that blowing, fricative sound; and *brbrbr* (raspberries) for the car sound. These sounds are very different from one another in rhythm, intonation, and in consonant and vowel content.

- I say each of the target sounds two or three times and then print each one on a piece of paper. Sara repeats each sound as I print it.
- I say each sound and ask Sara to repeat it and then stamp a happy face beside the corresponding letter(s).

Sara identifies all sounds except /m/, which she confuses with /ah/, so we practice discriminating /m/ from /ah/. For this task:

- I say the sounds /m/ and /ah/, and then print the letters *m* and *a*.
- I give Sara a felt marker and ask her to print the sound she has heard.
- She listens, repeats the sound, and then prints the appropriate letter.

Sara is able to perform this task correctly. Using the same task format, she is also able to discriminate /sh/ from /s/!

Parent Guidance

✔ Every day, do the *a*/*m* discrimination task as a warm-up, followed by the phoneme identification task with all suggested phonemes, including /s/. If mastered, add whispered /p/ /p/ /p/ and /ee/.

✔ Use the *auditory sandwich* technique (audition/vision/audition) if Sara is unable to identify a sound by audition alone:

  - say the sound a few times for Sara to process by *audition* alone, then ask her to repeat it. If she is unable to do so...
  - use a *visual* cue, such as lipreading or printing the sound while saying it. Ask her to repeat the sound.
  - say the sound again immediately, for processing by *audition*. Encourage Sara to repeat it.

✔ Use familiar words containing target sounds. For example, to reinforce /m/, use *Mama, mine, me,* and *more.*

Responding to Her Name

The goal of this activity is to help Sara learn to identify when her name is being called. I use a fun pop-up stacking toy with six rings. This procedure is similar to the auditory conditioning task:

- Sara holds a stacking ring up to her ear and then I say *Listen!* I mime to her that when she hears *Sara* and turns towards me, she can put a ring on the pop-up toy.

- From a distance of one foot behind Sara, I call her name.
- She turns to me. I congratulate her and give her a stacking ring.
- We repeat steps 2 and 3 as I call her from two, three, six, eight, and finally 10 feet away.

Sara celebrates by activating the lever that sends the rings flying up into the air. She turns to her name even at a distance of 10 feet. To increase the level of difficulty, I try calling her name unexpectedly. She is less consistent at this unless I am very close, about one foot away. I also make the original task more difficult in a different way, by turning it into a discrimination activity with the words *Sara* and *Mama*, as follows:

- I place five beads in front of her mother and five in front of Sara.
- I explain and demonstrate: *When I say Sara, you put a bead on the string and when I say Mama, Mama will put a bead on.*
- I call their names in random order.
- Each person places a bead on the string when her name is called, until all beads are strung.

Sara performs this activity successfully.

Parent Guidance

✔ From behind, about two feet away from her, call Sara's name unexpectedly. If she turns to you, congratulate her, and then call her from slightly farther away. If she does not turn to you, try again at one foot. If she does not respond at this distance, tap her on the shoulder, tell her you were calling *Sara!*, and call her name again at this distance with her turned away from you. Repeat at distances of two or three feet. Praise lavishly when she turns to you. As a rule, it is best to have a good reason for calling her, such as a forthcoming treat, or outing, or a meal, so that she doesn't decide to tune you out for being annoying.

✔ Since Sara was able to discriminate *Mama* from *Sara*, add the name *Papa* with whispered, exaggerated *p*'s. If Sara is able to choose correctly among these three, add *Abdallah* (Sara's brother), using a sing-song intonation for his name.

✔ Frequently, call other family members within Sara's earshot. Also have her call them, when appropriate.

Identification of Simple Expressive Phrases

I use a set of cartoon drawings that represent a variety of common phrases, mounted on construction paper, designed specifically for this activity. As a reinforcer I use a mechanical apple from which a worm darts to grab a penny. I have chosen the phrases *Shut the door; Ow! That hurts; Sit down;* and *Put it in the garbage,* which have different rhythm and intonation patterns. To make these phrases still more different from one another, I use *acoustic highlighting* techniques such as lengthening the /sh/ of *Shut the door* and the *Ow!* of *Ow! That hurts,* using a sing-song intonation for *Sit down,* and emphasizing the staccato rhythm of *Put it in the garbage.*

- Hiding each drawing, I say the associated phrase a couple of times, showing Sara the drawing and asking her to say the phrase. She then places a penny on the drawing. I introduce the first two drawings this way and then Mother introduces the others.
- I cue Sara to *Listen!* and then say one of the phrases.
- Sara repeats the phrase, then removes a penny from the corresponding drawing and feeds it to the worm.
- Mother and/or I continue the second and third steps until the activity is completed.

Sara is able to identify these phrases correctly, so I add a very abrupt *Stop!* and a long, enthusiastic *Hi!* She begins to confuse *Stop!* with *Sit down,* so I ask her to discriminate between an even more curt *Stop!* and a slower, more sing-song *Sit down.* She is probably confused by the newly salient /s/, which she has been unaccustomed to hearing well in these expressions. When I highlight other features of these words, as above, and reduce the number of choices to only two, Sara is successful.

Parent Guidance

✔ Practice the same task at home, using the cartoon drawings provided.

✔ Make a point of using these expressions frequently during the day. Post these and other targets on your fridge or in some other convenient spot.

✔ As soon as Sara can identify a word or phrase by listening in a structured exercise, expect her to do this by audition throughout the day in as many settings as possible.

(cont'd on next page)

> **Parent Guidance** *(cont'd)*
>
> ✔ When necessary, use the *auditory sandwich* technique (audition/vision/audition). Tell her, for example, *Shut the door* through audition alone a couple of times. If she does not respond appropriately, use lipreading and/or a gesture if necessary, while saying *Shut the door* again. Finally, say *Shut the door* once or twice again through audition alone. In this way, you are providing visual support while still reinforcing audition. As Sara acquires more auditory experience, she will be more likely to identify phrases by listening alone.

Identification of a Few Basic Verbs

I use a colorful toy furniture set and a toy girl. Sara has to make the girl *Sit down; Sh! Go to sleep; Go up, up, up the stairs* or *Wash, wash, wash, wash* upon request.

- I say each verb once, then I ask her mother to say the target verb once. I produce the appropriate prop and encourage Sara to repeat the target verb.
- When the chair, the bed, the stairs, and the sink are all in front of Sara, I cue her to *Listen!* and I say, *Go up, up, up the stairs.*
- Sara indicates which verb she has identified by repeating it after me, then chooses the right prop and makes the girl perform the appropriate action.

Sara has no difficulty with the first three verbs except *wash*. She tends to confuse it with *Sh! Go to sleep*. She is probably hearing the /sh/ sound much more strongly than before her implant and is distracted by it. I make the two verbs as acoustically different as possible by lengthening the /sh/ of *Sh! Go to sleep* and by saying *Wash, wash, wash, wash* as rhythmically as possible with no extra emphasis on the /sh/. Sara is then able to identify *wash* correctly.

Identification of Familiar Nouns

For this activity, the materials are rubber picture stamps, an ink pad, and a large piece of paper on which I have drawn the outline of a house and a few pieces of furniture. The target words are *baby, hat, shoe,* and *flower* because their different vowels, consonants, and number of syllables make them easier to hear. I *acoustically highlight*: for *baby* I use a sing-song intonation. I lengthen the /h/ in hat and both

---

Parent Guidance

✔ Practice the structured verb-identification activity every day. Use real or toy props. Gradually try to shorten the /sh/ of *Sh! Go to sleep* and reduce the number of repetitions of *wash*.

✔ Use these verbs at every opportunity during the day. If Sara does not identify them, use the *auditory sandwich* technique.

✔ Play a variation of Charades: take turns ordering each other to mime a particular verb.

---

the /sh/ and /oo/ of *shoe*. I lengthen *flower* and use a gently rising, then falling intonation.

- Hiding each stamp, I say the target word a couple of times, followed by mother. I produce the stamp, Sara repeats the target word, is handed the stamp, and then places it in front of her.
- When all stamps are displayed, I cue Sara to *Listen!* and ask *Where's the... ?*
- Sara repeats the target noun and then selects the appropriate stamp. I ask her where she is going to put it and why. She then stamps it wherever she chooses in the house picture.

Sara selects all nouns correctly, so now I will increase the difficulty of the task by exaggerating the words a bit less and/or increasing the set size from four to five or six.

Parent Guidance

✔ Play Memory (also known as Concentration) using pairs of the target words, to give Sara experience listening to them. A customized, home-made version can be made with file cards cut in half and pictures drawn or glued on.

✔ With crayons and paper in front of each of you and a barrier such as a tray between you, take turns telling each other, *Draw a...* while drawing one of the target nouns on your paper. Compare drawings.

✔ Add more challenge by increasing the set size to six nouns, adding, for example, *apple* and *man* and/or reducing the exaggeration of the target words.

GOALS

Speech:

Sara has already mastered most vowels and simple consonants. In this session, the main focus is to reinforce a selection of previously mastered speech targets in order to give her practice listening to them with her new implant. These include nasal consonant /m/, fricative (blowing) consonant /s/, vowels /ah/, /oo/, and /ee/, and diphthongs *ah-oo* (*Ow!*) and *ah-ee* (*eye*). I chose /m/ because it is one of the sounds Sara had trouble with in the phoneme identification activity, and /s/ because it is a new sound for her. She had been able to detect it with her frequency-transposition hearing aid, but now it will sound quite different. Finally, since accurate identification of vowels has always been a problem, we're practicing front-vowel /ee/, mid-vowel /ah/, and back-vowel /oo/ to ensure that Sara acquires lots of experience listening to them.

First, I ask Sara to imitate several series of repeated babbled syllables containing the target sounds. As she is very fashion-conscious, I use a create-your-own-outfit puzzle (Amanda's Closet™ from Discovery Toys), which she assembles piece by piece after each set of a few babbled syllables.

Speech Targets:

- **/s/**
    - Sara listens to /s/ in isolation, then repeats after me.
    - Sara listens to *sasasa* or *seeseesee* or *soosoosoo,* then repeats after me.
    - I reinforce Sara's correct imitations with verbal praise and by providing a puzzle piece for her to place.

If she had been unable to repeat a particular babbled syllable string I would have used the audition/vision/audition *auditory sandwich* technique, followed by reinforcement.

- **/m/**
    - Same procedure as for /s/, using babbled syllables *mamama, meemeemee* but not *moomoomoo,* as the acoustic similarity between /m/ and /oo/, known to be problematic for Sara, would likely cause her to fail at this syllable string.
    - Sara tends to confuse /m/ with /w/, a liquid sound very similar to /oo/. To focus on the difference between /m/ and /w/, I use a discrimination task. I print *mamama* and

wawawa on a piece of paper, saying each one as I print it. I lengthen the /m/ and use a more sing-song intonation for the *oo-ah* of *wa*. I then say *mamama* and *wawawa* in random order.

Sara repeats each syllable string after me and successfully puts a check mark under the appropriate letters.

- **oo, ah, ee in isolation**
  - I encourage Sara to imitate a single *oo* or *ah* or *ee*. I use slightly rising, then falling intonation for each one.

She confuses *oo* with /m/ until I specify that we are working on vowels only.

- **oo, ah, ee in babbled syllables**
  - Same procedure as for /s/ in babbled syllables, above, using *bahbahbah, boobooboo, beebeebee.*

Sara correctly imitates all syllable strings with /b/. She has more difficulty with the /sh/ syllable strings *shahshahshah, shooshooshoo,* and *sheesheeshee.* I first say the /sh/ in isolation to cue Sara to the consonant sound. Then I slow down the syllable strings and lengthen the vowels. Sara is then able to imitate them.

- **ah-oo and ah-ee in isolation**
  - Same procedure as for vowels in isolation, above.

Sara produces *ah-oo* as *ah-m* until I print the two target diphthongs for her. She then discriminates them correctly.

- **ah-oo and ah-ee in babbled syllables**
  - I use *bowbowbow* and *byebyebye.*

Sara has difficulty here, so I slow down, lengthen the diphthongs, and place more emphasis on the /oo/ and /ee/ parts of each one. Sara then correctly achieves them.

Word Games

For the word games, I use a board game and incorporate the target speech sounds /m/ and /s/ into it by means of a set of articulation cards (Articu-cards™ from Communication Skill Builders). Before rolling the die each time, Sara turns up a card and says, *That's a...* (using an

> **Parent Guidance**
>
> ✔ Play a board game, that requires Sara to imitate a babbled syllable string or use a target m- or s-word in a sentence, before each turn.

m-word such as *man, mouse, mitten, moon, mask* or an s-word such as *sun, school, sock, sandals*).

GOALS

Language:
Sara had already acquired many language skills before she received her implant. In this session, the goal is to help her to identify easy-to-hear, beginner-level language targets. The long-term objective is to progress grammatical item by grammatical item, following a developmental hierarchy, occasionally adapted to ensure that targets are audible. For example, if /s/ was not yet detected, we would postpone working on the plural noun marker /s/.

Language Targets:
- to discriminate *in* from *under.*
- to identify question forms *What's he doing?* and *What's that?*

Discriminate *In* from *Under*
I use my favorite activity for teaching basic prepositions. The materials include bean bags, a large toy car, and a playhouse.

- I put the large toy car on the table, point to it and then ask Sara to put a beanbag *in.* Then I ask her to put another beanbag *under.* To emphasize the difference between the two words, I exaggerate and lengthen the /n/ of *in* and vary my intonation from a high /un/ to a low /der/ with *under.*
- Then I ask her which one is *in.* She selects it and then gets to throw it into a tub far across the room. I replace the *in* beanbag and ask which one is *under,* followed by the same reinforcer. I ask which one is *in/under* a few more times.
- For variation I repeat the same overall procedure with the house instead of the car. By the end of the activity Sara is able, with close listening, to discriminate *in/under* consistently, so I will

increase the level of difficulty to *in the car* versus *under the car* or add a third preposition, *beside.*

Identify Question Forms *What's He Doing?* and *What's That?*

I reinforce these question forms separately several times first, then mix and match them. For the question form *What's that?,* I use picture cards and a feely-meely bag containing corresponding objects.

- I show Sara six pictures, asking *What's that?* Each time Sara answers correctly, I place the picture on the table.
- As Sara reaches into the bag, I ask *What's that?* She identifies the simple objects by feeling them and says, *That's a...* She removes the object from the bag to see if she has guessed correctly.
- Her mom or I take a turn, alternating with Sara until all objects have been identified.

For the question *What's he doing?,* I use the verb cards from Creatures and Critters™ (available from Communication Skill Builders). These cards portray cute frogs and turtles performing human activities.

- Sara picks a card from a pile.
- I cue her to *Listen!* and then ask, *What's he/she doing?*
- Sara answers the question.
- Her mom or I pick a card, listen to Sara ask the question, and then one of us answers it.
- We continue until we have used up five cards.
- For the combined activity, we continue with the verb cards using the same procedure described above, occasionally asking each other, *What's that?* to identify one of the frog's or turtle's quirky accessories.

Sara requires a bit of prompting to listen to the question asked, as opposed to the question expected.

Parent Guidance

✔ When you are reading a picture book to Sara, often ask her these two target questions.

✔ Throughout the day, ask her these two questions whenever an opportunity arises.

Mom's Notebook

As Sara's mother has now attended auditory-verbal therapy sessions for three years, she has the knowledge and experience to carry out therapy goals at home. Throughout the session, between activities, I provide activity suggestions to her mom, who jots them down in a small notebook. At the end of the session, we quickly review the assigned targets.

Conclusion

Sara's implant has now been switched on for about one month. After two weeks of wearing the implant, her ability to understand familiar words and phrases, through listening alone, reached her preimplant level. Her ability to identify high-frequency sounds /s/ and /f/ is superior to her preimplant levels. She is beginning to make the hard-to-hear place differentiation among front-plosive consonant /p/, mid-plosive /t/, and back-plosive /k/. Sara can now identify most vowels and diphthongs. We continue to work on identification of low-frequency phonemes /oo/ and /m/ because they are still confused. Distance listening is dramatically better in that Sara can hear her name being called from across a 20-foot room or even from an adjacent room. Her ability to understand spontaneous spoken language through audition, at the time of this lesson, was as weak as before she received her cochlear implant. She has now started to improve and can occasionally piece together enough words to capture the gist of an impromptu remark. Sara loves her new implant and exclaims repeatedly that it's better than her hearing aids.

To date, Sara's performance with her cochlear implant has been excellent. With further refining of her cochlear implant MAP and continued listening practice throughout the day, her parents and I are optimistic that she will eventually be able to understand most spoken language through listening.

Lesson Plan For Evan

Sally Tannenbaum, M.Ed., C.E.D., Cert. AVT

Evan is now two years and eight months old. At three months of age his hearing loss, of unknown etiology, was first suspected and at eight months he received hearing aids. His parents were told that he had a left-corner audiogram with no responses past 2000 Hz in either ear. His mother reports an unremarkable pregnancy and delivery, and there is no history of hearing loss in the family. It took several months for Evan to wear hearing aids consistently.

When Evan was 11 months old he and his family enrolled in their school district's parent-infant program, which they attended twice a week until Evan was two years old. They began to use sign language, and Evan wore both his hearing aids throughout this period. According to his parents, however, he received little benefit from his amplification and did not turn to his name nor to any environmental sounds. They reported that Evan responded about the same whether or not he was wearing his hearing aids.

Evan began to use sign language at 12 months old, when he also became very quiet and made few vocalizations. His signing increased, and by two years of age he was putting two signed words together. At that time Evan's parents started to gather information about the cochlear implant by reading the literature and meeting with families whose children had an implant. After comprehensive evaluations, the implant center recommended Evan as a candidate.

In November 1995, at two years, four months of age, Evan received a cochlear implant. His parents report that he loved the implant from the beginning and asked for it to be put on. He does not wear a hearing aid in the contralateral ear. Evan and his family enrolled in an auditory-verbal program when he was aged two years, eight months, and therapy began immediately.

Parent Orientation Session

Prior to beginning therapy, the parents and I review the audiological information and discuss the principles and goals of an auditory-verbal program. I try to address any questions and concerns. Evan's parents want to know how to move from a total communication (TC) program to an auditory-verbal approach, and how I will react when Evan uses sign language in therapy. This is a very valid concern, since Evan's

Parent Guidance

In order to create a *listening environment* at home throughout Evan's waking hours:

✔ Stay close to Evan while talking and singing to him.

✔ Reduce ambient background noise.

✔ Get Evan's attention through listening.

✔ Point to your ear and say *Listen!*

✔ Ensure that Evan wears his cochlear implant during all waking hours.

✔ Speak in a natural voice and sing songs throughout the day.

✔ Use meaningful situations to encourage Evan to pay attention to the environment.

✔ When one of you comes home from work, knock on the front door and wait. The other parent needs to call Evan's attention to the sound and say: "Listen, I hear Mommy knocking on the door, let's go open the door for Mommy." Mommy can give Evan a special greeting such as: "Hi, Evan; you heard me knocking on the door."

✔ Use the *learning to listen* sounds; these show up on placemats, clothing, dishes, books, puzzles, and even on diapers! Using these sounds throughout Evan's day will provide repetition and help him process what he is hearing.

✔ Skills such as blowing, lip smacking, tongue clicking, licking, and blowing "raspberries" are prerequisites for developing speech. *Blowing* helps a child to whisper and develop voiceless consonants such as /p/ and /t/. *Chewing* and *swallowing* help develop the muscles necessary for speech production. Many of the *learning to listen* sounds incorporate these pre-speech skills.

primary mode of communication was sign language. A young child with a cochlear implant receives a great deal of auditory information, and as listening and language goals are achieved the amount of sign language is usually reduced.

I demonstrate a variety of ways to use the *learning to listen* sounds, explaining that the big vehicles and animals make a loud sound while the smaller ones make a quieter sound.

Evan's parents learn to listen carefully to his vocalizations. I discuss early developing sounds of young children and review the vowels and diphthongs that are informally learned through everyday applications of the *learning to listen* sounds. I encourage them to keep a diary of Evan's development and bring this book to all sessions. They are to record what Evan is hearing, any sounds to which he is not responding, his vocalizations, and the language Evan understands without visual cues. I need to know if Evan is turning when called, or if he points or looks at Mommy when asked, *Where's mommy?*

We discuss everything about Evan so that I know his daily schedule and routines, favorite toys, television shows, pets, friends, and family. This helps me to incorporate familiar topics and situations into the therapy sessions.

Introduction to the Lesson

I am in private practice and my therapy room is located downstairs in my house. It is a relaxed place for children and parents where we have fun *learning to listen.*

My lesson starts the moment Evan and his family arrive in the neighborhood. I want to *hear* them coming down the street. Therapy is not an isolated session that takes place at a table. I encourage parents to march, run fast, walk slowly, jump, skip, walk backwards, or sing all the way to Sally's Gate. After they knock on my door and call my name, we exchange greetings. Then we talk about what we are wearing and what the weather is like. I take the time to talk about *what is happening.* The focus of the session is *structured around highlighting speech and language through listening,* with communication being closely related to Evan's interests.

The Freeze Dance

GOALS
- to create a relaxed and enjoyable listening environment.
- to give Evan a few minutes to adjust to the therapy room.
- to demonstrate the absence or presence of sound.
- to develop auditory attention.
- to encourage localizing the source of a sound.

ACTIVITY
Evan's mom holds him in her arms. I turn on my tape recorder and play the *Freeze Dance,* a child's song containing pauses throughout it. When

the music begins I start to dance and point to my ear and say, "I hear that, I hear the music." Evan's mom is a little shy about dancing and I tell her, "Come on, Mom, dance to the music." She begins to dance and Evan begins to smile. When the music pauses, we stop dancing, I point to my ear, shake my head and say, "Sh, it stopped! I don't hear it! It is all gone!" When it begins again, I point to the tape recorder and back to my ear and say, "I hear it, I hear the music." After a few times of stopping and starting I tell his mom, "Wait a few seconds to see what Evan does by himself when the music starts up again." Evan starts to move his body as if to say, "Come on, Mom." When the song is over I clap my hands and say, "It's over, it's all gone, I don't hear it."

ANALYSIS

The Freeze Dance is a great activity to start a first session with a small child. This is an activity we will do again in later sessions. Sometimes everyone has a bracelet of bells to shake while we are dancing, or puppets to move to the music. In this session both his mom and Evan enjoyed the dance, and Evan adjusted to the new environment.

Parent Guidance

✔ Play the Freeze Dance at home and encourage dancing to various songs.

✔ Sing to Evan; it will help him develop natural-sounding speech.

✔ Form a small marching band; each time you stop banging the drum, everyone must freeze.

✔ Be sure to point out the presence or absence of sound by saying, "I hear it" or "I don't hear it."

The Calling Game

GOALS
- to detect the presence of sound.
- to learn to listen to his name.
- to encourage vocalizing for attention.
- to develop greetings.
- to encourage turn-taking.

ACTIVITY

Evan's mom holds him with his back on her chest so they are both facing the same direction. I stand a couple feet behind them and using a sing-song voice call, "Evan." His mom turns around holding him, points to his ear and says, "I heard that."

I then put a Cookie Monster puppet on my hand and say, "Hi, Evan." Cookie tickles Evan to reward him for turning to his name.

"It's my turn to turn around," I say. "I am going to listen for my name."

I ask Evan's mom to count to 10 before she calls my name. This helps Evan to become aware of the absence of sound. During this absence I point to my ear, shake my head and say, "I don't hear anything."

His mom then calls my name and I immediately turn around and say, "Hi, I heard that."

We play the game a few more times. When I call his name again, his mom waits for few seconds before turning him around, but we see no indication that he heard his name. He does not blink his eyes or start to turn his body. This lack of response is typical at this early stage. Evan does vocalize, but not to get my attention. He wants to get down and starts to complain.

I immediately turn around when he vocalizes his complaint and say, "I heard that."

ANALYSIS

There has to be a good reason for Evan to turn to his name. Once he is turning to his name in this structured setting, I expect him to turn to his name in situations throughout the day. A typical two-year-old, however, does not always listen to his name being called. Any vocalization that Evan makes can be used to demonstrate that *sound can make things happen*. We need to *respond* to his vocalizations in order to develop the auditory feedback loop.

Parent Guidance

✔ Play the Calling Game at home with Evan's brother or Dad.

✔ Help Evan to watch others play the Calling Game. Once he is able to respond he will play variations of the game, such as standing on his own and listening to two different people call him (not at the same time) from various parts of the room. Evan will have to identify the location of the sound.

(cont'd on next page)

Parent Guidance *(cont'd)*

✔ Mom and Dad can take turns calling Evan; encourage him to identify the speaker.

✔ Be creative with the Calling Game: you can use a colorful box with a surprise inside to encourage Evan to turn to his name.

✔ When you call Evan, be certain to have a *good reason* for him to turn to you.

The Cat

GOALS

- to identify that sound has a specific meaning.
- to learn that vocalizing can make something happen.
- to encourage listening to suprasegmental and vowel information of this particular *learning to listen* sound.
- to encourage development of auditory feedback through imitation.

ACTIVITY

The first sessions with Evan always include the *learning to listen* sounds. These sounds can be presented in a variety of ways through puzzles, books, stuffed animals, small toys, and beanie babies.

I have a wooden feely box that I use to introduce the sound *meow*. I place a soft stuffed kitty inside the box and hold it under the table. I point to my ear and say, "Listen, I hear a kitty, meow, meow, I hear the kitty." I secure Evan's auditory attention when I say "meow." He becomes very still and looks at me as if to say, "I hear that."

I put the box on the table and continue to say the kitty sound. I give Evan's mom a turn calling the kitty. After she says *meow,* I bring the kitty out of the box. Next, it is Evan's turn to call the kitty. I put the kitty back in the box and hold it in front of Evan, waiting for him to vocalize.

Evan does vocalize an /ee/ sound which I immediately reinforce by having the kitty come out of the box. I say, "I heard that, you called the kitty, meow."

The kitty has eyes that open and close, so I put it on the table and say in a very soft voice, "Sh, kitty is sleeping." Evan immediately responds to the /sh/ sound by turning to the sound. I then tell the kitty to WAKE UP! in a very loud voice. We all take turns saying *Night, night* and *Wake up!*

ANALYSIS

I picked the sound *meow* first because it has good suprasegmental information and I know that Evan has a cat at home.

It is important to wait for Evan to vocalize. I still need to remind myself to wait!

I reinforce any vocalization Evan makes to show him that language can make things happen. If Evan did not vocalize, which is not unusual in the first session, his mom would have had another turn to call the kitty.

My primary goal here is to evaluate how Evan responds to the *learning to listen* sounds, but I also target comprehension while playing with the cat. Evan turned each time I said the /sh/ sound, which indicates that he is hearing up to 2000 Hz.

Parent Guidance

✔ Point out all the cats you hear and see in your neighborhood. Say *meow* each time you see a cat.

✔ Evan needs a lot of repetition.

✔ Visit a pet shop with Evan.

✔ Use a variety of materials to reinforce the *learning to listen* sounds, such as: puzzles, books, stuffed animals, clothing, stickers, labels, and of course the real things!

✔ Present the *learning to listen* sounds through *listening first*. Say the sound, point to your ear to get Evan's attention, and say the sound again. Help him find the sound in the book or puzzle if he can't find the sound himself.

✔ Put toys aside in a *learning to listen* basket. Use these toys for a week or two and then switch them with some other toys to keep his interest.

✔ Evan is very young, so give him a lot of time to play with the toys.

Sound Conditioning

GOAL
• to encourage auditory detection of a variety of sounds.

ACTIVITY
Since this is Evan's first session I ask his mom to model this activity. I stand beside his mom where Evan can watch both of us. Mom holds a bean bag up to her ear. When she hears the clicker she drops the bean bag in the bucket. She smiles and says, "I hear that."

ANALYSIS
Evan indicates he is hearing the clicker by turning to it and then turning back to his mom as if to say, *You can drop the bean bag now.* Putting blocks in a container, pegs in a pegboard, and objects into play dough are good reinforcers for this important structured activity. Within a few sessions Evan is expected to pick up the bean bag on his own and drop it in the bucket by himself. If Evan shows no auditory response to the clicker, I try a drum or another noisemaker.

Then, I move on to the Ling Six-Sound Test (/ah/, /oo/, /e/, /sh/, /s/, and /m/). Once Evan is conditioned to these sounds, I add distance to the task and encourage him to repeat the sounds he hears and learn to identify them. When Evan can do this task for the MAPping procedure of the cochlear implant, his audiologist can obtain important information.

I carefully document what Evan is hearing and at what distance. Each change in his MAP may result in different auditory responses. As a team, the parents and I will inform the audiologist about Evan's listening performance.

Parent Guidance
✔ At this level Evan is watching the activity closely, so it is important to have more than one person present. If you are alone and drop the object and present the sound at the same time, Evan will imitate what he has observed. Thus, he will hold up a bean bag, perhaps make a sound, and drop the bean bag. This is not the goal. Evan is required to listen for the sound and, upon hearing it, drop the bean bag into the bucket.

(cont'd on next page)

Parent Guidance *(cont'd)*

✔ Model *sound conditioning* with Evan's dad or his brother while Evan is watching.

✔ You might try some other reinforcers. These reinforcers, however, should not be *too* interesting, so that Evan gets right to the task instead of playing with the reinforcers.

The Airplane

GOALS
- to listen to the sound /ah/ for the airplane.
- to identify that a sound has a specific meaning.
- to develop vocalization with adequate breath flow (vocalize /ah/ with a sustained breath stream).
- to encourage the use of vocal play (the use of voice patterns varying in intensity, duration, and pitch).

ACTIVITY
I point to my ear, calling Evan's attention to the sound and say, "Listen, /ah/. I hear an airplane." The airplane is hidden inside a plastic egg. I bring out the egg and say /ah/. I hold the container near Mom's mouth and she says the sound.

Next, I hold the container near Evan's mouth and wait for him to say the sound. Evan is quiet and doesn't repeat the sound. I hold it near my mouth and say the sound again. Next, I shake the egg, point to my ear and say, "I hear that, it is an airplane. /Ah/." I shake the egg near his mom's ear, she points to her ear and says: "I hear that; /ah/, it is an airplane." I shake the container next to Evan's ear and he reaches for the container. We open the container and Evan finds the airplane. While he is playing with it I say the airplane sound again, varying my pitch. While the airplane is flying high I make the sound high, and as the plane comes down I lower my voice. When the airplane stops flying I say, "Sh, I don't hear it, it stopped."

I bring out two more airplanes, repeating the same pattern. Evan does say /ah/ for the last airplane.

I immediately reinforce this by repeating the sound and opening the egg, letting him find the airplane. I give one of the airplanes to his mom and the other one to Evan. We all fly the airplane while vocalizing /ah/. When it is time to put them away I ask his mom for her airplane and we say, "bye-bye." I repeat this with Evan's airplane and with my airplane. Evan does wave bye-bye to the airplanes, but he does not vocalize. I point to my ear and say, "I don't hear you saying bye-bye." I use the *hand cue* and say, "Bye-bye." I repeat this with his mom, who says, "Bye-bye," and then use the hand cue with Evan, who says, "Ba" and waves. I say, "I heard you say bye-bye."

ANALYSIS

Evan vocalizes /ah/ for the last airplane and is able to sustain the sound for a few seconds. In the next session I will use airplanes first to reinforce this sound and then quickly move on to talk about the airplane: *"The airplane goes up, up, up, and around and around and down."*

If Evan had not waved bye-bye I would have taken his hand and waved it for him. This is a childlike way to develop pattern perception of an often-heard phrase.

Parent Guidance

✔ Listen for airplanes throughout the day. When you hear one, point to your ear and say the airplane sound: "Listen, I hear an airplane. /Ah/. It's up in the sky. There it is. /Ah/. Bye-bye, airplane."

✔ Look at books about airplanes while reinforcing the sound /ah/.

✔ Make paper airplanes and fly them while saying the sound /ah/.

✔ Place a toy airplane or a picture of one in a couple of rooms at home. When entering the room say the sound /ah/ and ask Evan where the airplane is. If Evan looks in the direction of the airplane, he is beginning to identify what he is hearing.

✔ Work on duration by flying the airplane around while sustaining the sound /ah/. Contrast the sound /ah/ with short airplane trips: /ah/ /ah/ /ah/.

About Face

GOAL

- to develop the identification of a sound that is too loud or too quiet by listening to voices that are loud, quiet, and just right.

ACTIVITY

I bring out three pictures of faces. The first face is *huge* and is *shouting* Evan's name! I make a face and cover my ears and say, "It is too loud, I do not like it!" The next face is tiny and is calling Evan's name in the softest voice possible. "It is too quiet, I do not like it." The last picture is a face with a smile that, of course, is calling Evan's name in a pleasant voice. "It is just right, I like it." Next, I bring out a container of tokens. I hold up the picture and repeat each phrase, using the appropriate intensity, and place a token on a picture.

I ask Evan's mom to listen and, when I say the phrase, to pick up the token off the correct picture and drop it into the container. Evan watches and listens throughout this activity. When I put the pictures away I ask Evan for each picture one at a time. Evan's mom helps him select the correct picture, waves *bye-bye,* and puts it away.

Throughout the session, we use loud and quiet voices and point out when something is too loud, too soft, or just right. A truck goes by during the session and Evan puts his hands over his ears. His mom immediately reinforces this gesture by saying, "I hear the truck, it's too loud! Listen, I don't hear it. It went away. It's okay now."

ANALYSIS

Acoustic cues on vocal intensity occur throughout the range of speech frequencies. During this activity, Evan only observed. After a few more sessions I anticipate that he will identify loud and quiet voices. Identifying a sound as *too loud* or *too quiet* will help the audiologist MAP Evan's cochlear implant.

I will engage Evan in vocal play in which loud and quiet voices and high and low voices are contrasted.

Parent Guidance

✔ The story of *Goldilocks and the Three Bears* reinforces the goals of intensity, pitch, and duration, so this is a good time to enjoy it with Evan.

✔ Using the strategies of the About Face activity, point out *loud, quiet,* and *just right voices.*

✔ Pretend to go to sleep. It will take a *very loud voice* to wake you up!

The Car

GOALS

- to develop identification of the *learning to listen* sound for the car.
- to enhance prespeech skills and vocal play through blowing "raspberries" and the *beep-beep* sound as we play with the cars.
- to develop some early functional language.

ACTIVITY

I have a toy car hidden inside a small box. I say the car sound, *brrr beep-beep* while pointing to my ear. Evan's mom points to her ear and says, "I hear a car." I hold the box near my mouth and say the sound again. Using the box as a *hand cue,* I hold it near Mom's mouth and she says the car sound. When I hold the box near Evan's mouth he blows raspberries but does not say "beep-beep."

I repeat the sound correctly and tell Evan, "I hear the car."

He opens the box to discover a car with a dent in one door.

"Uh oh, the car is broken! It was in an accident," I say.

I bring out more cars and continue to say the car sound.

ANALYSIS

Speech skills are made meaningful through their use in spoken language. Evan imitated the "raspberries" while playing with the cars. In the next few sessions I anticipate that he will imitate the *beep-beep* sound following the *raspberries.* I document his imitations and spontaneous utterances and note his voice quality and vowel and syllable production. He imitated one syllable, produced the vowels /ah/ and /e/, and blew raspberries.

Parent Guidance

✔ Evan loves vehicles, so spend a lot of time on the vehicle sounds and present these in various ways. A feely box, a shoe box, and egg containers can provide interesting motivators.

✔ *Blowing raspberries* will stimulate Evan's strength and coordination for talking.

✔ Every time you get into a car you have a wonderful opportunity to say the *car sound.* So, go for car rides often, especially to a farm where many sounds live.

(cont'd on next page)

Blowing Bubbles

GOALS
- to develop blowing, a prerequisite for speech production.
- to develop vocalizing, vocal pitch, and duration.
- to promote language development by listening to meaningful phrases containing functional words.
- to develop self-esteem through positive reinforcement.

MATERIALS
Plastic bottle containing commercial bubble solution or home-made soap solution, plus a wand for stirring.

ACTIVITY
I talk about the bubbles before I present them. I say, "I have something to blow."

We practice blowing. I pretend the bubbles are floating in the air, and I start to pop them.

I say, "There is a bubble. Pop, pop, pop! Whee, the bubbles are coming down."

Then I present the bottle of bubbles to Evan. I show him the picture of the bubbles on the bottle. I hand the bottle to his mom and ask her to open it. I take the wand and stir the bubbles. Then, I take the wand out. His mom tells me to "blow the bubbles." We all take turns blowing and popping the bubbles.

Before I put the bottle away I talk about how wet the table is: "Uh oh, the table is all wet. We need to wipe it up. Here is a towel, wipe, wipe, wipe."

I give the towel to Evan's mom and she wipes the table in front of her. Then she shows Evan how his section of the table is wet, and gives him the towel to wipe it up. As Evan is wiping the table, his mom tells him what he is doing.

ANALYSIS

Evan was not able to blow the bubbles through the wand, which is not unusual for a child his age. *Blowing* is a prerequisite for developing speech. Evan needs a variety of things to blow, including ping-pong balls, feathers, cotton balls, and windmills. We will *pretend to blow* on hot food and tea.

Parent Guidance

✔ Bubbles are fun! Have a good time and enjoy the experience together.

✔ Play with the suprasegmental aspects of speech through vocalizing *Whee* and changing the pitch as the bubbles float down.

✔ When the bubbles spill, which is highly likely with a two-year-old, remember to make it a language experience!

✔ Listen for vowel production in the words: *blow, down, pop, wipe*.

✔ Watch how Evan visually tracks the bubbles. Does he follow them with his eyes?

✔ Pay attention to how Evan is communicating, both nonverbally and verbally. How does he communicate that he wants another turn to blow?

✔ Encourage Evan to blow a variety of things, such as ping-pong balls, feathers, cotton balls, windmills, paper, warm food, and water.

✔ Always finish your lesson at home with a smiling child. Playing with bubbles or play dough, doing a Freeze Dance, or reading a story can usually accomplish this.

Conclusion

At the end of the first session, I review the goals and activities with Evan's mom. I stress the need to provide Evan with numerous opportunities to engage in listening activities throughout his waking hours. Evan's mom records these suggestions in her notebook.

Evan responded well in his first session. He vocalized spontaneously and upon request. He watched intently and made good eye contact. He played appropriately with the toys and appeared interested in all the activities.

> ## Mom's Notebook
>
> ✓ Dance with Evan and point out the presence and absence of sound.
>
> ✓ Sing with Evan throughout the day.
>
> ✓ Play the Calling Game. Remember when calling him there must be a good reason for doing so!
>
> ✓ Play with the Learning to Listen sounds, especially the sounds of cats, airplanes, cars.
>
> ✓ Put together a basket of Learning to Listen sounds.
>
> ✓ Call Evan's attention to sounds that are too loud, too soft, and just right.
>
> ✓ Point out environmental sounds.
>
> ✓ Encourage Evan to watch and listen as we demonstrate the sound conditioning task.
>
> ✓ Encourage Evan to blow bubbles, warm food, cotton balls, and paper.
>
> ✓ Use functional phrases, such as: all gone, open the door, sit down in your chair, it's hot, don't touch.

My goals for Evan with a cochlear implant are not very different than if he was wearing hearing aids. I find that children with cochlear implants move through the early *learning to listen* stages quickly.

Each therapy session incorporates listening targets that are important for the cochlear implant MAPping process. Evan's listening goals include: sound conditioning, comprehending intensity, identifying spondee words (two-syllable words with equal accent on each syllable, such as *ice cream, airplane,* and *high chair*), and pattern perception.

Open communication with the implant team is critical, especially since Evan cannot tell the audiologist what he is hearing yet. This involves real teamwork! Evan's parents, the audiologists, and I work together to ensure that the cochlear implant is doing what it is supposed to do: helping Evan *learn to listen!*

Although he has a hearing impairment, Evan has the same needs as any child. Like any two-year-old, he wants to play and have a good time.

While we are reviewing the session, Evan starts to act mischievously. Mom gives him a loving hug and says, "You're so cool. I love you."

That's exactly what it is all about!

Lesson Plan for Jordon

Beth Walker, M.Ed., C.E.D., Cert. AVT

Jordon is two years, two months old. He is an only child and lives at home with young parents. His mother works part time and his father full time. He has a profound, bilateral sensorineural hearing loss which was diagnosed at age 13 months by a combination of auditory brainstem response (ABR) testing and behavioral testing. At the age of 15 months, Jordon received two powerful hearing aids. At this time, Jordon's mother and father chose the auditory-verbal approach. After two months of intensive auditory-verbal therapy and more audiological testing, Jordon demonstrated aided responses to sound only at 250 Hz and 500 Hz, outside the speech range.

Over the next three months, Jordon's audiologist increased the gain on his hearing aids to what she felt was the maximum allowable. Continued audiological testing revealed that Jordon had minimal hearing. Although Jordon's parents worked with him consistently and enthusiastically, he made little progress. When Jordon was 20 months old, his parents began an auditory-oral approach, and a recommendation was made to investigate cochlear implantation.

Jordon's parents proceeded with the assessments for cochlear implantation and he was confirmed as a candidate. Jordon had cochlear implant surgery shortly after his second birthday. All electrodes were inserted; the implant was hooked up when he was 25 months of age, and on the second day after initial stimulation, all electrodes were activated. He immediately wore the speech processor all day long, and the family rejoined the auditory-verbal center.

The following lesson plan took place one month after stimulation.

Introduction to the Lesson

Jordon and his mother began coming to the auditory-verbal center for weekly therapy sessions. His father was able to attend the sessions about once a month. During the first sessions Jordon and his mom would knock on the door and wait until I called, "Come in!" After a brief greeting, we moved towards a table where Jordon could immediately see an exciting toy in front of a high chair. This encouraged him into the chair, where he played with the toy while his mom and I discussed Jordon's progress since the last session. During this time I listened for any particular concerns and rejoiced in his progress. I also planned any adjustments I wanted to make in our time together that day, in case Jordon's mom had questions that could be addressed during the session. Questions requiring detailed answers are addressed at the end of the session or in a follow-up phone call.

On a typical visit, after the initial chat, we briefly discuss the goals of the first activity. I begin each activity with Jordon, modeling strategies used to reach the goals. Often, I explain the purpose for each strategy as I play. After the parents have watched for a few minutes, I turn the activity over to them, and they practice the strategies with my coaching until they are comfortable using them at home. Jordon usually stays in the high chair for the first few activities and then moves to the floor. Mom and Dad may take notes during the activity, or they may want to wait until the end of the session, when we summarize.

Since Jordon's parents know how to check the cochlear implant themselves, I take a moment to encourage Mom to check the speech processor to ensure that it is functioning.

I Hear That! Conditioned-Response Activity

GOALS

Audition:
- to prepare for audiologic testing to update the speech processor MAP.
- to detect the six Ling sounds.

Cognition:
- to attend to a task for one to two minutes.

RATIONALE
I begin the session with an important conditioning activity. As Jordon will learn language primarily through listening, the audiologist must be able to reMAP Jordon as often as needed to obtain the clearest auditory signal from the speech processor. Jordon must be able to do the

conditioned-response task consistently during the time of the audiological appointment. We do a conditioned-response activity at the beginning of every therapy session to determine which sounds he is hearing as he typically does.

ACTIVITY

Even though he must *play this game* when his parents or I ask him, we try to make it fun. Jordon is required to hold small rubber balls at his cheek and put them in a cup when he hears a speech sound (usually one of the six Ling sounds). After he has collected five or six balls, he can throw them into a plastic tub of water.

ANALYSIS

Jordon makes fairly consistent responses to five of the six Ling sounds (/ah/, /oo/, /ee/, /sh/, /m/). He is not showing a consistent response to /s/. We need to know if this is because he isn't receiving enough stimulation in the frequencies where /s/ has its energy, or whether he has not yet learned to pay attention to that sound. In order to make the /s/ more acoustically salient, we move closer to his microphone, present a slightly louder /s/ than we would at normal speaking level, pair it with a *whispered* /oo/ which slightly lowers the acoustic energy of the /s/, and pulse the /s/ (*ssoo — ssoo — ssoo,* rather than *ssss*). He does respond to this, so we begin to take away one modification at a time until he is responding consistently to a /s/ spoken at the level of natural conversation.

Parent Guidance

✔ Modify the /s/ in order to help Jordon respond. Use strategies modeled in the session. Write these down to share with his daddy.

✔ Practice a conditioning task for a few minutes each day until Jordon learns it and responds appropriately. A few suggestions for conditioning-task reinforcers are: breaking up branches and sticking them in dirt, rolling cars down a ramp, tossing tub toys into the sink, and throwing dirty clothes, one at a time, into the washer.

✔ Check responses to the six-sound test daily.

One Frog Too Many

GOALS

Audition:
- to identify common phrases given through audition.
- to attend to the *learning to listen* sounds.

Speech:
- to imitate duration of common phrases.

Language:
- to comprehend a core of common phrases.
- to develop basic turn-taking skills.
- to initiate communication about Jordon's own ideas.

Cognition:
- to develop response to the hand cue.
- to attend to a short story.
- to learn how to interact with books (right side up, page turning from left to right).
- to recall what happens on the next page of a familiar story.

RATIONALE

I use the same book we had in last week's session. This activity is to encourage Jordon's parents to *share* a book *with* him, instead of reading *to* him. Jordon's parents have been frustrated because Jordon hasn't seemed to enjoy stories. In our last session, we discussed sharing books. In this session I want to demonstrate a variety of ways to share books, to extend Jordon's interest in books, and to integrate language and auditory targets in the process. I use *One Frog Too Many*, a wordless picture book by Mercer Mayer (New York: Dial Books, 1975). As there are no words, there is no "right" way to tell the story. These books are especially good for parents who tend to *read at* rather than *with* children.

ACTIVITY

I say, "Listen, Jordon!" Then I make a quiet rustling noise with a plastic grocery bag. I say, "I have something that goes 'hop hop hop.' Wanna see?" I encourage him to take the frog prop out of the bag. We proceed in a similar way with the other props, which include a second smaller frog, a dog, a boy, a turtle, and a boat. I get his attention through listening by making a soft sound with the bag, and then call his attention to the *learning to listen* sound for each prop. Then Jordon plays with the toys. We act out the story together, using all the props.

I share the first few pages with Jordon, acoustically highlighting the common phrases associated with each picture. He plays with the props, acting out the pictures and making up some of his own actions.

I then hold the book facing me so that Jordon can see neither my mouth nor the pictures, and I tell Mom about the next picture. I again use a common phrase associated with the picture: "The frog said, 'Ow! That hurts!'" I acoustically highlight the common phrase. I let Mom see the picture and say, "Let's tell Jordon the frog said, 'Ow! That hurts!'" I used the hand cue when I say, "Ow! That hurts!" to prompt Mom to imitate the phrase.

As Jordon is looking at that picture, I encourage Mom to read the next page to Jordon and to encourage him to tell me about it by imitating the common phrase. We continue reading pages to each other and acting out the story.

When we reach the next-to-last page, I hold the book back, look questioningly at his mom, and ask her to recall what happened on that page by telling me and using the props. On the final page, I make the same request of Jordon. Mom helps him act out the final page with the props.

ANALYSIS

Jordon alerts to the soft sound of the rustling bag after three presentations. He needs continued exposure to soft environmental sounds in order to respond consistently.

His excitement when manipulating the story props indicates that he *does* enjoy books as we follow his lead and encourage him to take a turn. Other ways of using props will increase his interest in stories and extend his dramatic play skills.

As Jordon plays with the props, he spontaneously imitates the *learning to listen* sounds twice, when the sound is paired with movement, such as accompanying each hopping movement with the word *hop.* He approximates both the duration and the vowel. His initial imitation of the dog's sound, *woofwoof,* is one long *uuhhh,* indicating perception of the *length of the two syllables* together, not of two distinct syllables. When prompted slightly, however, to make the break between the two syllables more obvious (*woof—woof*), Jordon spontaneously imitates a closer approximation of duration.

Developing perceptual skills are indicated by Jordon's vocal approximation of the duration patterns in the phrases *No! no!* and *That hurts!,* including approximations of *ah* and *uh*. Approximations of early developing consonants (/p/, /b/, /m/, /h/, /w/) are expected as he continues to learn language through listening.

Parent Guidance

✔ The main purpose of reading with Jordon is to create a love of books.

✔ Share stories he enjoys over and over *with* him. Use props to maintain interest and generate the foundations of conversation. Encourage Jordon to initiate play and act out story elements with the props.

✔ Encourage use of the *learning to listen* sounds and imitation of common phrases.

✔ When encouraging imitation, remember that later, Jordon will be paying closer attention to vowel and consonant features. He is just beginning to focus on differences in duration, intensity, and pitch.

✔ Act out and tell the story of *One Frog Too Many.*

✔ Begin collecting props for other books.

✔ Bring a book and props to our next session and *read* to me.

Ride a Horsie!

GOALS

Audition:
- to attend to the abundant prosodic features in nursery rhymes.

Speech:
- to encourage spontaneous vocalizing.
- to encourage spontaneous use of varied suprasegmentals.
- to develop approximations of varied suprasegmentals through imitation in vocal play.

Language:
- to demonstrate understanding that spoken language has meaning through production of a higher rate of speech-like vocalizations.

Cognition:
- to create an interest in the rhythmic patterns of spoken language.
- to respond to the hand cue when encouraged to imitate on demand.

Communication Development:
- to develop basic turn-taking skills.

RATIONALE

Jordon has been sitting in the high chair for awhile and this nursery rhyme activity provides an opportunity for *active* interaction. The activity is short and highly motivational. Jordon will want to play it again and again, providing many opportunities to encourage him to initiate the game repeatedly through vocalizing. This activity is so much fun that it usually causes the child to raise vocal pitch and change intensity spontaneously. This provides an opportunity for the stimulation of varied suprasegmentals through vocal play.

ACTIVITY

I explain the main goals of the activity and then ask Jordon, "Wanna *get down?*" I wait for him to respond and when he does not, I repeat the question, holding my hands out to him, and wait again. When he begins to move back and forth in the seat, I ask his mom, "Yes?" and use the hand cue to prompt a *yes* response.

I quickly get Jordon out of the seat and begin to bounce him on my knees while saying the *ride-a-horsie* rhyme. I bounce him in rhythm first, with the faster first part of the rhyme, and then slow the bouncing towards the end as my voice slows ("youuu'll faalll..."). When I get to the last word, "dowwwn!" I lean him way back to protect him from falling. I imitate his squeal of delight and look at him expectantly, hoping he will imitate the squeal again. When he does not, I squeal to his mom, and she squeals back. I tell her I'll play one more time before her turn. I pull Jordon back up to a sitting position on my knees and wait, looking at him expectantly, as if to say, *Do you want something?* He just smiles back at me so I ask his mom, "Do you want Jordon to play *some more?*"

She says, "Yes, some more!" and I begin the rhyme again. I want Jordon to associate Mom's talking with the fun's beginning. He squeals a bit, so I repeat his squeal and he squeals again! Mom holds Jordon and waits for him to vocalize to initiate the rhyme. When he does not, I model the *more-play scenario,* and his mom starts over again. The next time she begins the rhyme she waits, looks expectantly, asks him if he wants more, and uses the hand cue. Jordon vocalizes a little bit.

ANALYSIS

Waiting and looking expectantly prompted fewer spontaneous vocal-izations than I had anticipated and consequently, I used other strategies to encourage vocalization. First, I established an expectation for repeat-ed activity in the game and then waited for Jordon to initiate another round. Second, I paused and looked expectantly, as if to say, *Is there something you want?* Then, I asked his mom to model the response vocally, and finally I prompted with the hand cue.

Jordon's voice quality was quite weak, owing to infrequent vocal-izing. He will do more listening than talking during these first weeks of cochlear implant use. Consistent use of strategies to prompt listening and talking in conjunction with excellent technological management are critical for spoken communication development.

The repeated actions and rhyme did provide several opportunities for vocal play, and Jordon's repeated squealing indicates development of his auditory feedback loop.

Parent Guidance

✔ Jordon's use of his new hearing potential should increase vocalization, thereby improving his voice quality.

✔ Help Jordon pay attention to the frequency of and variation in the new signal from the cochlear implant.

✔ Initiate activities where motion is associated with *Jordon's talking*. Repeat the activity a couple of times, and *wait* for Jordon to initiate it again by vocalizing.

✔ Play *active* games to encourage spontaneous use of variation in duration, intensity, and pitch (suprasegmentals). Imitate playfully when he makes sounds. This develops auditory *self-monitoring* (listening to his own voice).

(cont'd on next page)

Parent Guidance *(cont'd)*

✔ Tickle games, roughhousing, water play, and stacking up and knocking over blocks are good activities to enrich suprasegmental behaviors.

✔ To encourage communication, use strategies such as *looking expectantly, pausing, waiting, using another person to model talking, and using the hand cue.*

Swinging Sounds!

GOALS

Audition:
- to attend to a soft environmental sound.
- to provide exposure to a variety of *learning to listen* sounds.

Speech:
- to encourage imitation of suprasegmental features.

Language:
- to help Jordon attach meaning to the *learning to listen* sounds.
- to encourage comprehension of a few functional words.

Cognition:
- to encourage memory for where things belong.
- to match a picture to an object.

Communication:
- to help Jordon to initiate a *conversation* by verbal or nonverbal means.
- to develop turn-taking.

RATIONALE

Although Jordon had a good deal of exposure to the *learning to listen* sounds prior to receiving his implant, we have begun this process all over again to help him pay attention to and begin to derive meaning from the information provided through the implant. The *learning to listen* sounds provide opportunities for a variety of suprasegmental features. His parents had grown weary of playing with the *learning to listen* sounds during the months Jordon wore hearing aids because they observed no responses. In this session, I create an interesting play scenario with the *learning to listen* sound toys. As it requires little preparation, it can easily be replicated at home.

ACTIVITY

Before the session I tie one end of a long, thin rope to the handle of a plastic bucket, put the bucket on a nearby filing cabinet (up high and out of sight), and tie the other end to a hook in the ceiling. When I pull back on the bucket and then let it go, it swings back and forth. Mom picks up Jordon and walks near the spot where I have put the bucket. I ask her to distract him for a second while I pick up the bucket containing a toy and put it behind me.

I say, "Listen!" and when I have his attention, make a soft sound by tapping a toy cow on the side of the plastic bucket.

I say, "You heard that! It was a toy cow that says 'mooo!'" I wait and say, "Wanna see the cow that says moooo?" When he nods, I help him to pull the cow out of the bucket. After he pulls it out he is not interested in playing with it further until I say, "Let's swing the cow over to Mommy." I show him what we will do by pulling back on the bucket and then looking at his mom. She steps back and Jordon and I pull the cow "up-up-up" and then I say, "gooooo!" and the bucket swings over to his mom. She dumps out the *cow that says moo* and chats a bit more about it. When she swings the bucket back to Jordon and me, I repeat the entire sequence, beginning with the soft tapping of a different *learning to listen* sound toy. Jordon delights in swinging the bucket back and forth, so we are able to play with several *learning to listen* sounds. After the swinging is over, I take two toys out of the bucket and ask Jordon to put them back, matching them to pictures in a segmented box. I continue to take toys out, two at a time, choosing sounds that are very different acoustically (*moo* and *bububu,* rather than *moo* and *ahhhh*). Finally, I bring out a new *learning to listen* toy, the top, and I sing its accompanying song from *Hear & Listen! Talk & Sing!* (Estabrooks and Birkenshaw-Fleming, 1994). Mom practices singing with me so that she can sing it at home.

ANALYSIS

Similar to his responses to soft environmental sounds during the *One Frog Too Many* activity, Jordon required several presentations before he detected the tapping on the bucket. We will continue to expose him to a variety of soft sounds and expect him to respond.

The technique of *waiting* yielded verbal and nonverbal responses to questions and also prompted Jordon to direct the course of the activity. After the second sequence, Jordon understood the routine and indicated that he wanted to do the swinging himself by imitating the swinging motion of the bucket. After the fourth sequence, he indicated that he wanted to switch roles with his mom by vocalizing and pointing at her.

One month after Jordon's implant was hooked up, I had *reintroduced* eight of the *learning to listen* sounds (cow, bus, airplane, car, dog, pig, baby, and boat). Jordon benefits greatly from exposure to *learning to listen* sounds, which contain a broad range of acoustic information across the speech frequencies.

Jordon's developing perceptual skills are confirmed by his repeatedly choosing the correct *learning to listen* sound from a set of two when putting away toys.

A big challenge in this game is *distance,* because one adult involved in the conversation is sometimes across the room and we need to be within Jordon's critical listening distance (within *earshot*).

Parent Guidance

✔   There are many ways of making the *learning to listen* sounds fun again both for you and Jordon.

- Repeating mini *field trips* to see real *learning to listen* sounds in action at a nearby farm, the airport, or a pond.
- Pulling the *learning to listen* sound toys out of unlikely objects such as socks and pillowcases.
- Making a sneaky game of putting the *learning to listen* sound pictures in unlikely places, such as on the ceiling, under chairs, or in shoes.
- Taping paper flaps over the *learning to listen* sound pictures in Jordon's room.
- Repeating the Swinging Sounds game at home.

✔   Get Jordon's attention before providing verbal language for the *learning to listen* sounds.

✔   Introduce the new sound and song for *round and round* with anything that goes around such as tops, wheels, and circles drawn on paper with crayons.

(cont'd on next page)

Parent Guidance *(cont'd)*

✔ Jordon successfully identified the *learning to listen* sounds from a set of two different durational patterns, so increase the set to three.

✔ Jordon is receiving a clear signal with the implant. There is no need to test his perception skills constantly. He is learning language through listening, and this is encouraging.

✔ Sing *learning to listen* songs from *Hear & Listen! Talk & Sing!* Use the accompanying audiotape to help memorize the songs.

✔ Call Jordon's attention to a variety of quiet sounds throughout the day.

Wash the Baby

GOALS

Audition:
* to identify common words and phrases through audition.
* to expand *auditory attention*.

Speech:
* to practice prespeech behaviors.

Language:
* to comprehend a core of common phrases.
* to comprehend functional words.
* to initiate actions.

Cognition:
* to problem-solve.

RATIONALE

This activity replicates a typical play scenario for young children and utilizes household objects. Jordon's parents have the idea that fancy toys are more interesting and will promote language development faster than ordinary objects in his environment. I emphasize that fancy toys are not necessary to develop language. Like other activities, this one combines several goals and provides opportunity for interaction, development of prespeech skills, and exposure to common words and phrases.

ACTIVITY

With Jordon's mom's knowledge, I have hidden a *dirty* baby doll in the corner of the room before Jordon comes to the therapy session. We will find the baby, pretend to be upset that it is dirty, and wait for Jordon to initiate some action.

"Waa! Waa! Listen, Jordon! I hear a baby!" I say, and then repeat it softly. Jordon *attends* to the auditory stimulus for about 15 seconds and then looks around for the source of the sound. Together, Mom and Jordon find the baby. Mom and I playfully feign being upset, and Mom says, "Ooooo — she's dirty!" Jordon begins to wipe the dirt off the baby's face.

I say, "Good idea, Jordon; let's wash the baby!" I acoustically highlight the phrase *wash the baby*.

All the items needed for washing the baby (wash cloth, pitcher of water, and liquid soap) are in a cupboard in my therapy room. The items are in small plastic bags in a cardboard box so that we have to *take them out* one at a time and then *open* each one, providing many opportunities to hear these functional words. We then wash the baby.

The conversation during each part of this activity provides much opportunity for repetition of common phrases and functional words. We pour a little water into the tub (*pour it*), a little at a time (*more water*), until Jordon indicates by gesture or vocalization that we have enough (*stop!*). The water is *all gone* from the pitcher. We put the baby in the tub (*put her in*) and pretend that she is cold (*Brrrr! It's cold!*). We frequently comment, "Oooo, she's dirty!" When Jordon tires of washing we are *all done.* I use thick liquid soap, which bubbles easily. We scoop the bubbles in our hands and playfully blow them towards each other (*blow it!*). There is a big wet spot on the floor (*uh-oh!*), so we wipe up the floor (*wipe, wipe, wipe it up*) and put all the materials back in their containers (*put it away*).

ANALYSIS

Jordon attended to the auditory input of the baby's cry for more than a few seconds *only* when I accompanied it with a lot of facial expression and drama. Extended attention to auditory stimuli is a target.

After Jordon's mother commented, "Oooooh, she's dirty!" Jordon stopped, looked to his mother and waited 15–20 seconds before he wiped the baby's face. Jordon's mother initially appeared uncomfortable when I asked her to *wait*. Solving problems for Jordon is a normal reaction, but he is capable of indicating his own desires and generating solutions to small problems when encouraged.

Jordon waited for several seconds after listening to simple directions before he could follow through. This is typical of children soon after the initial stimulation of the implant. He will require *context* to process directions over the next few weeks but I expect his follow-through time to reduce. As his parents *wait* for Jordon's response, he will process phrases more quickly. Jordon's parents have heard the erroneous analogy that a child who is deaf or hard of hearing is like a vessel and if adults pour language in, it will eventually come spilling out the top. Consequently, adults often monopolize potential interactions and neglect critical *wait time*.

Jordon's blowing was initially more like spitting, but after a few turns he began to approximate blowing. He had demonstrated neither imitated nor spontaneous blowing at home.

Parent Guidance

✔ *Wait* for Jordon to initiate actions and problem-solve whenever possible. He will be motivated to use spoken language if he is given opportunities to initiate actions and events on his own. In your notebook list times when this would be appropriate, e.g., when milk is spilled, shoes need tying, toys get broken, doors need opening.

✔ Talk with Jordon about what he is thinking, feeling, and doing. Talk in phrases rather than single words. There is much more acoustic information in a phrase.

✔ Jordon will demonstrate understanding of language by the rate, rhythm, and stress patterns of phrases *before* he understands actual words.

✔ Create opportunities for Jordon to hear the repetition of common phrases such as, *Uh oh — fall down!, Pick it up, All gone, Take it out, Open it.* He will begin to make sense out of the *strings of words* he hears.

✔ List daily home activities during which common phrases occur naturally. Detailed notes help you *follow through*. This is especially important when both parents cannot come to each session.

Conclusion

Prior to receiving the cochlear implant, Jordon did not respond consistently to loud sounds, vocalized infrequently, and understood very little language without accompanying gestures. Since receiving the implant, he consistently stops activity upon hearing loud and moderately loud sounds in a quiet environment. He often puts his hand to his ear to indicate he has heard something. He responds by looking up when his name is called on the first or second call when the environment is quiet, and when he is not highly involved in an activity. He detects five sounds in the six-sound test (/ah/, /oo/, /ee/, /sh/, and /m/) most of the time and sometimes /s/. I expect him to detect all these sounds, both at close range and at varying distances within the next few weeks. We will encourage consistent alerting responses to soft sounds such as quiet knocking, whispering, quiet whistling, and talking from another room when the environment is quiet. We will look for him to respond consistently to his name in a variety of situations.

Jordon currently identifies several *learning to listen* sounds from a set of two that differ in duration, and he can identify a few common words and phrases with abundant contextual support. We will develop identification of all of the *learning to listen* sounds and more common phrases with minimal contextual support.

Prior to the implant, Jordon had few vocalizations. Now he vocalizes more frequently, though not abundantly. Most vocalizations approximate the vowels *ah* and *uh,* and his voice quality is still breathy. He sometimes uses his voice to attract attention and he imitates some duration patterns, but does not yet imitate or spontaneously vary intensity or pitch. Although he does not imitate consistently in response to the hand cue, his *spontaneous imitations* are increasing. We will encourage imitations varying in duration, intensity, and pitch and stimulate production of back and front vowels. We will help him develop blowing.

Prior to receiving the cochlear implant, Jordon communicated by gesture, pointing, crying, and pulling adults towards desired items. Though his parents attempted to gain his attention via sound, they had to resort to touch. Jordon understood his parents only when they used gestures, such as pointing to a chair to indicate that he was to sit down or holding up his plate when it was time to eat.

Jordon now communicates his needs and wants by gesture sometimes accompanied by vocalization. He is beginning to understand that sound is used for communication. His parents are able to gain his attention through sound and he can move farther from their view without constant need for supervision. We anticipate that Jordon will learn to use his voice consistently for communication.

Before the cochlear implant, Jordon demonstrated comprehension of one *learning to listen* sound, the cow, when he was able to speechread, and showed no interest in nursery rhymes or singing. He now *attaches meaning* to several *learning to listen* sounds. He comprehends a few simple words and common phrases and is attentive when his parents sing to him. We will encourage comprehension of common phrases and functional words through listening, and imitation of familiar nursery rhymes and songs.

Prior to the cochlear implant, Jordon demonstrated cognitive skills typical for his age except in areas related to language. Current goals include enjoyment when sharing books with parents, attention to spoken language for longer periods, acting out stories with props, response to the hand cue, and matching pictures to objects.

Jordon's progress since receiving the cochlear implant demonstrates the powerful combination of technology and parent-centered therapy. Jordon's parents are delighted that he responds to sound and is beginning to make sense out of spoken language. Because he had been virtually silent before the implant, they rejoice in each uttered sound! They believe he has the potential to develop spoken language and to participate academically, socially, and emotionally with his friends and family. They plan for their son to have a happy childhood and fulfilling future, just like other kids!

References

Estabrooks, W., & Birkenshaw-Fleming, L. (1994). *Hear & Listen! Talk & Sing!* Toronto: Arisa.

Mayer, M. (1975). *One frog too many.* New York: Dial Books.

Lesson Plan for Joey

Jo Acree, M.S., CCC-A, Cert. AVT

Joey was born a fraternal twin, the result of a normal full-term pregnancy, in 1987. He was diagnosed with sensorineural hearing impairment at 20 months of age, despite reported parental suspicion of hearing difficulties at 12 months. He was plagued by chronic ear infections throughout his infant and toddler years and was noted to exhibit fluctuating sensorineural impairment as well. His first set of PE ventilating tubes were inserted at 19 months of age.

Joey was initially given Phonak Superfront PPC2 hearing aids. Owing to the fluctuating nature of his hearing impairment it was difficult to determine the benefit he received from this amplification. Once Joey's hearing stabilized in the right ear, his aided responses were consistently in the moderate range of hearing loss (40–60 dB HL).

Joey and his family were involved in an oral program for children who are deaf or hard of hearing that included home visits, an oral preschool, and therapy with a speech-language pathologist. He was enrolled in an auditory-verbal therapy program in March 1993.

In August 1994, Joey received Unitron US80PPL hearing aids, and his aided responses improved to 25–45 dB HL from 250–4000 Hz. Despite the improvement, the left hearing aid provided no benefit because of fluctuations and poor discrimination ability. Joey has been using only the right hearing aid since February 1995. He continued to show excellent benefit from amplification in the right ear, with speech sounds accessible from 250–4000 Hz, a spondee threshold (identification of familiar two-syllable words with equal stress on each syllable) of 40 dB HL, and a speech discrimination score of 60 percent (auditory only) on the *Word Intelligibility by Picture Identification (WIPI)*. Joey was making slow progress in all areas but he struggled, as listening and learning language did not come easily.

During a visit with his mom, I suggested that Joey might be a candidate for a cochlear implant, as the protocol was changing. Although he would not have been a candidate several years ago because of his better ear, I believed the difficulties Joey was having were sufficient to pursue investigation of the cochlear implant. His left ear provided no speech recognition with amplification, and his right ear, although appropriately aided, was not carrying the load. Less than a month later Joey's mother called our clinic requesting all the information we could send about cochlear implants. The family had decided that if the implant could improve Joey's quality of life, then they would go for it!

Preimplant assessments were scheduled. Things didn't look promising at first, as some members of the implant team felt Joey's auditory skills were "too good" to consider him. He was receiving good benefit from the hearing aid in his right ear, with 60 percent speech discrimination in a closed set of four pictures. Also, the team was evaluating his better ear for the implant without considering his poorer ear. Our intention was not to replace the benefit he received from amplification, but to supplement it with an implant in his other ear. Joey's mom reported feeling "penalized for working so hard with Joey" because he had achieved some success with his hearing aids. Once the team began to evaluate the poorer ear, candidacy was considered, albeit with hesitation. The auditory integrity of the nerve was questioned, as Joey hadn't worn a hearing aid on that ear for nearly two years. Also, as he had rejected the hearing aid, it was feared he might reject the implant as well. These were all questions with no definitive answers.

After considerable assessment and debate, the team recommended the implant, barring no medical contraindications. The final approval came early in July 1996, and Joey had successful surgery two weeks later. There were no complications, and all electrodes were fully inserted. Joey continues to wear a hearing aid on his right ear.

Introduction to the Lesson

All the activities in the following lesson (one month after initial MAPing) are conducted with Joey wearing the cochlear implant only. All information is presented through audition without visual cues, and goals for language development are incorporated into the auditory goals. Joey is a "listening child" who used his residual hearing to the best of his ability prior to the implant, and he has always communicated through spoken language.

Ling Six-Sound Test

GOALS

Audition:
*   to evaluate MAPped benefit for hearing *and* the understanding of speech.

Language:

- to develop comprehension of a variety of question forms (i.e., "Can it...?," "Does it....?," How does it...?," etc.).
- to encourage and reinforce more variety in Joey's expressive questions.
- to reinforce academics.

ACTIVITY

Throw slimy creatures and insects into water in response to hearing the Ling speech sounds (/oo/, /ee/, /ah/, /sh/, /s/, /m/). The Ling sounds span the frequency range of speech; a child's responses to these sounds provide information about the speech he is able to hear in a quiet setting. Joey listens with the slimy creatures, holding them to his ear until he detects a presented speech sound, then throws them in the water. He especially enjoys providing Mom with a view of the creatures, up close and personal!

We use a large Tupperware™ container and fill it about one-third full of water; sometimes we use food coloring in the water to make it more interesting. For the first few minutes of the activity Joey is asked to respond only if he hears or detects the sound and then to detect them all at a distance of three feet, six feet, and 10 feet. To determine if he actually understands or discriminates the six sounds he must repeat them. Joey exhibits confusion between /oo/ and /m/, often producing /m/ when hearing /oo/. He has no difficulty identifying the other sounds, including /s/ at 10 feet!

Throughout this activity, Mom incorporates vocabulary and language targets from a current science study, as Joey has been having difficulty with the advanced vocabulary. She asks, "Is this an amphibian or a reptile?," "How do you know?," and "What's the difference?" This is an excellent example of how auditory and language goals overlap.

ANALYSIS

This activity is crucial to determine Joey's ability to utilize the cochlear implant for hearing and processing speech. The measure of *appropriate MAPping* is to maximize the speech signal. We need to know what Joey is hearing and, more importantly, what speech sounds like to him. For instance, Joey is able to *detect* all six Ling sounds. When asked to repeat them, however, /oo/ and /m/ sound the same to him. These are difficult to discriminate even though he *hears* them. This provides us with information about his MAP. He is probably not getting enough information in the low frequencies to detect the nasal murmur and therefore is not able to discriminate /oo/ from /m/. As we fine-tune his MAP we will know to evaluate his responses closely to the apical (high-number) electrodes. "What can we do in the meantime?" asks his mom.

Prior to the implant Joey could detect /s/ inconsistently and had great difficulty discriminating /oo/, /ee/, /m/. His greatest difficulty was discriminating /oo/ versus /ee/, as he was lacking access to high-frequency sounds. The primary difference between the two sounds is a peak of energy in the high frequencies that is present for /ee/, but not for /oo/. In addition, He could identify these sounds only at close range (six inches to three feet), certainly not at 10 feet!

Parent Guidance

We need to help Joey develop his ability to hear the difference between /oo/ and /m/ in isolation.

✔ His mom and Joey practice discrimination drills with the two sounds at home. They write the two sounds on a piece of paper in columns (also reinforcing the concept of *column*) and place Smarties™ candies under each sound. Joey listens as his mom randomly produces the two sounds. With each production Joey removes a candy and places it into a cup. If he makes a mistake and chooses a candy under the /oo/ when his mom has said /m/, he must replace it and listen again.

✔ Since Joey is able to produce both these sounds with ease, he is encouraged to repeat after his mom, thereby building an *auditory feed-back loop* for the sounds. This means that after he hears the sound, he repeats it and then hears his own production and is able to compare the two, recognizing when they match. He also builds his auditory memory of the sounds as he produces them.

✔ This activity can be done in a variety of ways to discriminate any sounds or words of particular difficulty. For example, since Joey confuses "cat" and "cap," we can do syllable drills for the pair /at, ap/. We begin with a different vowel to help identify the difference (/at, oop/), then increase the difficulty by using the same vowel but with varying durations (/at, aaaaap/), and finally drill the original pair (/at, ap/). Joey enjoys the brief two-minute drill because of the variety of ways it can be accomplished; he can simply repeat the sounds /at-ap/, choose pegs from cups (/at/ = blue,

(cont'd on next page)

Parent Guidance *(cont'd)*

/ap/ = yellow), or set up headers on a sheet of paper as in the following example and put a check mark or star under each one as it is heard:

am	ap
✓	✓
✓	✓
✓	✓
☆	☆
☆	☆

Joey can:
- place or remove bingo chips from beneath the correct sound.
- use a rubber stamp beneath the sound heard.
- remove Cheerios™ and then eat them.
- make checks with glue and then apply glitter.

Joey's mom also notes several speech errors that indicate difficulty with the nasal sounds /m/, /n/ that were not evident prior to receiving the implant. Joey's responses to warble tones in the soundbooth, with his implant alone, revealed elevated thresholds in the low frequencies. The goal of the next MAPping session will be to expand Joey's range in the low frequency (apical electrodes) and perhaps change the frequency allocation table to provide more low-frequency information. As the family is familiar with use of the Ling sounds for checking the function of hearing aids, Joey can now utilize them to verify the function of his implant by repeating those sounds to himself as he puts on the implant every morning.

Listening for Minor Differences in Speech

GOALS

Audition:
- to identify and discriminate the final consonant sound in paired words, e.g., *cloud/clown, boat/bowl, plane/plate* (in phrases).

Language:
- to expand vocabulary, reinforce prepositions, and improve the ability to give directions.

ACTIVITY

Joey will follow directions using paired objects with final consonant differences. We will begin with three or four of the target words in each direction and increase the number according to his success.

Each player (parent/child) has a matched set of objects hidden behind a barrier. Each set includes paired objects that differ in the final consonant sound only. Joey's mom goes first, so that Joey has a solid example to follow. This is especially important with new activities. His mom sets up a situation with the objects on her side of the barrier. She says, "The *cow* is going to play the *horn* and sit on the *cloud.*" Joey matches his objects according to the directions he heard and the barrier is lifted. They compare to see if the objects match. Joey follows the direction correctly without discrimination errors. Now it is his turn.

Joey says "The *plane, cow, horse* under *plate.*"

His mom is practicing asking for clarification when Joey's sentences are not complete. She says, "Pardon me?"

Joey repeats his instruction: "Put *plane, cow, horse* under the *plate.*" He has improved the language structure, although it is not yet perfect. Mom accepts it and follows through.

Then the ante goes up and the instructions become more complicated, for example, "Put the *cloud* between the *plane* and the *horse* and the *horse* beside the *plate.*" A variety of prepositions are also reinforced. Joey places the clown between the plane and the horse and the horse beside the plate. "Oops, not the clown!" says his mom.

Joey follows the instructions throughout the activity almost perfectly, with minimal requests for repetition. His mom will continue to reinforce this goal at home, as he did make a few errors. Joey enjoys this activity as it is competitive, has an element of suspense, and allows him to give very tricky instructions to his parents.

ANALYSIS

We want Joey to be able to discriminate small differences in words through listening whenever possible. In the real world he will be expected to draw upon his skills from context, or knowing the subject matter, to listen for key words and to use strategies to obtain information he doesn't understand. Fine-tuning his discrimination abilities will help in many circumstances and will take the guesswork out of listening.

Joey was in the early stages of developing the ability to discriminate final consonant differences before getting the implant. He was selecting one object from a group of eight to 10, presented at the end of a sentence, e.g., "Give the little girl the *horse.*" In the examples above, he is discriminating at least four of the paired objects in embedded sentences, a significant improvement.

We should remember to incorporate new language skills when

giving directions. For example, Joey has recently learned the concept "row"; use a direction such as, "Put the *horse, couch,* and *clown* in a row." Be careful to use concepts that he already understands, and not completely new concepts. We want to teach one thing at a time, and to reinforce new concepts. In this task you are teaching Joey to listen for minor differences of speech.

Parent Guidance

✔ You can integrate this goal into daily activities by cutting out paired-word pictures with differing final consonants and taping them on your salt and pepper shakers. At the dinner table, everyone must ask for the salt and/or pepper according to the picture: "Please pass the *can.*" Changing the pictures every couple of days provides a variety of listening experiences and introduces new vocabulary.

✔ Play the I Spy game and include paired words. For example, say, "I spy something funny that sounds like *cloud* but ends with 'n'" (*clown*). Joey is hearing so much better with his cochlear implant now that he can probably even play this game in the car!

✔ Joey needs to improve his ability to give directions, so the family will play lots of games, taking turns being the teacher. A good game for following directions is to have Joey give directions to a particular destination while in the car and have the driver follow his directions. If you don't end up at the ice cream parlor but at the landfill, it will stress the importance of giving proper directions; if you make it to the ice cream parlor, you have a built-in reward. Imagine the possibilities!

Listen to Short Tape-Recorded Directions

GOALS

Audition:
- to develop auditory skills for listening in a difficult listening situation (tape recording) with no visual cues.

Language:
- to develop strategies to obtain linguistic information.
- to reinforce concepts and categories.

ACTIVITY

Short two- to four-item directions were prerecorded. Joey is presented with a grid of 20 pictures and a set of colored pencils. He listens to each tape-recorded direction and then follows the instruction. This is a new activity, and Joey initially lacks confidence.

"Listen to the tape; here's the first one," I say.

"Circle the *frog* with *blue."*

"What?" he asks.

"What did you hear?" I respond.

"Put circle on the frog?" he replies, hesitantly.

"Yes! That's very close. Now what do you need to know?"

"What color?"

"Great! How do you find out?"

"What color you say to use?"

I play the tape again and he hears, "Circle the frog with *blue."* This time he gets it and is ready for the next one.

"Turn it on!" Joey demands.

Gradually, each direction becomes more difficult, e.g., "Find the *animal* in the *first row* and *underline* it with any *color."* Joey's confidence increases and he rarely asks for repetition or clarification. This is very exciting because not only is Joey hearing the tape, he is following the directions *and* he is enthusiastic.

ANALYSIS

Listening to tape-recorded information is difficult for two reasons. First, there are *absolutely no visual cues.* Even when one covers one's mouth to reduce speechreading cues, there are clues to be obtained through facial expressions; some kids report they can even "cheek read." These types of cues are not available when using a tape recorder. Secondly, the reproduction of voice is not exact on a tape recorder; the frequency range is much narrower and distortion is usually present. Listening to mechanically reproduced speech is an excellent way to prepare Joey to use the telephone, which has a similar tonal quality.

This activity also helps Joey develop strategies to obtain information that he "didn't catch the first time." He is encouraged to repeat what he did hear or to ask for the specific portion of the phrase or direction he missed, such as, "What color did you say?" or "Put the horse where?" Expect him to use complete sentences. When Joey uses incomplete sentences, ask him for clarification.

Joey could not have been successful with taped information without a cochlear implant. With his hearing aids alone he was still exhibiting difficulty following detailed directions at close range when presented in a quiet environment. This was accompanied with reluctance and protests. At present Joey is very willing to listen to tape-recorded information.

Parent Guidance

The tape recorder can be used for a variety of activities. The goal is always the same: to develop listening skills in adverse acoustic situations.

✔ You can tape descriptions and/or riddles. Presenting actual objects or pictures to select will make this easier. A fun family game is to place a bell in the middle of the table and to declare that the winner of each round will be the first one to ring the bell *and* identify the item.

✔ You can leave Joey a tape to listen to when he gets home from school, explaining his chores and the snacks he can have. Following tape-recorded stories (tracking) helps reinforce reading, language structures and listening.

✔ A family member can record a selection from a book, perhaps one or two pages, and Joey can follow the text in the book. Stop the tape periodically and ask him to indicate *exactly* where it stopped. Be sure to give Joey the opportunity to record himself. This will help to develop speech clarity. Don't do any story comprehension on tape yet; Joey is developing this skill in easier listening environments first.

Summary

This was an excellent lesson for Joey, his mother, and me. We began with simple detection of specific speech sounds and advanced to tape-recorded directions containing five or six key words. The taped activity was not in my original lesson plan, but he was responding so well to other listening activities that I added it. I think the greatest benefit of the tape-recorded directions was that Joey gained confidence from this activity. It is obvious that he is using his cochlear implant successfully and already is able to perform auditory tasks that he could not do with his hearing aids alone. His achievements provide excellent information about future goals for Joey.

Joey needs to improve discrimination of minor differences in vowels and consonants by place of production (consonants produced in the same manner — stop, fricative, nasal — but the tongue/lip placement differs, e.g., /p, t/, /m, n/, /f, s/), based on the errors he made in both the first and second activities. Knowing his discrimination errors helps us to set realistic expectations in conversational speech.

It is also evident from samples of Joey's expressive language that he continues to omit many auxiliaries and small words in his sentences. His mom will continue to model *and* to expect more complete sentences. Also, in the second activity, Joey's difficulty in giving clear and concise directions was evident. Specific receptive language goals to provide Joey with a stronger language base include understanding a greater variety of question forms, vocabulary development, expansion of concepts, and figurative language such as idioms and metaphors.

Joey, his mother, and I are very pleased by his success with the cochlear implant. He continues to make excellent progress in his listening, language, and speech. "He's hearing better and more easily than before, and the difference it makes in his energy level at the end of the day is unbelievable," reports Mom. His twin brother reports that he is concerned that Joey "is using the implant for evil and not for good" because Joey has much more time to aggravate his family!

Lesson Plan for Lilly

Amy McConkey Robbins, M.S.

The youngest of five children, Lilly was born with a profound hearing loss and the etiology was Waardenburg's syndrome. The loss was identified at 11 months of age, and Lilly is the only member of her family with a hearing impairment. She was subsequently given hearing aids and participated in a parent-infant program using Pidgin Signed English (PSE) for two years.

At age three years, three months, Lilly came to our center with a vocabulary of only 50 formal signs. Her primary means of communication were gestures and pantomime, and she exhibited numerous behavioral problems, including tantrums and noncompliance with daily home routines. At the time of the initial visit, her mother stated, "Lilly runs our home." In spite of the two previous years of intervention, Lilly demonstrated only rudimentary speech skills and no functional listening skills.

We gave Lilly a seven-channel Tactaid 7 device and followed the TARGO, a tactile learning curriculum (Robbins, Hesketh, & Bivins, 1993). We also emphasized a total communication (TC) approach, utilizing spoken English and Signing Exact English (SEE2) (Gustason & Zawolkow, 1993). In this signing system, every word in English may be represented on the hands, including all grammatical endings such as -ing and -ed. Lilly mastered a number of goals, including compliance with adult requests which was essential to her future success: She had to recognize authority in order to benefit from her therapy sessions. Her lexicon of signs grew rapidly in six months to include 250 signs and two-sign combinations. Using the Tactaid 7, Lilly learned to vocalize on demand and to tell the difference between long and short tactile patterns. She also developed a conditioned tactile response. Few other auditory or speech goals were met. Lilly consistently vocalized using a "creaky voice," a very low-pitched voice with a gravelly quality, and could not modify this even with training and feedback.

After six months of training with the Tactaid 7 and positive candidacy for the cochlear implant, Lilly received a Nucleus 22-channel implant in her right ear with a full insertion of 22 electrodes. She was three years, 10 months old at the time. She also received a Spectra mini speech processor with the SPEAK encoding strategy.

Audiologic Information

Prior to receiving her implant, Lilly demonstrated an unaided pure-tone average (the average of her responses at 500, 1000, and 2000 Hz) of 103 dB HL in the left (better) ear, with no response above 1500 Hz. Her aided responses in her left ear were 65–70 dB HL, again with no response above 1500 Hz. In her right ear, she had an unaided PTA of 113 dB HL, with no response above 1500 Hz. Aided thresholds in the right ear were similar to those in the left, falling at 65–70 dB HL, with no aided responses above 1500 Hz. The right ear was chosen for cochlear implantation. After receiving the implant, Lilly demonstrated a flat soundfield audiogram to warble tones with thresholds at 30–35 dB HL through 4000 Hz.

Introduction to the Lesson

For many children who have learned through the oral approach, using minimal auditory cues, the information transmitted by the implant is a vast improvement over what the child previously heard. However, a child who has learned through total communication requires a radical refocusing of goals, along with substantial changes in parent and teacher expectations, before he or she can become an auditory learner using a cochlear implant. Expectations for listening and speech production, at home and in school, must be maintained consistently, or nothing may change.

Our philosophy of therapy is to teach parents the skills needed to continue the work with their child in natural contexts. The time spent in therapy is simply too brief to teach all the required skills and, in fact, the best venue for mastering these is in play and daily activities. The aim of therapy is not to teach children every skill they need, but to select targets that will *generalize* to other skills.

Most of the "listening-only" tasks described in the following session are carried out using an acoustic screen. This consists of two thicknesses of black speaker mesh stretched between the rings of an embroidery hoop. Although speechreading cues are eliminated, the fidelity of the speech signal is still high. The most natural way to reduce speechreading cues is to position oneself next to or slightly behind the child. For children who use TC, however, this may be problematic, as they are accustomed to reading signs in a face-to-face orientation, making the acoustic screen a preferred option.

Throughout the session, auditory "sabotage" is used as a means to encourage generalization of skills (Robbins & Kirk, 1996). Sabotage involves presenting a different auditory stimulus than the one the child expects to hear. The stimuli used as sabotage are carefully selected in order to achieve specific goals. At this early stage of implant use, the sabotage used is silence, because we want Lilly to tell us reliably when she *doesn't* hear anything. This skill is an important building block in giving accurate implant thresholds and learning to report device malfunction or nonfunction. The primary goal of sabotage is to teach the child that most sounds occur in the real world without any warning. The next stimulus used for sabotage will be Lilly's name, as she must learn to recognize it even when she doesn't expect to hear it.

Following are the therapy goals and activities for Lilly at two intervals. At the first interval, *one month post implant,* she was four years, one month of age. A follow-up on Lilly at *four years post implant* is also included, when she was eight years, five months of age.

GOALS

Speech:
- use of normal voice (as opposed to "creaky voice") when vocalizing.
- production of /w/ and /b/ before vowels; production of /m/ following vowels.
- use of outward airstream for /b/.
- production of the vowels /ah/, /ee/, /oo/.
- replication of rhythm and inflection patterns (suprasegmentals).

Language:
- comprehension and use of three-word combinations (signed + spoken), especially Adjective + Noun + Verb; Verb + Adjective + Object; and Subject + Verb + Object.
- new vocabulary: *need, place, mug, fill, full, empty, tray, belong, both, a few.*
- synonyms for overused words/signs: *quit* for *finish; mug* for *cup; small* for *little.*
- transfer of known vocabulary from sign to spoken words.

Audition:
- spontaneous report of "Nothing" when sabotaged with silence in listening activities.
- discrimination of her name.
- recognition of suprasegmental and segmental patterns.

Cognition:
- temporal sequencing, both nonverbally and through language *(first, last, next, then).*

Spoken Communication:
- calling "Mom" or clinician's name when seeking our attention.
- communicative turn-taking.
- use of speech alone for appropriate social routines (greeting people, saying good-bye).

Ling Six-Sound Test
This activity is performed to ensure that the implant is functioning properly. I produce /ah/, /ee/, /oo/, /sh/, /s/, /m/ in random order,

using the acoustic screen. Lilly raises her hand when she hears, and attempts to identify and repeat each sound. At four weeks after initial stimulation of her implant, she should detect them all, but may identify only /sh/. Lilly's limited preimplant hearing was not adequate for her to form auditory representations of these sounds. I ask her to try to identify them, however, and thus convey the expectation that she eventually will do so. I also clarify each one for her visually. Lilly attempts to repeat each sound after it is presented, receiving production practice within this perception task. As Lilly is learning to report reliably when she hears nothing, I raise the screen but say nothing once during the test, praising her for not being tricked by this sabotage. If Lilly uses a "witch's voice" (vocal fry or creaky voice), I label it as such and say/sign, "You used a witch's voice when you said 'ah'; here is a pretty-voice 'ah'. Not 'ah' (vocal fry) but 'ah' (normal voice)." Mother is instructed to continue applying the Ling test at home whenever Lilly first puts on her device or if a problem is suspected.

Speech Work

A short syllabic drill follows, for intensive motor practice. Lilly imitates the targets /b/ and /w/ preceding the vowels /ah/, /ee/, /oo/, and these vowels followed by /m/ (Ling, 1976). I use a nonfunctioning microphone as the prop, as Lilly pretends she is "performing" and puts forth her best effort. I control the microphone, modeling and eliciting targets very rapidly. Instructions are given to Lilly in speech and signs, but the syllables themselves are modeled and repeated with no manual support. I say, "Let's practice our speech sounds: 'ba' [Lilly imitates]; 'ba' [Lilly imitates]; 'ba' [Lilly imitates]." We use an expansion-reduction technique, so that when Lilly is successful, we make the task more demanding; when she is unsuccessful, we reduce the demands. As Lilly is successful with the single-syllable production for this sound, I then model repeated syllables, "ba ba" [Lilly imitates], "ba ba" [Lilly imitates], "ba ba" [Lilly imitates], paying particular attention to her tendency to produce the /b/ sound while sucking in air instead of blowing out. This results in a popping quality and is a habit I want to eliminate. When this occurs, I contrast the correct syllable with the incorrect one, both through audition ("Listen to the difference: you said Ba" [sucking sound]; "I want to hear ba" [correct sound]) and with tactile cues. The latter is done by producing the two sounds on the back of her hand so that she can feel the airstream that occurs when the sound is produced correctly.

The next target syllable is *bee*. Lilly's production of the /ee/ is inaccurate, so I try several techniques to elicit the correct production. These include modeling the sound through listening alone, then providing visual cues and reminding her to produce the "smiling" vowel. As Lilly cannot produce a single-syllable production of *bee* correctly, we do not attempt any multisyllabic productions with this vowel. I move on to *boo,* continuing this procedure until we have covered the speech targets for this session. I reinforce Lilly with verbal praise, and periodically, as a reinforcer, she moves a climbing figure up the hill on a Tornado Rex™ game board. When the speech activity is ended, Lilly may set the tornado spinner loose, watching it career down the mountain. The more she has done, the higher the climber is on the board, and the more destruction the tornado causes! This helps motivate Lilly to be highly productive during the activity, which lasts only five to eight minutes. As Lilly uses TC, I encourage Mother to repeat the speech activity near the end of the session. This allows me to see how comfortable she is when working on speech targets and gives me an opportunity to coach her about specific techniques to use at home. Many parents of children who use TC have never been advised or helped on ways to work on speech production and have little knowledge or confidence about how to begin. With guided practice at this initial stage of implant use, these parents can become proficient and creative in helping their child with speech production.

Mirror-Mirror Game (Name Discrimination)

For this I instruct Lilly in speech and sign that when she hears her name, she should look in a hand-held mirror and say, "That's me" and ignore all other stimuli. The mirror prop was chosen because of Lilly's fascination with Snow White. Mother and I take turns presenting the stimuli, using an acoustic screen. This is a discrimination task (Erber, 1982). It is easier than a recognition task because Lilly is required to hold only one auditory image in memory ("Lilly") and does not have to identify the other stimuli, just ignore them. I say, "Lilly... dinosaur... Lilly... Lilly... I'm thirsty... birthday cake... Lilly," and Lilly picks up the mirror and says, "That's me," only when she hears her name. The stimuli are presented with speech alone. The foils are grossly different in syllable number and sound pattern than the target, "Lilly." If she is successful with these, I make the task more difficult by choosing foils more similar to the target, such as other two-syllable words, "shoelace," "treetops," "cupcakes," whose sound patterns are quite different from "Lilly."

Lilly is being taught to use a response when she hears her name ("That's me") that is different from the way she responds to all other stimuli (Robbins & Kirk, 1996), a technique recommended for children who use TC. This ensures our ability to know if she recognizes *her* name or simply detects sound when her name is called. Once we are certain of her name-recognition ability, we modify the "That's me" response, changing to "Yes?" or "What?"

This activity is used only after a child demonstrates consistent detection of sound within a listening set, a prerequisite to discrimination activities. Additionally, this activity was used only after Lilly was already familiar with her name visually and tactually. With this task, we are working towards *structured* name recognition through audition alone, and then to *spontaneous* name recognition. The latter, along with the ability to recognize silence, is considered one of the early hallmarks for success in auditory learning (Robbins & Kirk, 1996). Name recognition is emphasized in home activities: Lilly will draw an outline of her face on a piece of paper. Each time she successfully discriminates her name from other stimuli, she adds another feature to the drawing. The activity ends when Lilly's portrait of herself is complete. In addition, the parents will continue to call Lilly's name when they want her attention, even though she rarely responds. The parent encourages her after securing her attention, by saying, "Lilly! I was calling your name. I said Li-lly!"

Identification and Production of Onomatopoeic Sounds

From a large set of about 30 objects, I produce the corresponding ono-matopoeic sounds one by one, *before* showing Lilly the object associated with that sound. This is carried out first with listening alone; lipreading is added if Lilly is unsuccessful. As Lilly has previously worked with these sounds using her Tactaid 7, she is familiar with many of them, visually and tactually, but is now learning the auditory correlates of these. She spontaneously attempts to imitate the adult model. Her mom and I praise Lilly for her attempts and use mirror modeling (Robbins, 1994) to shape a more accurate production. For example, if Lilly uses a central vowel /uuu/ for the expression used when going down a slide, the therapist replies, "You said *'wuuuuuu'*; let's try *'weeee.'*" Lilly receives feedback about her witch's voice when she uses vocal fry. A perception task is incorporated by grouping a few objects and presenting them individually through listening alone. Lilly must select the corresponding object. If she is successful, more items are introduced to the set, and she must select the object based on listening alone. If she is unsuccessful, the set size is reduced, or confusable items are reviewed. Items with the /b/ sound are highlighted, such as *bu bu bu* for bus and *ba-a-a- a* for sheep, with emphasis on outward motion of air rather than a sucking or popping sound. As noted during the speech activity, feedback and practice to help Lilly to contrast the two airstream motions for the /b/ sound.

Teaching recognition and production of onomatopoeic sounds is a commonly used and helpful technique. Most onomatopoeic sounds have multiple segments with highly characteristic suprasegmental patterns, such as great fluctuations in pitch contour or repeated syllables. These are quite audible and contain much more acoustic information than do single words. The repeated use of a set of onomatopoeic sounds, such as those described by Estabrooks (1994), teaches the child a representative sample of early-developing consonants and vowels, including /ah/, /ee/, /oo/, which are produced with maximum excursion of the tongue in three directions. Teaching these three vowels is recommended as a first step by Ling (1976). Once these are mastered, the child can be taught the other vowels that "fill in" the vowel circle. Also, onomatopoeic targets function as "protowords," helping the child to understand the consistent link between an object (for example, a hen) and a series of spoken sounds ("bak, bak, bak"). These protowords are a stepping stone towards the use of real words which are more abstract than protowords.

Hit Parade

Lilly and I sign and sing together two familiar songs that have very different melodies and rhythmic patterns, such as "Jingle Bells" versus "Three Blind Mice." A Christmas bell is associated with the first song; a small box with three tiny mice is associated with the second. After reviewing these, I sing the first line of one of the songs, using an acoustic screen. Through listening alone, Lilly determines which song I sang, selects its corresponding object, and sings the first line. If she is successful, a third song with yet a different pattern is added, and so on. The parents continue work on music at home, initially singing the same songs that Lilly has enjoyed in therapy. This helps her "overlearn" these songs and increases her confidence. Later, the parents may try different songs, including lullabies or meaningful hymns.

Listening Walk

Although speech, not environmental sounds, should be the primary focus of auditory learning activities, environmental sounds are also important. Lilly, her mother, and I leave the therapy room and take a short walk in the hallway to listen to sounds. We use signs and speech to discuss what we have heard. The purpose of this activity is threefold: first, it demonstrates to the parent how to go for a Listening Walk, which should be a daily activity with children who use TC, during the initial weeks after stimulation of the implant, to expose them to the many meaningful sounds in their environment. Second, it takes the child out of the structured and sometimes contrived setting of the therapy room, serving as a "bridging activity" (Robbins, 1990). Third, it provides a break in the therapy routine for a young child who needs frequent changes during a one-hour session.

I enter responses on a Listening Walk Record as follows:

Listening Walk Record

Date	Sound	Detected Y/N	Spontaneous Y/N	Comments
May 30	*Door slamming	*Y	*Y	*Startle response
" "	Therapist calling her name from behind	Y	Y	Lilly pointed to her ear, signed "Listen," but could not identify what the sound was
" "	Footsteps in hallway	Y	Y	Could be tactile
" "	PA system	Y	N	Mother cued with hand-to-ear response, "I hear something!"
" "	Name called from 15 feet	N	N	Distance too great
" "	Water fountain gurgling	Y	N	Lilly described as "soft" from 6 feet away and "OK" from 2 feet away
" "	Fingers striking computer keyboard	Y	Y	Said she liked this sound!
" "	Rustling paper	Y	N	Said she heard it "a little bit"

*Items from this line down are written in by the parent or therapist during the walk.

Under the *Detected* column, I record whether or not the sound was audible to Lilly. Under the *Spontaneous* column, I record whether each response was spontaneous or whether it had to be pointed out by an adult. For example, although Lilly detected a speaker's announcement over the PA system, this was called to her attention by Mother. The number of *spontaneous* responses to sound should increase over time. Having had no functional hearing prior to receiving her implant, Lilly may be surprised to learn that some things in the environment produce sound almost constantly, and that these sounds help people know about their surroundings. This is a special moment for children who have used TC prior to receiving a cochlear implant because their world is organized almost entirely through vision. Lilly's family continues their daily Listening Walks, which are taken in the home or outside, and they bring their completed record to each therapy session. From time to time, we also read the book called *The Listening Walk* (Showers, 1961).

Tea Party

The goals of this activity include communicative turn taking, comprehension, and production of phrases with three critical elements (such as "Give *Wes a blue napkin*"), and production of the high front vowel /ee/. The game follows several therapeutic principles previously outlined by Robbins (1994), including the use of dialog, and the child playing teacher. A picnic basket full of dishes and pretend food is presented. Our task is to set the table for the tea party. A teddy bear, "Wes," joins the party so that we can refer to him with pronouns (*he, him,* and *his*). Lilly is familiar with many of the single-word vocabulary items in sign, which we review. Each one is presented first with the sign/spoken label, then through listening alone. The rationale for this order of presentation is to reinforce Lilly's existing signed representations of words, and then to add the new, corresponding auditory representations. At this early stage, Lilly's confidence in listening is limited. As she expands her auditory capabilities, information will increasingly be presented through listening first.

Lilly shows detection of /ee/, but produces it inconsistently, often substituting a central vowel such as /u/ in *cup,* and nasalizing it. As recommended in a phonological training program known as the Cycles approach (Hodsen & Paden, 1992), *auditory bombardment* is used first to provide repeated exposure of the /ee/ vowel in words, with no demand for production at this stage. For auditory bombardment, I isolate a group of items that contain /ee/ and tell Lilly, "Listen to these /ee/

words: *tea, me, eat, treat,"* presenting them through listening alone. I acoustically highlight other /ee/ words throughout the tea party. Ten new relevant vocabulary words, such as *place, mug, fill, empty,* and *tray,* were introduced during the previous session and assigned for home carryover; I use them again as we set out the items, and check Lilly's comprehension and production of them. I say, "I'll put this cup at my *place.* Look! The teapot is *empty.* Lilly, what is this?" (showing her a tray).

Language comprehension and production are incorporated into the game by giving commands in signed and spoken form: "Get a green plate," "Mommy needs sugar," "She needs a napkin," again acoustically highlighting the /ee/ vowel when appropriate. We focus on current grammatical structures such as verb + adjective + object ("Eat the round cookie"); synonyms ("That plate is *little;* it's really *small"*); and vocabulary expansion ("That's a *cup;* this is a *mug"*). Name recognition is also reinforced, as the therapist begins each request by using the acoustic screen and calling either "Mom" or "Lilly" to indicate whose turn it is. Occasionally, sabotage is used and nothing is presented. If Lilly recognizes this silence, identifying it as "nothing," she receives praise from both adults. The ability to recognize silence when expecting to hear sound is a critical early step in auditory learning with the cochlear implant. It is the basis for other skills, such as the ability to report device malfunction or nonfunction reliably, and for adequate setting of threshold levels. In addition, the absence of sound almost always occurs without warning. That is, no one tells the child, "Your device is going to malfunction in 10 minutes, so be prepared to hear nothing." Rather, a listener must discern the absence of sound with no prompting. Learning this skill early in implant use should help the child generalize this behavior to everyday listening situations. Silence could be used at this point because Lilly had already shown the ability to discriminate reliably between the presence and absence of sound.

The role of teacher is then delegated to Lilly's mother, and finally, to Lilly. When it is her turn to give the commands, Lilly must call my name or "Mom" to designate the listener. If she taps or pulls at us, the adults fail to make eye contact, saying and signing to her, "You must say 'Mom.'" We also identify a few words or phrases that will be said without signing during the game, including "please," "thank you," and "you're welcome." It is essential to start this practice immediately after the implant is first stimulated in order to give the child who uses TC experience with oral communication and to convey the concept that communication can occur through speech alone, which may come as a surprise to some children. Only through successful practice will children develop confidence to try their auditory and oral skills in other situations. Expressions such as "hello," "good-bye," "let's go," "time for bed," and "how are you?" can be used because they are common and predictable from the context. If the child does not understand the phrases through listening, even after several repetitions, the adult may sign for clarification. During natural conversation, it is better to sign all the words in a sentence or none of them, in order to provide a complete English-language model.

Book Worms

We end our session by sharing the book *One Frog Too Many* (Mayer & Mayer, 1975), a wordless picture book. Lilly is to comprehend and express the concept of ordering events (temporal sequencing). Vocabulary that conveys this concept, such as *then* and *next,* is modeled as Lilly narrates the story. We stop on each page and discuss the pictures, emphasizing question comprehension such as: "What animal was in the box?" or "Where is the boy leading the animals?" As Lilly's auditory skills expand using the cochlear implant, this "bookworm time" will include more listening activities. In the story "The Three Bears," for example, I will ask Lilly to identify the characters, through listening alone, as I use a deep-pitched voice for Papa Bear, a breathy voice for Mama Bear, and a high-pitched voice for Baby Bear. At a more complex level, I will ask Lilly to identify whether I said, "I do not like that Sam-I-am" or "I do not like green eggs and ham" in the book *Green Eggs and Ham* (Geisel, 1988). These two sentences have identical rhythmic and syllabic patterns, but vary slightly in the words used at the end of sentences. This is good practice to help children maintain auditory attention to the completion of sentences, where critical information may occur.

Summary

After only four weeks of using the cochlear implant, Lilly is building the first foundations of listening. Most of her skills, however, are tied to *structured* listening situations and need to be developed in *spontaneous* listening responses (carryover or generalization of effect). Eventually, it is hoped that Lilly's auditory skills will allow her to learn vicariously from the world around her, rather than being dependent upon direct instruction.

Considerable time is spent interacting with Lilly's teachers. During a school visit that occurred shortly after this session, Lilly and I conducted a mini-therapy session in front of the school staff. The teachers expressed surprise at Lilly's developing auditory skills and noted that she did not demonstrate most of these at school. We discussed the urgent need for modifications in teacher expectations in order to cultivate Lilly's listening in the classroom. The teachers realized they should no longer use visual or tactile cues to get Lilly's attention, but should try consistently to secure her attention through audition first, even though this skill was still emerging. The staff identified phrases that were used routinely during the day and which could be spoken to Lilly without signs. As we talked through her therapy goals, the teachers thought of numerous applications of these within the classroom. Further interaction with the school staff continues via phone calls, weekly faxing of lesson plans, and sharing videotapes of therapy sessions.

The cochlear implant provides new listening potential for the child who uses TC. It also presents the risk that auditory behaviors will be developed in a rote fashion and as subskills unrelated to overall communication. If such "greenhousing" of auditory skills occurs (Robbins & Kirk, 1996) the child's listening ability may never be in synchrony with other communicative abilities. Auditory skill development in isolation is not an appropriate goal for children who use TC, in the initial stages of learning to use their newly acquired listening potential. The ultimate goal is communicative competence, where the use of audition takes a rightful place in helping children to interpret their world.

Four Years Later: Lilly at Age Eight Years, Five Months

After receiving her cochlear implant, Lilly attended a self-contained TC preschool. Her kindergarten program consisted of a morning TC class and a mainstream afternoon kindergarten class with a SEE2 interpreter. In first grade, her full-day placement was in a regular classroom with a SEE2 interpreter. The role of the interpreter has changed dramatically since Lilly received her cochlear implant, requiring considerable adjustment by the school staff. At four years post implant, Lilly uses signs only for receptive clarification. She reports that this is particularly helpful for academic material, given her recent placement in a classroom for gifted and talented students. The teachers continually assess Lilly's need for interpreting. When she is able to function well in a subject without an interpreter, she does so. A lesson in phonics or rhyming, for example, may be vastly altered when manual interpreting is used because the skills being taught are highly auditory in nature. Lilly has never used an interpreter for such lessons.

One of the challenges of giving a cochlear implant to a child who uses TC is to find a balance between the amount of visual versus auditory information provided to the child. As the child gains more experience through listening, she moves from being a visual learner to being an auditory learner as much as possible. Using her implant, Lilly is progressing well towards complete competence in oral communication.

After two years of use, Lilly's internal device failed. She received another, which was reactivated within 12 weeks. Her listening development continued to progress, with no apparent plateau.

GOALS

Speech:
- production of consonant cluster *sk-*.
- improvement in her cul-de-sac (nasal) resonance.
- coarticulation (overlapping of articulation across sounds) during running conversation.

Language:
- providing definitions for words.
- linguistic problem solving.
- comprehension and use of complex syntactic structures.
- reading meaning between the lines for semantic understanding.

Audition:
- open-set (no choices available) comprehension of complex information.
- manipulation of small units in words to change meaning.
- comparison and contrast of fine difference in temporal sequencing.
- self-monitoring of conversation.

Cognition:
- class inclusion/exclusion (knowing whether items belong in a set).
- use of spoken communication repair strategies.

Ling Six-Sound Test
This test is carried out as outlined earlier. Lilly now identifies all six sounds, even at a distance of nine feet, so any change in her respons-

es prompts me to check her equipment and to query her about other factors such as fatigue, illness, and the use of certain medications.

Speech Work

I start *sk-* with some imitative motor practice, then move on to real words. I say, "Repeat after me: skah, skah, skah [Lilly imitates]; skah, skah, skah [Lilly imitates]; skah, skah, skah [Lilly imitates]." When Lilly is successful with all these, I move to other vowels: *skee, skee, skee* [Lilly repeats three times], *skoo, skoo, skoo,* then *skay, skay, skay,* and on through a variety of vowels. This helps Lilly develop a strong orosensory-motor image of the correct production; she hears and feels the clusters over and over, much as a pianist practices a few notes of a difficult passage many times until it feels and sounds natural. When the cluster is correct with a given vowel, I quickly put the sounds into real words. For the *skoo* sound, we practice *school, scoop, scooter,* first in isolation, then with a carrier phrase such as, *That's a school; that's a scoop; that's a scooter.* At the next level, I require Lilly to deviate from the specified carrier phrase. I show her pictures of the target items and ask, "Is that a school?" Her response is, "Yes, that's a school" or "No, that's a scoop." If she makes an error, such as, "Yes, that's a *shool,"* I use the expansion-reduction technique, reducing the phrase to, "a school, a school" (she repeats), then "That's a school, That's a school" (she repeats). If she makes no errors, I embed the target words in longer sentences. My goal is for Lilly to use accurate production of the consonant clusters, even in a context with high linguistic and articulatory demands. When she can do this, I have confidence that her production of the clusters is stable.

We make a list of the words that contain the target consonant clusters we have worked on. I ask the parents to put the list on the refrigerator or in another prominent place in the home, so that everyone is reminded of them. The parents agree to give Lilly feedback when she uses these words, providing either praise for accurate productions or correction (such as, "Not *shool,* Lilly, *school"*) for inaccurate productions. These target words are also sent to school, so that the staff there can reinforce them.

"Less Is More" Speech Monitoring

This is less a separate activity and more a monitoring process that takes place throughout the session. I identify specific speech targets that will be monitored during the session. I choose targets that Lilly produces well in isolation but misarticulates in conversation.

The target for this session is *sitting,* which Lilly often produces as *stitting* in conversation. I write the word SITTING at the top of a dry-erase board and remind Lilly that she will receive only a + or 0 on the board, each time she says the word. Anytime Lilly uses that word, I put either a + or 0 on the board, without stopping conversation. The + marks go in a column on the left, the 0 marks on the right. If Lilly receives a 0, she may self-correct, but the original rating is not changed. Use of good resonance during speaking is also a goal.

This activity follows the principles of a "less is more" technique (Robbins, 1994), which argues that speech carryover may occur faster if fewer targets are corrected *every time they occur,* than if multiple targets are corrected only haphazardly. Moreover, it is also consistent with the Hodsen and Paden (1992) approach. It assumes that Lilly does not need more motor practice for the word in isolation, but needs to have a more accurate production during coarticulation within sentences. In other words, she knows how to produce the word correctly, but fails to do so when the linguistic demands are higher, suggesting incomplete automaticity (Ling, 1976). For this reason, explanations about her error productions are unnecessary ("You said stitting instead of sitting"). Rather, with an immediate reminder about her error, Lilly is able to self-correct rapidly.

What Is It?

Worthley's (1978) *Sourcebook of Language Learning Activities* provides numerous stimuli for this game, or I create them myself. The object is to utilize multiple sentence-length clues to determine what "it" is. All clues are provided initially through listening alone. Using the acoustic screen, the therapist says, "What is it? It is soft. (Pause.) It keeps you warm. (Pause.) It is made of cotton or wool. (Pause.) It goes on a bed." Lilly chooses to repeat each clue after it is given to ensure she has heard it correctly. If Lilly misunderstands a clue, we follow the hierarchy in Table 1. Clarification is first provided through listening alone by using repetition, acoustic highlighting, slowing of rate, clearer pronunciation, heightened intonation contrasts, or rephrasing. If these are unsuccessful, speechreading cues are given, and finally, manual cues, beginning with fingerspelling and moving to signs.

Which Number Was Said Twice?

This activity is a twist on the traditional "digit repetition task." Using an acoustic screen, I say a list of numerals, such as "4, 7, 2, 3, 4, 8."

Table 1. Hierarchy of cues during listening activities for a child who uses TC

(Use in descending order)

Auditory cues	Acoustic highlighting
	Repetition
	Slowing rate
	Clearer pronunciation
	Heightened intonation contrasts
	Rephrasing
Speechreading cues	One word
	A short phrase
	Part of the message
	Entire message
Manual cues	Fingerspell first letter
	Sign one word
	Sign a short phrase
	Sign part of message
	Sign entire message

Through listening alone, Lilly must decide which number was said twice. She must hold all the numbers in memory, compare them, and decide which one was repeated. Rather than focusing on global linguistic meaning, this game requires Lilly to focus on the discrete differences between one- and two-syllable words. The activity is made more difficult with a longer list, easier with a shorter list. Sabotage may be used, such as "8, 0, 9, 6, 3, 5." If Lilly can spontaneously report that no number was said twice, we have confidence in the fact that she is effectively processing this memory/cognitive task through listening alone.

Change a Sound

This listening/semantics game requires Lilly to manipulate a sound within a word in order to change its meaning. For example, I say, "Change a vowel in the word *pork* to make it mean a play area" [park], or "Change a vowel in the word *lame* to make it mean a citrus fruit" [lime]. Consonant changes may also be included, although these are more difficult for Lilly. Consonant distinctions involving place of articulation, such as /t/ versus /k/ or /f/ versus /th/, are particularly problematic. I sometimes find stimuli for this game in *Listening Games* (Maxwell, 1981). If Lilly is unsuccessful, I follow the hierarchy of cues described earlier. We then switch roles and Lilly presents the *sound changes* to me and I must fill in the target word. Since only one sound in a word is altered, Lilly's speech accuracy must convey the information. Lilly brings 10 word changes to the session (homework). In addition to providing speech and listening practice, this game builds vocabulary and word definitions.

Solve a Problem

During this discussion activity, Lilly uses language to solve a problem. We begin with listening only, adding lipreading cues or manual cues when needed. I pose a problem, sometimes with a picture or written description. Some problems may relate to current events, such as: "A woman in South Dakota drove on a country road in a blizzard and is now stranded in her car in a snowdrift. She has her cellular phone with her but doesn't know where she is. What can the rescuers do to find her?" Other problems relate to dilemmas relevant to Lilly's life, such as: "One of your parents' cars is in the shop for five days. You and your brothers have many extracurricular events this week, and your parents' jobs are 50 miles apart. How can your family solve its transportation problem?" I pose the problem using an acoustic screen, so that Lilly first receives the information through listening alone. I check her auditory comprehension by having her repeat each part of the problem as I pose it.

Newspaper: City of Venice

In this session, we read a short newspaper article about the city of Venice, Italy, which is sinking into the ocean. Lilly becomes familiar with the topic and sorts out some of the difficult vocabulary. I then describe the problem through listening alone, using the acoustic screen. I say, "The city of Venice is endangered."

Lilly repeats, "The city of Venice is endangered."

I say, "The islands have sunk almost to sea level."

Lilly responds, "The islands have *shrunk* almost to sea level."

I clarify, "No, the islands haven't *shrunk,* they have *sunk,* they are *sinking.*"

Lilly corrects herself, "Oh, the islands have *sunk.*"

"Almost to sea level," I continue.

Lilly repeats, "almost to sea level."

I add, "A main source of the problem is that people have tapped the underground water supplies."

Lilly questions, "People have done what to the underground water?"

I answer, "They have tapped it; *tapped* into it. They want to pump it out."

"Oh, they've tapped the underground water," she nods. This process continues until the entire problem has been posed and I am confident she understands it.

Then we begin the problem-solving discussion. I no longer want Lilly to repeat what I say; I want us to engage in reciprocal dialog. I ask, "How can the people of Venice get fresh water if underground tapping is so harmful?"

She responds to clarify, "Did you ask how the people of Venice can get fresh water without tapping underground?"

"Yes," I answer.

Lilly replies, "They need a water source that will not affect the height... you know, the level of the land."

I query, "But what would that water source be? Venice is really just a cluster of tiny islands." At this point, Lilly encounters some difficulty, which cannot be resolved through auditory cues. She says she does not understand my question and asks me to repeat. I do so.

Lilly says, "What would the new source of water be? What did you say about Venice?"

"That it is really just a cluster of tiny islands," I repeat.

"Venice is *cluttered* with something?" she asks.

"No," I respond, "it is just a *cluster* of tiny *islands*. You know, islands are land completely surrounded by water."

Lilly nods, "Oh, islands. Venice is *cluttered* with islands?" I attempt several other auditory cues but cannot get this word across.

I repeat, "Venice is just a cluster of tiny islands," removing the acoustic screen for the phrase, "a cluster of tiny islands." This allows her to speechread the problematic words. However, as visual cues are not particularly helpful in discriminating *cluster* from *clutter,* I then finger-spell c-l-u-s-t-e-r, and she recognizes her error. I don't spend too much time on individual words because the goal of this activity is meaningful problem solving through dialog and comprehension of the total message.

As we continue our discussion, Lilly suggests that water be piped in from the mainland. "They could use mountain water from the Alps," she offers, so we talk about the use of an aqueduct for that purpose.

In this activity, Lilly has an opportunity to *put it all together,* learning about current events and newsworthy information. I am able to evaluate Lilly's expressive syntax, depth of vocabulary knowledge, articulation, and conversational skills. Most of the discussion occurs in spoken English, although I provide sign support for troublesome information, and fingerspell a number of foreign words, as Lilly requires more manual support when encountering an unfamiliar topic.

Hit Parade

We end the session with a song. Lilly is very motivated to listen to and understand current pop and country-and-western songs, largely because her hearing peers and older siblings do. We review new vocabulary in songs and discuss hidden meanings in the lyrics by "reading between the lines." We sing the chorus and first verse of a country-western song, "I Thank God for Unanswered Prayers." I ask Lilly why the songwriter would be thankful for prayers that went unanswered. She explains, "Because he prayed that a certain woman would love him but she didn't. Then later, he met a perfect woman, and now they are very happy in love." Idioms are identified in the lyric, too, such as "the man upstairs." After sorting through the details of the language, we play a tape of the song, singing along and enjoying the musical experience as a whole. For home carryover, Lilly agrees to listen to this song several times and to write a verse of her own for it. Understanding and enjoying music are culturally important experiences for Lilly.

Summary

Lilly's auditory skills have progressed to a level where she is able to process much complex information through listening alone. The total communication method allows her the option to receive speechreading or manual cues to augment auditory ones. A goal in therapy is to reduce the number and extent of these additional cues, although I willingly provide them when they are needed for successful communication.

Lilly's parents understand very well that she needs to practice more complex listening without visual cues. Initially, they did not welcome this suggestion because they felt that, even though she was capable of using audition alone for simple tasks, she needed signs for complex ones. It was necessary to demonstrate to them what Lilly could accomplish with her hearing, and to show them that, without intensive practice, we would never know the extent of her auditory potential. Ultimately, they were pleasantly surprised at her learning abilities through listening and have actively supported our efforts with consistent home carryover. The parents continue to use signs at home when they are carrying on family dialog. This creates no need to stop and explain, and does not exclude Lilly from any part of the discussion, when Lilly does not fully understand the conversation.

Lilly's case demonstrates the potential that exists for many children who learn TC before receiving a cochlear implant. Her auditory success has depended on a combination of factors, without which this success would be unlikely. These include a strong family commitment to maximizing the auditory component within a TC approach, the school's willingness to adjust their expectations and teaching priorities, and Lilly's own *x-factors* of personality, intelligence, and temperament, which combine uniquely to form this special child.

Acknowledgments
I wish to thank Allyson Imber Riley, my colleague and partner in working with Lilly; Linette Caldwell, for manuscript preparation; Susan Sehgal, for editorial comment; and Mary Pat Moeller, for her mentorship.

References
Erber, N. (1982). *Auditory training.* Washington, DC: A.G. Bell Association for the Deaf.

Estabrooks, W. (1994). A*uditory-verbal therapy for parents and professionals.* Washington, DC: A.G. Bell Association for the Deaf.

Geisel, T. (1988). *Green eggs and ham.* New York: Beginner Books.

Gustason, G., & Zawolkow, E. (1993). *Signing exact English.* Los Alamitos, CA: Modern Signs Press.

Hodsen, B., & Paden, E. (1992). *Targeting intelligible speech* (2nd ed.). Austin, TX: Pro-Ed.

Ling, D. (1976). *Speech and the hearing-impaired child: Theory and practice.* Washington, DC: A.G. Bell Association for the Deaf.

Maxwell, M. (1981). *Listening games.* Washington, DC: Acropolis Books.

Mayer, M., & Mayer, M. (1975). *One frog too many.* New York: Dial Books.

Robbins, A.M. (1990). Developing meaningful auditory integration in children with cochlear implants. *Volta Review, 92* (6), 361–370.

Robbins, A.M. (1994). Guidelines for developing oral communication skills in children with cochlear implants. In A. Geers & J. Moog (Eds.),

Effectiveness of cochlear implants and tactile aids for deaf children. *Volta Review, 96* (5), 75–82.

Robbins, A.M., Hesketh, L., & Bivins, C. (1993). *Tactaid reference guide and orientation* (TARGO), Somerville, MA: Audiological Engineering Corporation.

Robbins, A.M., & Kirk, K.I. (1996). Speech perception assessment and performance in pediatric cochlear implant users. *Seminars in Hearing, 17* (4), 353–369.

Showers, P. (1961). *The listening walk.* New York: HarperCollins.

Worthley, W. (1978). *Sourcebook of language learning activities.* Boston: Little, Brown.

Lesson Plan for Chris

Judith I. Simser, O.Ont., B.Ed., Cert. AVT

Chris's profound sensorineural hearing impairment was diagnosed when he was 13 months old. An auditory brainstem response (ABR) test yielded no response. After 14 months of diagnostic therapy with effective parent participation following the auditory-verbal approach, it was determined that Chris had very little hearing potential. He had some difficulty doing play audiometry, and the only thresholds obtained indicated vibrotactile responses. Both the parents and our professional team felt that Chris and his family would benefit from a total communication (TC) approach. It was suggested that the family consult the local school for the deaf, where they began a home visiting program using TC. When he turned three, Chris attended a class for children who were deaf at a public school in his city. Chris's parents took sign language classes, and they and their son became fluent in sign as their primary mode of communication.

With the advent of cochlear implants in Ontario, Chris's parents became interested in the device. He was assessed and judged to be a candidate. When he was four and a half years of age, Chris had cochlear implant surgery in Toronto, receiving a full insertion of 22 electrodes. Six weeks later, the device was switched on, and Chris continued with the same self-contained program he had attended for the past two years.

Chris's aided thresholds with his cochlear implant were:

Frequency:	250 Hz	500 Hz	1000 Hz	2000 Hz	4000 Hz
Threshold:	30 dB HL	35 dB HL	35 dB HL	30 dB HL	35 dB HL

Chris used sign language to communicate with his parents and others who knew how to sign. Even after six months of cochlear implant use, however, his parents saw that Chris continued to use sign language and spoke only neutral vowels to communicate. In their concern to maximize his newly acquired hearing potential they requested that Chris rejoin the auditory-verbal program.

Chris's parents and I discussed the following options:

- continue the TC program, in the expectation that sign language would probably be Chris's preferred mode of communication, as he would still be learning visually.
- integrate Chris into a segregated oral class, where he would learn through speechreading, with audition as a supplement.
- reenter the auditory-verbal program with the goal of transition from sign language to the development of spoken language through listening.

Because this was an important decision, they were asked to consider the options and return a week later. They chose the third option. We agreed upon a three-month trial, after which we would reevaluate the chosen option.

Auditory-Verbal Plan at One Month
This is an early lesson plan that we used one month after Chris returned to the auditory-verbal program. He was five years, one month old and seven months post implant.

DISCUSSION
As Chris was unable to hear for the first four and a half years of his life, he had naturally learned to rely on a visual mode of communication. Because of his inability to respond to listening targets, he had become unreceptive to auditory teaching. Chris's parents need to develop confidence in their son's ability to learn through listening. In developing his goals, it is imperative that auditory tasks follow a hierarchy, progressing from easy to more difficult to hear. His parents should know that some children have been unable to develop confidence in using the cochlear implant because the initial auditory targets were far too advanced and difficult, causing a feeling of failure.

Parent Guidance

✔ Always provide an optimal acoustic environment. Reduce background noise by turning off the radio and the television unless it is being watched. Be aware of the noise of air conditioners and refrigerators; close windows to minimize outside environmental noises. Sit beside Chris on the side of his implanted ear when providing speech stimuli.

✔ Remember to talk in ways that increase the audibility of speech in order for Chris to have the best opportunity to learn to listen: Use clear speech; speak in simple two- to four-word phrases; use various rhythm and pitch contrasts, increase repetitions, and emphasize key words.

✔ Use the hand cue to alert Chris to listen and to emphasize listening rather than lipreading. In the early stages, the hand cue should be used especially when there is a situational cue. Tell him, while you are putting on your coat, "Put on your coat; we're going in the car. Get your coat." Also use the hand cue when you are reinforcing weekly targets integrated into your daily routines and play.

✔ Reduce use of sign language. In situations involving complex language, offer lipreading in combination with listening. We want to reduce reliance on signing and lipreading while simultaneously developing spoken language skills through listening.

GOALS

Audition:
- to demonstrate consistent response to his name.
- to learn to identify vowels /au/, /ah/, /o/, and /ee/ and to identify consonants varying in manner cues: /m/, /b/ or /p/, and /h/.
- to develop the ability to process one-item auditory memory tasks:
  - in phrases containing repetition of sound-word associations, such as, "The ball goes *bounce, bounce, bounce,*"
  - with single objects representing nouns, verbs, adjectives and adverbs that vary in vowel content, number of syllables, and suprasegmental features (e.g., "Do you want an *apple,* here's an *apple,*" "Where are your *shoes,* go get your *shoes,*" "*Cut, cut, cut* the paper.")
  - with a known word presented at the end of the sentence (e.g., "Where are the *bananas?*")
  - with a known word presented in the middle or beginning of the sentence (e.g., "Please put the *spoons* on the table.")

- to try *selection by description;* to teach Chris to attend to longer segments of information and to extract familiar words necessary for comprehension:
  - where the familiar word or sound-word is used repeatedly (e.g., "It goes *up, up, up* in the sky; it goes *a-a-a-a;* you ride in it; what is it?")
  - where known words are in a single repetition in the description (e.g., "It has *four* legs; it *hops;* it swims in the *water;* it's *green;* what is it?")
- to identify expressive phrases that have different rhythms and contain identifiable phonemes and/or words (e.g., *"Mmmm,* that's good!" *"Shhhhh,* Daddy's sleeping," *"Bye, bye,* Chris," and *"Ow,* that hurts").
- to encourage the development of a listening attitude by drawing Chris's attention to sounds and speech throughout the day and by stressing the development of listening through alerting Chris to sound by saying, "Listen! Listen! I hear that!"

Speech:
- to develop differences in duration, pitch, and intensity using sound-word associations (e.g., rising and lowering *oo-oo-oo* for a train, and short phrases, *"oh, oh,* it fell down").
- to reinforce voiced versus voiceless phonemes (e.g., *m→* vs. *h,h,h,* repeated).
- to extend vowel production to higher-frequency vowels (e.g., *aye,* /i/ as in *hit,* and /ee/).
- to alternate known vowels (e.g., *ah-oo* and *o-o-ah, oo-w-ah* to create *wa-wa-wa*).
- to improve /m/ in syllabic babble with a variety of vowels (e.g., *um→, um→; ummu-ummu; m→u, m→u; m→oo, m→oo*).
- to reinforce /p/ /p/ /p/ and /h/ /h/ /h/ (whisper these and alternate them).
- once syllables are developed, to alternate those varying in manner cues (e.g., *ma-ma, bo-bo*).
- to expect Chris to use speech to attract attention and to communicate.

Language:
- to develop fundamental vocabulary containing a variety of parts of speech.

- to develop comprehension and expression of frequently used phrases.
- to begin using negatives such as *no* and *not the*.
- to develop verbs as directives (e.g., *Wash your hands, Open the door*).
- to identify family names such as *Mommy, Daddy, the baby,* and familiar animals such as *dog* and *cat* to prepare for noun-verb phrases.
- to develop comprehension and use of question forms, *What's that?* and *What's he doing?*
- to capitalize on everyday situations to reinforce listening and language development.

Communication:
- to acknowledge Chris's attempts to communicate through gestures and/or sign language and to provide three- to four-word spoken phrases to encourage and reinforce verbal interaction.
- to develop and expect use of greetings and courtesy language.
- to encourage Chris to listen at all times but especially in natural situations (e.g., when the table is set and you've come out from the kitchen: *"It's time for dinner"*).

Cognition:
- to arrange objects in categories.
- to select objects that don't belong (from a set of four).
- to sequence a four-part story.
- to associate objects with pictures.
- to identify three to four letters.
- to reinforce number concepts to five.

Introduction to the Lesson

Chris and his mother arrive at the clinic and I go to the waiting room to call him. He is playing with a toy and does not respond to his name. I gesture to his mom not to touch him. I go behind him close to the microphone of the cochlear implant and call him three times. No response! So I visually cue him to listen, go behind him again and practice the same task twice more.

I remind his mom to expect him to respond when she calls him and to teach him to respond in this way. At this stage, she should try not to call him to test his response, but to call only when she has something specific that she wants or needs.

Outside the therapy room, within reach of the children, there are coat hooks with pictures above them. Chris takes off his coat, and I ask him to hang it *on the cat that says meow, meow.* Then, while he is holding his boots in his hand, I ask him to put them *under the fish.* I tell Mom that these auditory tasks are considered a single-item auditory memory because Chris has the objects in his hands. That is, Chris only has to listen to *where* to put the objects. In the future we will expand by creating a two- to six-item memory, e.g., "Put your *coat* on the *frog,*" "Put your *boots* under the *ball* and your *hat* on the *dog.*" Instead of saying, "Good boy," I suggest that there is more auditory reinforcement in saying, "Right, you hung your coat on the fish."

As Chris can say a form of *sit down,* his mom knows to wait beside her chair until Chris tells her to do so. She expands the phrase to, *Thank you, I'll sit down on the chair.*

Phonetic Identification Game

The object of this game is to practice the auditory perception of early phonemes or speech sounds. Chris's auditory level is below his cognitive level; the use of enjoyable games is highly motivational. The game Probe™ uses a long plastic strip onto which you can insert an equally long strip of paper. It has little covers that snap over the strip of paper where you can put stickers or pictures, or write letters inside each little compartment to conceal them. Chris is an early listener, so I write down a *closed set* of five letters from the auditory targets. We take turns choosing and writing one letter. While the players try to guess the hidden letter, Chris has practice *listening to the phonics of speech sounds and identifying them.* We keep score of the number of tries for each person to guess the hidden letter correctly, low score being the winner.

Mum's turn: "Is there a /p/, *puh. Puh. Puh. Puh?*"

I use the hand cue to prompt Chris to imitate what he heard. This eliminates guesswork and promotes auditory feedback. I do this only if I know that he can produce a reasonable imitation of the phoneme. This avoids poor or inaccurate auditory feedback. He may need further experience in listening to the phoneme before he is able to produce it.

Chris: (Shakes his head to indicate a negative response.)
Judy: "You say to Mommy, no-no" (I use a hand cue to prompt imitation). "It's my turn."

This activity can also be practiced by hiding a letter written on a piece of paper in a container, by writing letters on a whiteboard, identifying them and then erasing them, by using letter stamps or magnetic letters, or by hiding papers with letters on them around the room and asking him to find a specific one. Many hints can be given through listening (e.g., "It's near the door. Open the door").

Tactile Game

In this activity, Chris is to select a single object by listening to familiar vocabulary. To add motivation for listening, once Chris has selected a picture of the item requested, he will try to find it hidden among other objects within the box, by his sense of touch.

I have about six objects known to Chris, and I put them into a shoe box with a rectangular hole in one end, one at a time. To prompt answering the question, "What's that?" I ask his mom to turn around so that she cannot see the objects. She asks Chris the identity of each object as I hand them to him.

Mom: "What's that?"

Mom asks me the same question and I answer briefly, "A shoe."

Chris: "Wa ah?" He attempts to imitate, rather than answer, the question.

When children don't know how to answer questions, the answers need to be modeled without repeating any components of the question in order to be a natural part of expressive language. The question should be highlighted or emphasized by repeatedly asking the same question with many different known objects. To make it meaningful, the answer should not be known to the person asking the question.

Once I have placed all the objects in the box, I ask Chris to put the pictures representing the objects on the table in front of him. He is to select the picture requested to indicate a correct response (e.g., "Where's the ball that goes *bounce, bounce, bounce?*"), then see if he can find it in the box without looking, but by feeling only. While he is feeling the objects, his mother has the opportunity to expand receptive language by saying, "Can you find the *ball?*" "No, no, no, that's *not the ball,*" promoting the negative form. This game can also be used to reinforce other parts of speech using *verb and/or adjective pictures* and objects associated with them (e.g., soap for *washing,* scissors for *cutting,* a candle stuck in play dough for *hot,* some tape for *sticky*).

More Games

To reinforce the perception and production of speech targets I give Chris a choice between the games, Hungry Hippos™ or Mr. Mouth™, both manufactured by Milton Bradley. It is important to give a choice whenever possible so that the child has a feeling of control. Almost any game can be used to develop almost any target. Chris chooses Hungry Hippos. To play this game you need to place about 15 colored balls into the center area of the game. As Chris is motivated, he is eager to imitate speech sounds to obtain the balls from me. In the early stages of practice the child must have a reason to imitate sounds; you must have something that he wants.

I whisper, *"hhhh-hhhhh-hhhhh"* and use a hand cue to prompt Chris to imitate.

Chris produces a *voiced* guttural noise.

"Listen," I say, then I *repeat the phoneme,* use the hand cue to prompt *Mom to imitate,* and then *give Chris a turn.* It is important for the child to know whether his production of the phoneme is right or wrong. The use of Mom's voice improves Chris's attention to the speech sound (a different voice adds additional cues). If he does not respond correctly, I may give a kinesthetic cue, such as feeling the breath stream on his hand, but then we all take turns *producing it repeatedly through hearing* to develop the auditory feedback loop. This practice enhances Chris's perception and production of the phoneme in the future.

I hand Chris the balls and, in order to practice a single-item auditory task, ask him to put four on the game.

We *reinforce unvoiced /p-p-p-p/* which Chris produces well and then *alternate unvoiced phoneme /p/ with /m/* to improve the perception and production of voiced versus unvoiced speech sounds.

Mom says, *"/p/ /p/ /p/ (pause), m→," /p/ /p/ m→"* and Chris imitates. This time I give him six balls and tell him to give them *to Mommy.* As this is not the obvious thing to do, he does not understand, so Mom says, *"Give them to me"* a few times, and I glance in her direction. If we give Chris a directional cue, we repeat the verbal request a few times to confirm what we are asking.

Chris's production of the phoneme /m/ is weak in the initial position, and he frequently substitutes /b/ probably because of lipreading. Previously, when Chris relied on lipreading, the phonemes /m/, /b/ and /p/ looked similar on the lips. Because he could not hear them, he often interchanged these speech sounds. I model for Mom to produce /m/ in the final position as I give her the balls to the game to continue this speech babble activity.

Mom covers her mouth and says: *"um→, um."* Chris listens and produces it well.

I whisper to Mom to try *um→mu* to move the phoneme /m/ into the middle position. Chris produces the /m/, but follows it with a nasalized vowel.

I say, "Try /h/ before the second vowel: *um→hu.*" This works! We continue the game.

We put the rest of the balls in the center and use lots of natural language during play (e.g., "I want the green hippo," "Wait for Mom to say 1,2,3, go," "How many balls did you get?" "Do you want to play again?" "You dropped a ball. It's under the table").

The incidental language used while preparing the activity is often more important than the activity itself, as it shows how to integrate targets into whatever you do during the day.

Photographs

I have many personal photographs to use for a variety of listening targets such as descriptions, question forms, prepositions, and sequence stories. Children often prefer them to commercially prepared materials. My cat has been photographed while wearing a Santa hat, drinking water, hiding under the table, even crouching in a paper bag!

While looking at a photo hidden from the others' view, I say, *"Shhhh, Daddy's sleeping.* What do you see, Mom?" She looks at the photo and repeats the phrase. Chris listens and tries to imitate, *"Shhh."* Once we have reviewed four pictures and they are spread on the table, I ask Chris to listen to a short phrase and select each one to put away. There are many reinforcers that can be used; for example, paper clips can be attached to each photo and the pictures can be picked up with a magnet.

DISCUSSION

Discussion between the therapist and parent occurs throughout the therapy session. It is an integral part of each session. If there is a family concern, discussion may consume the whole session while the child plays. The parents' level of understanding and feelings of competence are paramount to helping their child learn. The therapist teaches, guides, and supports the family in creating a listening, language-enriched communicative environment inside and outside their home.

In her notebook, Chris's mother records the activities that she practiced and the targets outlined during the session. She, therefore, has a good understanding of her objectives.

Parent Guidance

Audition:

✔ Continue *one-item memory tasks* as outlined in the lesson goals, but choose meaningful *new vocabulary to highlight* throughout the week. Remember, once Chris knows a word or phrase, always *expand to include some new information.*

✔ Begin *two-item memory* in its simplest form, two nouns or verbs in repetition (e.g., "Where's the *cow* that goes *moo, moo, moo* and the *car* that goes *brrbrrrrrr?"*). You might use two separate containers of water or two circles of play dough so Chris sees that there are to be two items, one for each container. Model with someone else first and remember to have them confirm what they heard. Practice this in a formal way as well as integrating it into daily routines (e.g., "Get the *spoons* and *cups,"* "Where are your *shoes* and *hat?"*). To ensure Chris's success in listening, the objects requested must be part of his known vocabulary.

✔ Continue step one in *selection by description* and *expand your sentences to describe objects* a little more (e.g., "The dog is drinking water; oh, he's wagging his tail. Look at his tail.")

✔ Expect Chris to turn and *respond to his name.* Reinforce him for doing so by saying, "Good, you heard me call you. Do you want some *hot chocolate?"*

Speech:

✔ Keep speech babble practice brief and motivating. If Chris experiences difficulty with certain phonemes, then do not reinforce them. Record the problems and wait until the next session. Otherwise, you will be reinforcing incorrect production.

✔ Produce /m/ in the medial position and move to initial position (e.g., *"ummu, mmhu, mmu, mmu").*

✔ Beginners often require more auditory input to produce the higher-frequency vowel /ee/ than the lower-frequency vowels, so do not be concerned if this takes more time. Just provide many opportunities for Chris to hear the vowel /ee/ as in *"ee, ee, ee,"* for a monkey, *"squeak, squeak, squeak"* for a mouse, *"weeee,"* as he goes down a metal or wooden slide (not plastic, as static electricity can erase his MAP). At this stage, listening is more important than production.

(cont'd on next page)

Parent Guidance *(cont'd)*

✔ Alternate /b/ and /p/ with different vowels that he can already produce (e.g., *"ba, ba, ba, [pause and change direction of pitch] boo, boo, boo, puh, puh, puh,… po, po, po"*).

✔ Develop /h/ in long duration to differentiate it from /p/ (whispered), *h h h h h, h h h h h.*

Language:

✔ Continue to record and assess new vocabulary that Chris develops through listening, and check that it contains a variety of parts of speech. We do not communicate by nouns alone. By developing varied parts of speech, Chris will gain the foundations for spoken language. Stress the pronouns *mine* and *me*, beginning routine verbs, early developing adjectives and adverbs, and the prepositions *on* and *under* (contrast acoustically).

✔ Once Chris comprehends short, meaningful phrases, encourage their expressive use in everyday experiences. In therapy sessions, invite Chris to play the role of the teacher, and ask his mom to select a picture depicting a phrase. She may understand the phrase only by the rhythm and vowel
content but this is fine at this stage.

✔ Do not press Chris for clear speech at this time.

✔ Practice listening to and identifying family names, as we did not have time to work on this activity. A structured activity you might try is to put out photos or little play people that depict Mommy, Daddy, and Chris's siblings including the baby, Elizabeth. From a cloth bag containing interesting objects, pick one, conceal it, and say, "Baby wants it, where's baby?" Once Chris shows you the baby, have him put the object on or near the baby. This is preparation for two-item auditory tasks (e.g., *Daddy is washing,* as Chris puts a little play man in a bathtub).

✔ Reinforce family names all day long.

✔ Use the same highlighting techniques in speaking to other family members as you would to Chris. The baby will benefit from the language stimulation, and there is a lot for Chris to learn while you interact with others.

(cont'd on next page)

Parent Guidance *(cont'd)*

Communication:

✔ Practice and reinforce turn-taking skills! Chris cannot hear if he is vocalizing and trying to monopolize the conversation at the same time. Turn-taking is best practiced in games. If Chris doesn't wait until you have finished talking, turn away from him while you talk, using a hand cue to indicate you are talking. When you finish talking, turn back, and indicate that it is now his turn.

✔ *Catch him listening and talking!* Reinforce the behaviors that you want. Listen actively! Stop what you are doing, and reinforce his verbal attempts. We will deal with his attention-getting behaviors later, when he has learned to talk.

✔ Continue to provide phrases as substitutes for his signs. It is your goal that signing gradually be replaced by verbal communication as Chris gains confidence in listening and talking.

Chris Today

Chris is now six years old and 1.6 years post implant. What a difference a year can make! He converses using intelligible speech, understands conversations through listening, is integrated in a mainstream class in his local school, and no longer uses sign language. On a recent standardized test of language, Chris scored only one year behind his hearing peers.

Chris's parents have developed a way of life that reinforces listening in all interactions. The choice of a cochlear implant and the auditory-verbal approach have provided Chris with his own choice of communication strategies.

Lesson Plan for Heather

Teresa Caruso, M.Sc.(A), Aud.(C), Cert. AVT

Heather is a five-year-old girl who was initially diagnosed with a significant hearing impairment at four months of age. She was assessed at this early age because of parental concern and a positive family history of hearing impairment. Heather's 11-year-old brother has a severe-to-profound hearing impairment.

Initial auditory brainstem response (ABR) testing suggested a moderately-severe-to-severe hearing impairment in the left ear and a severe-to-profound hearing impairment in the right ear. Based on this information, binaural Widex ES2HA hearing aids were prescribed and Heather was enrolled in an auditory-verbal program.

A follow-up aided audiological assessment was carried out, at which time no definite responses could be measured. Impedance audiometry suggested abnormal middle-ear function, and a consultation with the ENT doctor was recommended. The physician recommended a myringotomy and the insertion of PE tubes. An ABR was carried out following the myringotomy, which revealed no response at the limits of the equipment.

At further follow-up aided audiological assessments, there were no observable responses to auditory stimuli. More powerful hearing aids were prescribed and Heather experienced difficulty with feedback. She then received temporary binaural body aids, and later, powerful behind-the-ear hearing aids. Repeated audiological assessments revealed aided responses in the 80–90 dB HL range in the low-frequency spectrum, and her responses in therapy supported these audiological results. Although quite a vocal child, Heather was using primarily a neutral vowel sound such as / Λ / for "up." Her parents reported that she sometimes appeared to respond to her name at home when called loudly and within close proximity.

Discussions regarding cochlear implantation ensued, and the parents proceeded with the evaluation. Preimplant assessments indicated that Heather was a candidate.

Heather's middle-ear status continued to be abnormal, a concern regarding the surgery. Repeated myringotomies and placement of PE tubes did not clear the middle-ear disease. The implant surgeon required Heather to be free of middle-ear problems after removal of the tubes for six months prior to surgery. Once the tubes were removed, however, Heather suffered another bout of otitis. It was suggested that her parents look into the possibility of allergies and discuss the potential benefit of a tonsillectomy and adenoidectomy (T&A) with their physician. Heather was already a snorer and a mouth breather. The parents discovered that in some cases, children were relieved of middle-ear problems after the T&A surgery. As the ENT doctor did not agree with the procedure, the parents sought a physician who would conduct the surgery. After the T&A, Heather's left ear became disease free for six months without PE tubes. A year and a half after initial discussions, Heather underwent cochlear implant surgery. Heather has since had normal middle-ear function in the implanted left ear; her right ear has continued to have abnormal type B tympanograms (stiff eardrum mobility). Heather has been successfully using her Nucleus 22-channel cochlear implant for two years.

Heather's aided responses with the cochlear implant are in the 25–35 dB HL range and her speech processor is MAPped in common-ground mode.

Heather uses a cochlear implant on the left side but does not use a hearing aid on the right ear. Her residual hearing is such that she does not benefit from even a powerful hearing aid coupled to that ear.

Introduction to the Lesson

The goals for Heather's therapy session are separated into specific sections for clarity. In the auditory-verbal sessions, audition, speech, language, and cognition are interrelated in natural language contexts for overall development of spoken communication.

Audition:
- **Development of auditory memory for five items**

GOAL
- to follow a direction recalling five items, including the pronouns *she* versus *they*.

ACTIVITY
This activity involves acting out a story using toys. Various toys, including people, vehicles, playground toys (such as a slide and merry-go-round), and food, are placed on the table. Heather, parent, and therapist each have a turn playing teacher and student. The teacher will tell Heather a story about what the characters will do; Heather then selects the right people and enacts the story.

Heather's mom plays teacher first. She acoustically highlights (by stressing) the italicized words to help Heather focus on salient items, in this case the five items that Heather is encouraged to store in auditory memory.

"OK, Heather, are you ready?" her mom asks. Heather nods. *"She* is going to go for a ride in the *wagon* and *they* are going to go *swimming* in the turtle pool and then have *ice cream."*

Heather takes the girl to the wagon and the children to the swimming pool and then to the freezer for the ice cream. First she hesitates, repeating the stimulus silently, then follows through. To her delight, she carries out the direction and, with a grin, says, "There!"

"It my turn," Heather says. "Mommy listen. The girl wanted to go on merry-go-round and slide and daddy and the boy have to go on swing."

Heather's mom reinforces the pronouns *she* and *they* and models the phrase: "Oh, *she* wanted to go on the merry-go-round and the slide and *they* are going on the *swings."* She highlights the pronouns and the plural, which Heather deleted, by acoustically stressing them; then she carries out the direction.

"Good job, Mom," Heather says.

ANALYSIS

She versus *they* were contrasted in teaching these pronouns rather than *he* versus *she* because *she* and *they* are more acoustically different than *she* and *he.* As Heather develops her listening skills, it is important to follow a hierarchy of listening, from most audible spoken language to least audible.

Heather has good comprehension of the pronouns *she* and *they,* and these pronouns are being integrated into auditory memory tasks. We must ensure that Heather has the vocabulary necessary to do the task, otherwise it is not possible to determine whether the difficulty is in recalling five items or weak vocabulary. Heather does not use the pronoun *they* expressively and overgeneralizes the use of *she.* By encouraging her to play teacher, we can help her to integrate her language goals with an auditory activity. We are not simply asking Heather to recall five miscellaneous items. We are integrating her developing pronouns in what may appear to be a strictly listening-only activity. Mom is counseled that no activity ever targets listening, speech, *or* language; they all serve as a vehicle for one another and are interrelated.

Because we rely extensively on memory in everyday situations, it is important that Heather develop auditory memory skills. This is particularly important in the classroom, where teachers often unknowingly expect their students to follow a number of directions in sequence. For example, "Get your *red book* from your desk, turn to *page 18,* pick up your *pencil* and *wait* for further instructions." Auditory memory is critical in order to recall telephone numbers, addresses, and road directions. Heather needs strategies to help her recall information.

Parent Guidance
✔   Heather's parents might try having her visually scan the objects on the table, associated with the direction, to help develop her visual memory. They might also have her rehearse the direction silently ("in her head"), as one might do with a new telephone number.

Carryover:
✔   In daily routines, Heather's mom provides opportunities for Heather to develop her auditory memory skills. When setting the table, Heather is asked to get the *salt and pepper, napkins, forks,* and *juice.* In folding laundry, Heather picks up the *white socks, girls' underwear,* and *T-shirts.* Her mom removes the laundry from the dryer to avoid exposing Heather's implant to electrostatic electricity. Heather also helps to pack her own lunch and gets the *bread, peanut butter, jam, juice box,* and *cookies.*

✔   Heather loves paper-and-pencil activities and crafts. Using construction paper, glitter, and liquid glue, she traces the letters of her name with the glue. She then shakes different colors of glitter over the glue.
Integrating cognitive or thinking skills, Heather is asked to create a pattern with five colors and recall the order of these colors: "We'll do red, yellow, blue, green, and then orange... The letter 'h' will be red, the letter 'e' will be yellow," and so on. Then she does her mom's name and her brother's name. As they all contain more than five letters, she must repeat the pattern and begin with the first color again.

• Discrimination of phrases or sentences through imitation

GOAL
*   to help Heather to discriminate sentences of similar length and subsequently to encourage the development of expressive language.

ACTIVITY

This activity requires pictures or photographs that describe an event, and a container of play dough. Heather demonstrates discrimination of particular sentences by placing a ball of play dough on the correct picture. Examples of some of these sentences are: "Oh, shoot, I missed the ball!," "May I have some paper?," "Let's unload the dishwasher!," "Oh, it's pouring outside!"

Heather loves play dough. To expand her vocabulary of colors, we choose lime green and purple. This gives Heather two strategies from which to learn the new shade of green – coupling it with the known word green, and contrasting it with the color purple. In our lessons, we integrate one new color (word) with the colors Heather has acquired, to build vocabulary.

Her mom plays teacher first. She asks Heather to select the color of play dough and says, "May I have some paper?" Heather imitates the phrase and proceeds to place a ball of play dough on the correct picture. Heather is now the teacher.

"OK, you can have *line*... The lady going take dish out."

"Oh, I'll take the *lime* play dough and put it on the picture of the lady who is *unloading the dishwasher.*" Her mom has rephrased Heather's sentence using correct grammar. As Heather did not say *lime* correctly, her mom says, "But do you mean *lime?*"

"Yup," Heather says.

Her mom helps Heather to imitate "amamam, imimim, *lime*" (phonetic speech babble).

Heather produces the sound correctly, and her mom proceeds to place the lime play dough on the correct picture. As the activity proceeds, we incorporate the concepts of "a couple of," where Heather selects "a" versus "a couple of" play-dough balls.

As I commend her mom for assisting Heather in producing the word correctly, Heather says, "I'm waiting for you!"

"OK, sorry." I say to Heather, "The lady is peeling the oranges."

Heather scans the pictures and places her play dough on the correct picture. She doesn't select the picture of the lady peeling the orange, which demonstrates her discrimination of plurals.

"Heather, it's your turn to listen," her mom says. "Take a couple of balls of play dough and find the man washing the dresses."

Heather selects the picture of the man washing the dress, and places the couple of play-dough balls on the picture.

"Oh, there he is washing the *dress,*" I highlight. "Can you see where he is washing the *dresses?"* Heather does not follow through. "He's washing *two dresses,* see?" I highlight. Heather attends to the number two and takes the play dough to the correct picture.

ANALYSIS

The purpose of this activity is twofold: first, to improve Heather's discrimination skills and second, to teach the everyday phrases or sentences that are nonliteral. Her mom is guided to provide Heather with phrases that teach her to discriminate minor differences, such as *behind/beside, he/she,* being sure to incorporate rhyming words (*tea/key/pea*) and words that differ in final consonant only (*cap/cat, coat/coke, pen/pet, dog/doll,* etc.); for example, "The *lady doesn't* want to unload the dishwasher" versus "The *baby can't* unload the dishwasher." Heather is expected to make the manner discrimination between /l/ and /b/ in the rhyming pair *lady/baby.* Expressively, we are also encouraging Heather to use appropriate negation. Heather needs to improve her discrimination of words by place cues, such as in the *lime/line* example. Heather's discrimination error was due to the minor acoustic differences between the consonants /m/ and /n/.

Consonants are described according to the way in which they are produced, according to three articulatory dimensions (Ling, 1976): manner, place, and voicing. The acoustic energy related to these distinctions makes some consonants more audible than others. The consonants /m/ and /n/ differ in their place of production (*place cues*). The acoustic energy providing information on place of production lies in the mid-frequency and high-frequency range and occurs at relatively low intensity (loudness) levels. Most children with hearing losses have better hearing in the low- rather than high-pitch range and therefore, discrimination of consonants that differ in place of production are the most difficult. *Manner cues* occur in the lower-frequency range and are more readily audible. *Voicing* is related to vocal cord vibration: if the vocal cords vibrate as the sound is generated, the sound is voiced; if the vocal cords do not vibrate, it is voiceless. Cues for voicing are in the low-frequency range of hearing and are audible to children with even small amounts of residual hearing.

When her mom used phonetic speech babble to elicit the word *lime,* she did so for two reasons: to help Heather discriminate /m/ from /n/, and to help her use /m/ in meaningful communication in the word *lime.* As consonants that differ in place cues are the most difficult to discriminate, phonetic babble of specific consonants with specific vowels can help Heather improve discrimination of place cues.

Phonetic babble was also used to help Heather produce the target, *lime,* correctly. At a segmental level, phonetic speech babble involves imitation of vowels and consonants or consonant blends in single, repeated, or alternated syllables on demand. In the above lesson, Heather was asked to imitate the consonant /m/ in the vowel contexts of "ah," "oo," and "ee" in repetition. Phonetic babble is used to determine how automatically Heather is able to produce different speech patterns. If she has difficulty producing a speech pattern at this phonetic "babble" level, it is unlikely that she will be able to use it in everyday communication (phonology).

The second purpose of this activity is to help Heather learn everyday sentences and expressions that are not interpreted literally. When Heather imitates the sentence, she is also encouraged to expand the length of her utterances and to use the targeted expressions correctly. In the example above, Heather described the picture correctly but did not understand or use the phrase "unload the dishwasher" expressively. Imitation helps Heather to use the "little words" in language. She will often not hear these "little words" because of coarticulation and contractions.

Coarticulation occurs when the sounds of a word (acoustic properties) or the way it is produced (articulation) change depending on the words that precede or follow them. Speech is not produced by one sound at a time, like beads on a string; sounds overlap and flow into one continuously changing stream of sound. For example, in the phrase "picked it up," the "ed" at the end of the word "picked" is produced as a "t" sound whereas in the phrase, "picked the apple," the "ed" at the end of "picked" is not produced as a "t" sound at all.

A *contraction* is the shortening of a group of words, often marked with an apostrophe, for example, "I'll" for the words "I will," or "it's" for the words "it is." Contractions are difficult to hear because acoustic information is reduced. Acoustic highlighting can be used to overcome the reduction of acoustic information due to coarticulation and contractions.

Parent Guidance

✔ To improve Heather's discrimination skills, in worksheet activities she is asked to circle the *ball* or the *doll*. With sticker activities, Heather is asked to place the sticker "on *me*" or "on your *knee*." At dinnertime, various family members pass the *cheese* or the *peas*. At snack time, Heather can have an *orange* or a couple of *oranges*. In setting the table, Heather is asked to get a *glass* or the *glasses*.

✔ Heather and family members have many everyday routines where they may use figurative or nonliteral expressions such as *"pick up the mail," "stock the pantry," "put out the trash."* Her mom is guided to work on one idiom per week, using it appropriately in routines. Examples include: *"Get cracking," "Break a leg," "Let's boogie."* Her mom is also encouraged to use colloquialisms such as *"Oh, shoot," "Man oh man," "I can't believe it!"* As English is rich in figurative language, the understanding and use of it is necessary for natural communication.

Language:
- **Comprehension and expressive use of prepositions**

GOAL
- to evaluate Heather's understanding and use of the following prepositions: *behind, beside, between, in front of, next to, over.*

ACTIVITY
The activity involves "driving" a variety of vehicles along a "highway" and placing them in relation to other vehicles. The props necessary are an assortment of different vehicles and masking tape. The masking tape is cut into long and short pieces and stuck to the table to simulate a highway. Heather and her mom are challenged to come up with a way to create a highway given only the masking tape. In setting up this activity, a number of linguistic targets are identified:

- question forms — *"How could we make a highway?" "What does it look like?" "Why do we have tape?" "What's it for?" "Where do we put it?" "How many lanes should we make?" "How wide apart should we place the tape?"*

- concepts — *long, short, sticky, masking, beige* (to describe the tape), *edges, center* (to describe where to put the tape).
- verbs — *cut, rip* (to describe what to do with the tape).

The highway is created by placing two long pieces of tape along the edges of the table and several shorter pieces in the center to create the broken line for passing. A basket is pulled from under the table, revealing an array of colorful mini vehicles mixed with some dinosaurs. We discuss the dinosaurs, and decide they "don't belong." Heather's mom is selected to be first and models how to play.

"Mommy, you can go first. Find the yellow fire engine and put it *anywhere* on the highway," I say. Heather's mom proceeds by placing the fire engine in the center of the right lane.

I say, "My blue car is going to go *behind* the yellow fire engine."

I then instruct Heather to select a vehicle to travel *over* the high-way. "Heather, you find one that could go *over* the highway."

Heather does not select the airplane, nor does she "drive" her vehicle *over* the highway. I say, "Let's see, could a car go *over* the highway?" I pick up a car and pretend to fly it over the highway.

"No, that silly," Heather says.

"Oh. How about a school bus, could it go *over* the highway?" I demonstrate again as I did with the car.

"No way!" says Heather's mom.

"What do you think, Heather? Could you pick one that would go *over* the highway?" Heather selects the orange airplane. "That's right!" I say. "Airplanes can fly *over* highways."

"It's my turn," says Heather's mom. "The purple school bus is going to pass all the other vehicles and pull *in front of* the fire engine." She carries out her own directions.

"OK, Heather," I say. "You get the orange car." Heather selects the orange car. "Drive your car *between* the blue car and the yellow fire engine." Heather follows the instructions. "Good for you! Now you be the teacher and tell Mommy what she should do."

"Mom, take blue school bus and put *behind* the blue car." Her mom does so and Heather reinforces her, "Good job!"

ANALYSIS

These types of directions are appropriate for Heather as she has devel-oped an auditory memory for four items (color + noun, color + noun). During this activity, I determine that Heather is still having some difficulty discriminating *behind* from *beside*. When directed to place a vehicle *behind* another, she often placed it *beside* and vice versa. With acoustic highlighting techniques, Heather hears the difference. In fact, she uses both prepositions correctly. The following prepositions are targeted for development: *over, in front of,* and *next to*.

Prepositional concepts are used to describe spatial relationships. There are many different prepositions and prepositional phrases, and some describe the same spatial relationship, such as *next to* and *beside*. This is the challenge for Heather. Heather has learned *under,* and must now learn *underneath* and *below*. We first introduce *on* versus *under* (one syllable vs. two), and then *under* versus *behind*.

Parent Guidance

Integration of prepositions and prepositional phrases into daily routines is important.

✔ Her mom can hide things *under* Heather's pillow each night and have her look *under* her pillow to find the surprise. At breakfast, Heather looks *under* her cup or her plate to find a surprise. By hiding something unfamiliar, new vocabulary can be learned.

✔ In Heather's closet, her party dresses are kept *in the back* and her school clothes are kept *in the front.* Her mom asks Heather to slide her slippers *under* her bed and after her bed is made, her pajamas get tucked away *under* her pillow. She puts her schoolbag *behind* the sliding door in the hallway and her favorite toy *between* her teddy bears on her dresser.

✔ When loading the dishwasher, Heather might place the cups and glasses *above* the dishes. In the refrigerator, the drinks go *in the side of* the door.

✔ In getting into the car to go shopping, Heather is instructed to sit *behind* Mommy while her sister sits *next to* her in the *back* seat.

✔ Her mom and Heather discuss where her friends are seated in the classroom. Heather's best friend is seated *next to* her and Heather sits *in front of* the teacher.

✔ In placing stickers in her sticker book, Heather might place the seal sticker *below* the giraffe sticker or *to the right of* it.

Speech:

Formal speech teaching is carried out to develop speech sounds automatically, following the Ling Phonetic Level Evaluation as a guide. Speech sounds are presented through audition only, with visual or kinesthetic cues used to supplement *only if necessary,* followed by putting the production "back into hearing." That is, once Heather correctly produces a target phoneme that requires a tactile or visual cue, she is encouraged to listen to the phoneme and imitate it through audition only. This helps her to develop an auditory feedback loop.

Production of specific consonants should be expected in spontaneous speech consistently when they can be produced readily, without concentration on a phonetic level (speech babble). Sounds are always developed from the known (what Heather is able to produce) to the unknown (what she is developing). If Heather is able to produce a particular phoneme with a particular vowel or in a word, then that vowel or word can be used to facilitate production in other contexts.

Heather was working on the phoneme /g/. She was able to produce this phoneme only with the vowel /o/ as in "go go go!" In order to develop this phoneme with other vowels, speech babble was initiated with "go go go" and modified to "go go gah" "go go goo," and other vowel contexts. In this way, the phoneme /g/ can be transferred to other vowel contexts and developed in repetition ("gogogo gahgahgah geegeegee") and alternation ("gogahgoo gee googah") until Heather produces it effortlessly (to a level of automaticity).

Speech babble is conducted quickly and for short periods of time, and is performed using many specifically selected games that have many pieces or reinforcers. Games such as Operation™ (Hasbro Canada), Rockin' Robins™ (Irwin Toys), and Call the Plumber™ (Grand Toys) are excellent. Battery-operated games that vibrate, jiggle, and spin are highly motivating.

• Elicit production of the voiceless alveolar plosive /t/ in initial position

GOAL
*   to develop the phoneme /t/ for automatic production in initial positions and to use /t/ in everyday speech.

ACTIVITY
The Space War Ring Toss™ game consists of orange pegs and a yellow

Table 2. Target Phonemes

Therapist	Heather	Comments
"teeteetee"	"keekeekee"	• a discrimination error based on place cues is made, a "good" error
"t t t" (whispered)	"t t t" (whispered)	• I whisper the /t/ to help Heather hear it better
		• whispering increases audibility because the air stream is very easy to hear*
"teeteetee"	"keekeekee"	• same discrimination error
"t t t (whispered) teeteetee"	"t t t (whispered) teeteetee"	• I use the known (whispered form) and quickly pair it with the unknown ("teeteetee")
"teeteetee"	"teeteetee"	• after two presentations, Heather discriminates the phoneme correctly
"teeteetah"	"teeteetah"	• I use Heather's correct production of "teeteetee" to elicit its production with other vowels
"tahtahtah"	"tahtahtah"	• /t/ is produced in repetition in the context of the vowel "ah"

*Whispering intensifies voicelessness; voiced/voiceless cues are based on durational or timing cues, which are audible to children with even very little measurable residual hearing. Also, whispering intensifies consonants, not vowels, which are louder than consonants and can mask or cover them up.

one for the center, red rings, blue rings, and a gameboard. The board consists of two portals, which hold the rings for launching. The pegs get placed in a circle in the middle of the board, with the yellow peg in the center of the circle having the most worth. The object of the game is to launch one's ring from the portal and encircle one of the colored pegs. Each peg and ring is earned by producing the targeted phoneme, as illustrated in Table 2.

The /t/ is elicited in the same way with a variety of vowels. In reinforcing Heather's correct productions, players earn the pegs and the rings for playing the game. As Heather and her mom earn their rings, they place them in the portal and we all count backwards from five: "5, 4, 3, 2, 1, blast off!," and the players shoot. Sometimes we trick players by counting "5, 4, 3, 2, 1, 1, 1, 1, blast off!," encouraging Heather to listen for the go-ahead. After the shot, questions are asked, such as, "Who got more/less?" "How many does Mom need to catch up?" and "Who is keeping score?"

Parent Guidance

Speech is very challenging to teach. In developing the phoneme /t/, I guided Heather's mom with the following techniques:

✔ /t/ should initially be produced with /i/, since /t/ and /i/ are both produced at the front of the mouth. Less articulatory control is required to produce this combination than others.

✔ If Heather has difficulty with this phoneme, try to elicit it with a different vowel, such as "oo," "ah," or another vowel. The particular vowel will depend on which is easiest for Heather to say and which consonant-vowel combination can serve as an easy model for its development with other vowels.

✔ Consonants should be paired with a vowel and presented in repetition (which provides greater acoustic information and is easier to hear). *"Teeteetee"* is better than *"tee."*

✔ Consonant-vowel combinations should also be presented in alteration, for example, *"teetahtoo tahteetoe."*

✔ The acquired phoneme should be encouraged in expressive speech.

Carryover:

✔ In everyday interactions, use phonetic babble if Heather misproduces a word and to encourage it in spontaneous speech (phonology). For example, if Heather were to say, *"My koes are cold,"* her mom would elicit the correct production by presenting *"teeteetee teeteetoe My toes are cold."* This usually produces a correct utterance.

✔ When requesting gum, Heather says, *"I want dum, please,"* her mom elicits the correct production by modeling *"gogogo gogo gum I want gum, please."* Her mom provides a known form ("g" with "o") and transfers it to a context that is unknown ("g" with "u"). This encourages phonetic to phonologic transfer (Ling, 1976).

(cont'd on next page)

Parent Guidance *(cont'd)*

✔ Heather's mom does not do this for every speech articulation error. This would be frustrating, prevent natural communication, and discourage Heather's drive to use speech to communicate. Heather needs to develop the sound at the phonetic level and then transfer it to meaningful language. Rather than to correct speech incidentally, her mom is encouraged to babble Heather's speech targets for a few minutes four or five times per day and integrate the targets into Heather's routines. In Heather's lessons, we may work on a few targets at one time.

✔ Heather's mom is encouraged to promote this, but not necessarily to expect correct productions of a particular sound in communicative speech, until all the subskills (phonetic level) have been developed.

Conclusion

At the end of the lesson, a few minutes are spent reviewing the goals for the week and providing suggestions for integrating them into daily routines. This is extremely important. Heather's mom is her primary teacher and she actively participates in therapy to learn how to help Heather at home. Specific guidance is required. We review the notes that Heather's mom has taken during therapy. She keeps a "vocabulary box" in the bottom right-hand corner of the page, where she jots down any words that come up that Heather doesn't know. She will teach this vocabulary during the week.

Heather's mom will reinforce expressive use of the pronouns *she* and *they,* contrast the prepositions *over* and *in front of* (such as *in front of* the house, *in front of* your door), use three new nonliteral phrases (her mom suggests those most important for Heather), use the idiom *"Don't pull my leg!"* at meaningful opportunities (events can be contrived to provide opportunities to use these), and improve production of "t" and "sh." Family life and school progress are also discussed.

Heather has been using the implant successfully for approximately two and one-half years. Prior to receiving the implant, she was expressing herself by using limited verbal language, such as "up," "no," "pop up," and some sound-object associations. One year after initial stimulation of Heather's implant (hearing age = 1 year), her average sentence length was 3.5 words. She is now speaking in sentences and is understood by most people. On formal language assessments for children with typical hearing, Heather scores one standard deviation within the norm (fairly close to average). On the *Test of Auditory Comprehension of Language — Revised (TACL-R)* (DLM Teaching Resources), Heather obtained an age-equivalent score of 47–49 months when she was 59 months of age with a hearing age of only 19 months.

Heather is integrated in the kindergarten classroom at the local school. She actively participates in her community. She is able to have conversations with many people. She hears music and loves to sing along in Sunday school and church. The cochlear implant has changed Heather's life.

References

Gorman-Gard, K.A. (1992). *Figurative language: A comprehensive program.* Eau Claire, WI: Thinking Publications.

Ling, D. (1976). *Speech and the hearing impaired child: Theory and practice.* Washington, DC: A.G. Bell Association for the Deaf.

Lesson Plan for Ryan

Tina Olmstead, M.Sc., Cert. AVT

A first-born baby boy — what a lovely gift to receive on Christmas Eve. However, by the following Christmas, Ryan's profound sensorineural hearing loss had been detected, and he was given two powerful behind-the-ear hearing aids. Just before his first birthday, Ryan and his parents received a different kind of gift: the challenge of *learning to listen.*

Over the next three years, Ryan and his family attended weekly parent guidance sessions in which they learned to integrate listening activities into their daily routines. The parents can now recount those early years with the usual tales of joys and frustrations: the joy of success as the child learns to process auditory information and begins to say the all important first word; the frustrations of dealing with a two-year-old's temper tantrums and spending the therapy time discussing behavior rather than language development, all the while being reassured by the therapist that managing behavior is also part of the process of *learning to listen.*

After three years of using a hearing aid, Ryan was speaking in short phrases of three to four words. Although gains were being made, Ryan's parents and hearing management team confirmed that a cochlear implant could provide him with additional auditory information as he continued to learn to listen. Almost three years to the day after the initial diagnosis, Ryan was in the hospital for his implant surgery.

The new year signaled a new beginning for Ryan as the programming of his speech processor began. The three years of learning to listen with hearing aids provided a solid auditory base, as Ryan was able to transfer previously learned skills to his new form of hearing. He was able to respond to a variety of sounds across the speech range including /s/ and /th/. Shortly after the implant was switched on, Ryan's ease of acquiring language through listening was apparent.

Today marks the sixth year since Ryan's family received the news of his deafness and the third anniversary of his implant surgery. Everyone in the department anxiously awaits Ryan's arrival. There's a wide grin and a friendly hello for everyone whom he has come to know in the clinic.

"Ryan, are you ready?" I call... and it is off to another day of *learning to listen*.

Introduction to the Lesson

Ryan's lesson, like so many others in auditory-verbal programs, consists of goals in the areas of audition, speech, language, cognition, and academics, with a strong emphasis on parent guidance. All activities throughout the lesson incorporate components from each of these areas. Rarely is an activity designed to address only one specific element of the overall program. In short, we teach speech as part of the language lesson and language as part of speech lesson, using listening as the primary sense modality for instruction. Long-term plans, based on the individual child's needs, are generated at least yearly, and short-term goals translate into specific lesson plan goals.

GOALS

Audition:
- to follow a story and answer pertinent questions without pictures.
- to process six critical elements of information, including a variety of adjectives and time phrases such as *After lunch, the little boy rode his green bike*. Ryan must process the six concepts *after, little, boy, rode, green,* and *bike* in order to manipulate a group of objects correctly.

- to follow directions such as *Draw a pair of blue mittens on the smallest girl.*
- to reinforce word-final consonants: /st/ as in *fist,* /sk/ as in *ask,* /nd/ as in *hand,* and /snt/ as in *isn't.*

Storytelling

For this activity, I try to create an interesting tale that will capture the attention of the child, expand vocabulary, and reinforce specific language structures that have been recently taught. This activity also provides opportunities to discuss events that have happened or will happen outside the therapy room. For many children, talking about imaginary or abstract ideas is a challenge and this skill must be developed and practiced thoroughly. Depending on the age of the child, I may use a current event for the story, such as a report of a recent hurricane, a personal experience (as in *My Trip to Canada's Wonderland),* or a completely fabricated event starring the child, such as *Ryan's Pet Dinosaur.* After a year of my storytelling, most children know everything about my own family, our pets, and our adventures. In turn, the children begin to tell their own family stories.

Ryan, his mom, and I settle down in the familiar surroundings of our therapy room. Ryan's cochlear implant is on his left side so I sit to his left, and his mom sits to Ryan's right. Over the past several months, I have started Ryan's lesson with a story. He therefore asks, "Tina, are you going to tell me a story today?"

"Of course I'm going to tell you a story, and it is a very special one," I reply.

For Ryan's lesson, I have planned to add to a previously told story about my son's lizard. Ryan has been fascinated by the lizard and its many antics, so I'm sure he will listen attentively. The ground rules for the task were established long ago: Ryan listens to the passage in its entirety. At the end, he may be asked to retell the story and/or answer a set of questions related to its content. In the past, some stories have become the focal point of the whole session, and all goals for listening, speech, language, and cognition have centered around the story's events.

"OK, Ryan! Here is the story of *The Lost Lizard!*

"This morning, before I left home, I went into my son's room to wake him up. I noticed that the top to the lizard's cage was ajar, and the lizard was nowhere to be found.

"'Oh, no,' I screeched. 'The lizard is out!' Everyone came running.

I then remembered that my son had added crickets to the cage the night before. After he put the crickets into the cage, he had forgotten to put the lid back on tightly. Luckily, my son found the lizard hiding behind his backpack. After he trapped the lizard, he put it back into the cage, but the lizard had no breakfast! Poor Lizard!"

Questions for Ryan:
* What did I do before I went to work?
* What did I see?
* What do you think the word "ajar" means in *the top to the cage was ajar?*
* Where was the lizard?
* What happened after my son trapped the lizard?
* Why didn't the lizard have any breakfast?

The above story and questions were designed to reinforce the concepts of *before* and *after*, expand word knowledge, and develop Ryan's story-listening skills for lengthy passages of information. Through storytelling, other skills also develop, such as asking for clarification (Ryan asked about the word *ajar*), predicting outcomes (*How did the lizard get out?*), inferencing skills (*Why didn't the lizard have breakfast?*), and sequencing events for retelling the story to others.

Parent Guidance

Ryan's mom and I have discussed the importance of storytelling as an interesting and effective activity to build Ryan's ability to listen to lengthy passages of information. In a mainstream classroom, children are expected to listen to, interpret, and act upon information that is presented in stories, instructions, and conversations throughout the day.

✔ To reinforce this skill at home, his mom will ask Ryan to recount events of the school day by asking such questions as: *Tell me the funniest thing that happened at school today* or *Tell me all the things you played at recess.* I caution against the old favorite, *What did you do at school today?* because it almost always generates the standard response: *Nothing!*

✔ Mom will also ask Ryan to retell the Lost Lizard tale to his younger brother and then tell a story about one of their family pets.

✔ Finally, shelves filled with books at home contain a wealth of possibilities for storytelling!

Processing Six to Seven Critical Elements

By the time a student reaches the level of processing five to six critical elements, the listening exercise is familiar and the challenge for the therapist is to make the task fun and interesting. The child, at this level, enjoys the opportunity to be the instructor and makes every attempt to stump the therapist. The parent and therapist have many opportunities to model and highlight the often-missed function words contained in long sentences. For example, if the child says, *I'm going play hockey Saturday,* the parent will model and emphasize the missing words *to* and *on* and then ask the child to repeat the sentence with the additional words.

Using Playmobile™ figures, Ryan and I set up a small village complete with shops, schools, gas station, and a little lake. The following is a sample of auditory information given to Ryan: *The man with the beard and the lady with a hat went to the gas station before going fishing.*

Ryan repeats the instruction as he manipulates the figures. Although he attempts to repeat the sentence as presented, he misses a number of the small function words such as *with, the,* and *to.* I repeat the information in smaller chunks, giving special emphasis to the missing words. Then, I present the entire sentence again. Ryan successfully repeats the complete sentence without errors.

Ryan's mom adds the next piece of information: *After they got gas, they crossed the bridge and parked the car under the big tree.* I notice that Mom has used the word *crossed* rather than the simpler vocabulary of *went over* in the phrase *they crossed the bridge.*

Ryan asks for clarification by quizzically looking at his mom and asking, "They *what* the bridge?" Repetition of the word *crossed* does not solve the problem, so Mom substitutes *went over.* Mom is then guided to repeat the entire phrase again using the word *crossed.* The purpose of the repetition is to give Ryan another opportunity to hear the word *crossed* in context.

Even putting away the activity is a lesson in listening for a number of critical elements: *Before you put away all the people, put away the buildings and vehicles but not the plants.* I have included the names of the categories, *people, buildings,* and *vehicles* in order to review a previously taught skill. Ryan has no trouble removing the toys from the table.

Word-Final Consonants

For Ryan, an activity of using minimal pairs that vary in final consonants provides him with the challenge of listening to directions containing very fine consonant discriminations. We use a deck of picture cards for this activity, but a pail of objects could also be used. The words are *rain-rake; cat-cap; cloud-clown; pie-pipe; bone-boat.* Once we check that all the words are known to Ryan, the fun begins. We use the entire therapy room: for example, I may say, *Put the pipe behind the bookshelf and the rake under the table.* We do this activity quickly and, of course, everyone has a turn to be speaker and listener. Finding the cards again provides another opportunity to discriminate word-final consonants.

Parent Guidance

✔ I give Ryan's mom a set of pictures to take home and suggest that she and Ryan play the game during the week. I ask her to note any particular combinations that are difficult for Ryan to identify.

✔ Ryan's mom's list may become a great diagnostic indicator for planning strategies for remediation at next week's lesson. For example, if Ryan has made consistent errors with final /n/ versus final /t/, I will provide additional listening practice. I may have Ryan discriminate the nasal /n/ and the stop /t/ in syllables by associating /ununun.../ with his right hand and /ututut.../ with his left hand. As I produce the target sound, Ryan will raise the hand associated with the sound. The final nasal /n/ can be lengthened in production to highlight the acoustic information as opposed to the stop /t/, which is arrested abruptly. The sounds will be placed into words and sentences for further rehearsal.

GOALS

Language:
- to develop language of description.
- to develop comparative and superlative adjectives.
- to review comprehension of *how* and *when* question forms.

Identifying Picture Differences

There are a number of commercially made products for children that are aimed at developing the ability to identify the differences between two pictures visually. For children who have hearing impairments, the same materials can be used to develop spoken communication skills between partners. The object of the activity is to discover, without looking at the other's picture, the ways in which the two pictures are different. To find the differences, questions are asked that include a variety of adjectives and prepositions.

Pictures for this session feature two rodeo scenes that are generally quite similar but vary in detail. Ryan has one picture and I have the other. Ryan's mom is his assistant so that she can expand his vocabulary as well as model correct questioning, if required. The questioner continues asking questions until a difference is found.

Tina: Is there one horse in your picture?
Ryan: Yes.
T: Is the horse yellow?
R: No, my horse has brown and white spots.
T: My horse is yellow. Your horse is brown with white spots. Our horses are different!

At this point, Ryan begins to ask questions.

R: Do you have a clown in your picture?
T: Yes, I do.
R: Is your clown sitting in a barrel? (Mom helps with the word *barrel*.)
T: No, he isn't. He is walking in front of the bull. (His mom shows Ryan the bull in his picture and explains that we use the word *bull* to describe a male cow.)
R: Oh, I have two clowns. My other clown is walking in front of the bull. Is the clown wearing a red-and-yellow striped shirt?
T: No, my clown is wearing a yellow shirt with red polka dots.
R: The clowns are different!

We continue until we have found a few more differences. The activity gives us lots to discuss, including some general information about where one would have to go to see a rodeo, the events common to rodeos, and the names of the clothing items unique to a rodeo.

Comparative and Superlative Adjectives

Ryan enjoys vehicles, so I choose to introduce *-er* and *-est* endings by comparing the attributes of a number of vehicles. Many goals are incorporated into every activity, and this one gives us an opportunity to expand vocabulary by discussing transportation and how and when people need to use different types of vehicles. Ryan enjoys the humor as we imagine a trip to the clinic via rocket ship, and traveling to school in a hot-air balloon rather than the typical yellow school bus. A few

Parent Guidance

After completing the Picture Differences activity, we discuss ways in which the family can develop communication skills using details to explain how things are alike and different.

✔ Ryan's mom and dad can hide things around the home that are very similar, such as two toy cars. After a parent gives a detailed description of one of the cars (*I'm looking for the black car with red stripes along the sides*), Ryan can search for it. Roles are then reversed, and Ryan describes the object to be found.

✔ The family can also get in the habit of adding specific details to information in their daily conversations. Instead of saying, *Get your coat,* add details describing the coat: *Get your red-and-black plaid jacket.*

moments of fun provide a brief break and prepare Ryan for the next task.

Ryan selects a hot-air balloon and a helicopter from the pile. After discussing the characteristics including shape, size, and parts of the two vehicles, I ask, "Which one do you think is faster?" Ryan replies correctly. I then add a rocket to the other two and ask, "Which one is the fastest?" We have nearly 30 different vehicles, so we compare and contrast. There is lots of discussion including the words *farther, farthest, nearer, nearest, slower, slowest, heavier, heaviest,* and *bigger, biggest.*

Parent Guidance

✔ Throughout the day, there are endless opportunities to use -*er* and -*est* adjectives. One can compare the weight of backpacks, the distance to the homes of friends, the speed of cars, and the size of articles of clothing for family members. Ryan's mom was confident that she could find many chances over the week to use the comparative and superlative adjectives.

Photo Session

Over the years, parents have contributed photographs of their children doing just about everything a therapist could wish for in order to enrich language — from the simple routines of daily life to the exotic adventures of a trip to Australia. Young children are delighted as they talk about photos that illustrate such events: *The baby is washing; the girl is eating; or Mummy is sleeping.* Older children use the photos to expand their sentence structures, as in *The girl who is wearing a red hat is eating an ice cream cone.* The family photo album becomes an invaluable tool for reinforcing specific language goals at home. For this present lesson, the photos are an excellent resource for reviewing question forms with Ryan, including *when* and *how*. One photo of particular interest is Batman in his Batmobile, surrounded by children at a parade. I ask Ryan many questions, and I especially enjoy his description of how Batman helps people: *He beats up the bad guys!*

Parent Guidance

✔ Mom will reinforce *when* and *how* during daily conversations with Ryan. I also suggest that as she reads to Ryan each day, she include the target questions, such as: *How will the hero of the story resolve the problem? When does the hero ask for help?*

GOALS

Speech:
- to produce /r/ in repeated syllables.
- to alternate /l/ and /n/ with a variety of vowels.
- to use /ng/ in everyday speech.
- to develop word-final blends (/-st/, /-sk/, /-nd/, and /-snt/).

Incidental speech teaching is an integral component of every activity throughout the lesson. When Ryan spontaneously uses a recently learned target, he is positively reinforced for it. If he omits or substitutes a target phoneme, he is corrected either by modeling or by a quizzical look, which signals to him that something is missing; he then self-corrects. Mom and I always keep the target phonemes in mind so that opportune moments for correction are consistently seized without overly interrupting the flow of conversation. A thorough knowledge of the speech-teaching targets, subskills, and strategies, as outlined in *Speech for Hearing-Impaired Children: Theory and Practice* (Ling, 1976), can facilitate planning effective and appropriate speech programs for individual children.

Phonetic Drill

Phonetic practice should be kept brief but it is an important component to every lesson. As the child repeats or alternates particular phonetic patterns (e.g., /lalala.../or /lanalana.../), I analyze the quality and accuracy of the productions. I am able to determine phonetic contexts that require additional rehearsal, or identify phonemes that can be produced but are missing in conversational speech. Speech-teaching strategies are selected, modified, or initiated based upon the needs of the child.

In order to make the repetitive practice of speech drills interesting, the toy cupboard is filled with games and activities for speech reinforcement. There are countless ways to use stickers as reinforcers. Ryan loves ocean animals, so for this lesson I use a set of stickers that includes whales, dolphins and sharks.

I give a piece of white paper to Ryan and say, *"Draw a blue wavy line across the middle of the paper."* After he draws the line, we discuss that we are making an ocean for the animal stickers.

Through listening only, I ask Ryan to repeat /r/ with a number of vowels (e.g., *rarara...; rororo...; ririri...*). The only context that poses a problem for him is the context with the /i/ vowel. The /r/ becomes a /w/ as he spreads his lips for the /i/. The acoustic information is audible to Ryan through the implant, so I have him listen and compare /wi/ with /ri/. Ryan goes on to produce a lovely /r/ in the vowel context of /i/. Each time he produces the target phoneme, he selects an animal to put in his ocean. Of course, there is time to describe and compare the animals.

Parent Guidance

While Ryan is busy with his stickers, his mom and I have time to suggest ways in which she can evoke, rehearse and transfer speech skills into Ryan's everyday life.

✔   Ryan's mom will listen carefully to his everyday speech for accurate productions of /r/, /l/, and /n/. When needed, she will model productions for

---

Parent Guidance *(cont'd)*

Ryan or ask him to self-correct a word. I suggest a few games such as Go Fish, using pictures containing the target phonemes.

✔   Another good game is to place a common household object in a paper bag and describe it until Ryan guesses the identity. For Ryan, his mom may hide a reel, toy ladder, or a nail. A school photo of Ryan in the bag could provide a lot of fun and great motivation to produce a super /r/!

Phonologic Practice

The use of *going to* to express the future tense is one of many ways to practice the /ng/ in phonology. A set of picture cards showing people doing various activities is placed upside down on the table. I select one that shows a boy fishing.

I ask, "What is the boy *going to* catch?"

Ryan says, "The boy is *going to* catch a shark."

His mom selects a picture of a schoolgirl walking. She asks, "What is the girl *going to* do after school?" I reinforce Ryan's mom for being so clever because she has incorporated an earlier language target, *after,* into the activity.

When Ryan omits the /ng/, his mom reminds him by saying, "Where's your /ng/?"

The second time around Ryan responds, "The girl is *going* to play outside."

A quick way to rehearse recently learned sounds in phonology is to play *Where's the _____?* In this session, the game is *Where's the motorcycle?* Pictures containing word-final blends (*cups, hands, desk, ghost,* etc.) are placed face up on the table. Ryan then closes his eyes and turns around while I hide a sticker of a motorcycle under one of the cards.

Once the card is hidden, Ryan begins asking, "Is the motorcycle under the hands?"

I reply, "No, it isn't." He continues guessing until he finds the motorcycle and, as always, he gets to hide it for the next round. He must respond with, *"No, it isn't"* because *isn't* contains one of his final consonant-blend targets.

Parent Guidance

✔ I explain to Ryan's mom that many of the word-final blends occur in language contexts. The /st/ is common as a past-tense marker (e.g., *passed, kissed, raced*); the /nt/ is common in contractions (e.g., *don't, can't, won't*). It is helpful to point out the language contexts so that the parent tunes into the language structures as she listens to Ryan's chatter at home. Without specific guidance, the task of listening for the target phonemes in everyday speech may become an overwhelming job.

Time Flies

For Ryan, the time in the therapy room is spent playing game after game. For the parent and me, the time is spent building listening, speech, language, and thinking skills. Play and work together give Ryan the confidence he needs to communicate effectively through spoken language. Guidance to Ryan's mom gives her the confidence that she can continue the work outside the therapy room.

Before they leave, we quickly review Ryan's mom's notes. After six years of weekly trips to the clinic, Ryan's mom has become an expert at recording goals and incorporating them into the busy routines of daily life. The goals often overlap and can be rehearsed in just a few simple activities.

Mom's Notes

✓ Continue to use *before* and *after* in daily routines.

✓ Have Ryan retell the story of *The Lost Lizard* to younger brother.

✓ Use the word *ajar* at home.

✓ Follow directions with six or seven critical items.

✓ Use lots of adjectives.

✓ Listen for final consonants in speech.

✓ Use *-er* and *-est* endings, as in *faster* and *fastest*.

✓ Develop categories (buildings, plants, instruments, etc.).

✓ Review all question forms, especially *how* and *when*.

✓ Practice /r/, /l/, /n/, /ng/, and final blends.

The time with Ryan has flown by, and it is now time to say good-bye as he heads off for first grade in his neighborhood school. Ryan's mom will incorporate today's goals into lessons all week long.

Final Thoughts

As I enter my clinician's notes into Ryan's file, I quietly celebrate the third anniversary of his cochlear implant and the tremendous success he and his family have achieved. Christmas Eves will continue to come and go. The worries and anxieties of those early Christmas seasons have been replaced with joy and hope for a little boy who listens most of the time, and talks all the time!

References

Ling, D. (1976). *Speech and the hearing-impaired child: Theory and practice.* Washington, DC: A.G. Bell Association for the Deaf.

Lesson Plan for Nicholas

Janice Hutchison, M.A., Cert. AVT
Nancy S. Caleffe-Schenck, M.Ed., C.E.D., CCC-A, Cert. AVT

At the age of three years, Nicholas's progressive hearing loss was diagnosed and he was given hearing aids. Careful monitoring of his hearing indicated fluctuation; Nicholas's unaided hearing levels steadily ebbed downward until he presented with a left-corner audiogram. Aided responses at a number of frequencies were well below the *speech banana* for both ears. A thorough work-up by an otologist revealed a Mondini-type malformation. When fistula repair surgery did not improve Nicholas's hearing, his parents investigated the cochlear implant through our center.

The initial speech and language evaluation indicated that Nicholas had little receptive or expressive language and limited ability to imitate speech patterns. The sensorimotor integration evaluation suggested poor oral-motor planning and visual spatial difficulties. His parents had a strong commitment to using spoken language with Nicholas. The team and Nicholas's parents developed short- and long-term plans. Nicholas received his Nucleus 22 cochlear implant at age four and a half.

At Nicholas's first-year post-implant case conference, the team discussed his emerging spoken communication. There was concern about his slow growth in expressive language. This was attributed to his difficulties in oral-motor planning. The speech therapist on our team began to see Nicholas for therapy, and he continued to receive auditory-verbal therapy as well.

Two years after receiving his cochlear implant, Nicholas was learning language within several environments rather than having it taught in a structured fashion. His expressive language was improving. Auditory skills were documented: attention and response to spoken language, good distance hearing, auditory self-monitoring, auditory memory span, and processing. Nicholas's hearing engaged him in the world in which he lived. The team suggested that inclusion in a regular school might be appropriate. Although Nicholas's parents were initially reluctant to make the jump to the neighborhood school, school personnel assured them that the school's cooperative learning format would accommodate Nicholas's needs. Support services such as speech therapy and tutoring were available. Nicholas was thrilled to go to school, on his bike, with his brother!

This lesson, two and a half years after Nicholas received his implant, is based on his prerequisite skills and consists of four specific activities: *Nickel-Pickle, Take a Letter, Twenty Questions,* and *Learning Through Literature.*

PREREQUISITE SKILLS

- ability to imitate syllables and words from an auditory model.
- ability to hear information from a tape recorder or language master.
- ability to write letters and to recognize letter names.
- beginning spelling skills.
- reading skills such as a basic sight word vocabulary.
- 10 well-known category names such as *furniture, animals, clothing, machines.*
- ability to recognize yes-no questions from their intonation pattern.
- working knowledge of several auxiliary verbs such as *is, are, does, can;* others can be introduced within the context of the game (i.e., *Should* people be careful of this animal?).

MATERIALS

- cassette tape recorder.
- *The Book of Kids' Songs* by Nancy Cassidy, Klutz Press, Palo Alto, CA.

- the cassette that accompanies *The Book of Kids' Songs*.
- language master (EIKI available from audio-visual outlets).
- language master cards.
- chalkboard or erasable plastic surface.
- chalk or dry-erase markers.
- recorded songs.
- pencil and paper (for keeping track of the number of questions asked).
- a collection of pictures or objects representing familiar objects.

GOALS

Therapy is a combination of activities that promote the achievement of a number of different, yet incorporated goals. The therapy lesson includes goals from Nicholas's schoolwork, which are integrated into therapy targets.

Audition:
- to remember words in sequence.
- to remember four or five items in sequence.
- to process and understand taped words and sentences.
- to use auditory closure to complete sentences.
- to listen through an electronic source of sound.

Speech:
- to produce:
  - /l/ in words and sentences.
  - /t/ in words and sentences.
  - /z/ in words and sentences.

Language:
- to understand that two words can mean the same thing.
- to use /s/ for third-person singular verb tense.
- to expand vocabulary.
- to use questions that start with auxiliary verbs.
- to increase general knowledge through question games.

Cognition:
- to discover that printed words represent spoken words.
- to learn game strategies.

Conversation:

*   to use the question, *How do you spell _____?*
*   to request assistance.

Introduction to the Lesson

When Nicholas enters the office with his mother, he usually announces his presence by coming down the hallway, poking his head in through the doorway, and saying "Boo," then "Hi, Jan!" When I ask about his mother, he replies, "She talking to Ashley's mom." I respond, "She's talking. Okay, she'll catch up with us."

We chat as we enter the therapy room, and when Nicholas's mom joins us she tells me that Nicholas had a good week at school learning about coins and their value. The family spent time helping Nicholas count the money in his piggy bank. In addition, Nicholas did well on his spelling words, read *Brown Bear, Brown Bear* during story time, and remembered the class' sentence for the day. First grade is going well.

Nickel-Pickle — Making Words Rhyme

In this activity, Nicholas practices his speech targets and makes up words that rhyme. First graders are expected to be able to rhyme words, a tough task for someone with only two years of good hearing. The word *rhyme* is used and a silly song, *Willoughby, Wallaby, Woo* (from *The Book of Kids' Songs*) is used to develop this skill.

Jan: Nicholas, let's take a few minutes to practice some silly syllables. Then we'll put them into rhyming words. Here we go: *leeleelee-loolooloo.*

Nicholas: Leeleeleenoonoonoo

J: Listen to Mom, Nicholas.

Mom: Leeleeleeloolooloo

N: Leeleeleeloolooloo

J: Hot dog! You remembered to say the /l/ sound. Now try this one: leloooleloooleloo.

N: Leloooleloo. (He has a slight grin as he finds the correct motor pattern.)

J: Listen again: leloooleloooleloo.

N: Leloooleloooleloo.

J: (To Mom) As we know, Nicholas has come a long way in getting his tongue tip and sides to move smoothly and quickly. We know for sure that he hears the difference between /l/ and /n/, but maintaining the tongue motion with some vowels is difficult. Here I am asking him to maintain /l/ first with high- contrast vowels and then with vowels that are more alike in their tongue position. Nicholas has done a good job alternating these syllables. Now we'll put them into a set of real words.

(To Nicholas) Nicholas, listen to this one. *Let me look.*

N: Lemelook

J: Let me look

N: Let me look

J: Excellent work! Let me look at your book.

N: Let me look at your book.

J: Let me look at your cookbook.

N: Let me look at your cookbook.

J: I see that you are laughing. What's so funny?

N: Cookbook. The same words.

J: You're right! You found a rhyme. Can you say "rhyme?"

N: Whyme

J: Mom, did you hear that rhyme? We said cookbook.

Mom: I heard a rhyme. What about this? *Nickel-pickle.* That's a rhyme.

N: I know. Nickel-dime. (He hasn't quite distinguished categories of meaning from categories of sound similarity.) It a whyme?

J: No, you named money. Let's try something else. I have a funny song that uses rhymes and it's easy too, *Willoughby, Wallaby, Woo.*

(This song models a simple rhyming pattern in which the first sound of familiar names is replaced by a "w" and then the actual name is repeated. For example: Wommy for Mommy; Wicholas for Nicholas; Wyan for Ryan, and Waddy for Daddy.)

J: Willoughby, wallaby, woo, an elephant sat on you; willoughby wallaby, wee, an elephant sat on me.

(We look at the pictures in the book to see the silly context of the story. At the next turn I say "Wommy" while looking at Nicholas to see if his eyes indicate recognition of the name that was changed.)

J: (To Mom) If Nicholas can recognize which name we have changed, then we know that he is well on the way to sensing the patterns that make up rhymes. This time, I will use a different name and see if Nicholas can finish the rhyme. This is called *closure.* Willoughby, wallaby, waddy, an elephant sat on _____. (I pause and look hopefully at Nicholas, who pauses and then brightens up.)

N: Daddy!

J: That's a rhyme! Waddy-Daddy. That sounds pretty funny.

(The song continues for a few more rounds with Nicholas suggesting names and attempting to make the rhymes. Then, to round out the activity, we listen to the tape and follow along with the print.)

J: (To Mom) We don't yet want to introduce the idea of identical print patterns. Then the task or the idea of rhyming becomes based on print or look-alikes, not on hearing or sound-alikes.

For example, we eventually want Nicholas to understand that *knight* and *white* rhyme even though their spellings are different. If we get away from the idea of hearing the similarities and rely on seeing similar patterns of letters, Nicholas might logically tell us some day that *near* and *hear* rhyme, but *near* and *here* do not... Why do you think this was easy for Ryan to learn, but is harder for Nicholas?

Mom: Well, for one thing, Ryan always had normal hearing. But what I remember most was that at about age four, Ryan was just too silly to live with. He started making goofy rhymes with syllables. In a way, I suppose he was experimenting.

J: Well, that certainly was part of the process and we know what Nicholas was doing at age four — learning to detect sound. Even though that kind of silly rhyming is no longer age appropriate, we can try to recapture some of the influence it has in learning about auditory patterns. Actually, Nicholas's peers have gone on to learn chants and taunts that build on the idea of rhyming, things like *Cinderella, dressed in yella, went upstairs to kiss her fella* or *Hello, goodbye, stick your head in a cherry pie.* It's not exactly high level language, but certainly it shows ability to rhyme.

Parent Guidance

✔ Using familiar words, practice substituting another consonant for the initial consonant. Two-syllable words are easier than one-syllable words. **Example:** seven-peven — then say, "That rhymes."

✔ Give Nicholas three words to listen to and ask him if he can tell you which two rhyme. Be sure he says the words himself so that he begins to feel the similar motor patterns. **Example:** seven, me, heaven.

✔ If he doesn't know it already, sing the song *This Old Man* with him at home.

✔ Teach *Willoughby, Wallaby, Woo* to Nicholas's dad, grandma, and anyone else who will listen. Sing the song in the car and at home.

Take a Letter

This activity prepares Nicholas for the task of writing sentences from dictation, an important part of his first-grade curriculum. Nicholas listens to a simple sentence from a language master or cassette tape recorder and writes it down. He still needs guidance to integrate auditory information with print. Sentences, made especially for Nicholas, include a variety of challenges using some of his spelling words, one familiar word for which he does not know the spelling, and one word that is unfamiliar to him. The sentences have been recorded prior to the session by Jan, speaking at a slightly slower than usual rate. These sentences are directions for Nicholas to follow as soon as he "decodes" the message. As the adults analyze Nicholas's responses, we identify new goals and strategies.

Jan: Nicholas, you're getting to be such a good listener and writer these days now that you are in first grade. I have a message on this card and it tells you something very interesting. Listen to it and see if you can tell Mommy and me what it says.

(He runs the card through the language master and his eyes light up.)

Nicholas: *Money!* It say, *some money!*
J: I heard that too at the end. It says, *some money*. I wonder if there are some more words.

(Nicholas runs the card through again, and this time he gets the last three words.)

N: *For!* I hear it say *for. For some money.*
J: It *says* "For some money."
N: It *says* "For some money."
J: Here. Let me draw a line on this sheet for each of the words we've heard.

(I put three lines on the paper as I say the words, *for, some, money.*)

J: (To Mom) These lines are place holders so that Nicholas will have a reminder when it comes time to write the message. Our job is to watch him work and to note the strategies and problem-solving skills he uses. Then we are better prepared to help him at home and in therapy.

(To Nicholas) Nicholas! We don't have any lines for the other words. Shall we listen again?
N: Yeah.
Mom: Yes.

N: Yes. (He runs the card through again.) Ca-bi-ne? I don't know.

(Nicholas seems a little discouraged at finding an unfamiliar word and knowing that he will have to reproduce it in print. I note his predicament.)

J: It must be a new word. Let's listen again. (I play the card through and help Nicholas.) Ca-bi-net. That's what I heard.

(To Mom) Sometimes first graders think they are supposed to know everything and take it personally if they don't. We have to help him understand that not knowing is okay and that he has ways to deal with it.

N: Ca-bi-net! I don't know that. Mom, you know that?

Mom: Do I know that? Yes. We have one in our house. It's in the kitchen, but I think we call it a cupboard. It has doors and we keep cups and plates or boxes of food in it.

(Nicholas looks around the room and satisfies himself that he knows what a cabinet is. Then, he watches as I draw a line for the word *cabinet*.)

J: I think we need a pretty long line for *cabinet*.

N: Oh-huh-huh. It a big — long, long word.

J: You're right about that. Now I wonder what the other words are. (I draw three more lines in front of the others to help Nicholas along.) Let's see if you can get them.

(Nicholas listens again and follows along with his finger, pointing to each blank as he hears the words.)

J: (To Mom) One of the things Nicholas has to learn is that words might sound a little different when they're learned separately. For example, when we learn spelling words, we say them much more clearly than we do when they're strung together in sentences. As a result, children may get the idea that what we write doesn't necessarily relate to conversation. Also, Nicholas's teachers will expect him to do dictations by the end of the year. We'd like to get him familiar with the task before he's expected to do it in school.

(Meanwhile, Nicholas, working on his own, has figured out more of the sentence.)

N: Mom, Mom. I hear *"in the cabinet for some money."* (He points to all but one of the blanks.)

Mom: That's good. That's what I heard too.

N: I like it money at school. My teacher give me money for work.

J: Listen. My teacher *gives* me money for work at school.

N: My teacher *gives* me money for school.

J: What a deal. Now I see that you need to get one more word here. Did you listen to it?

N: Yeah, no. Let me one more time. (He listens.) I don't know. Nook?

J: Lalala look.

N: Lalalalook! *Look in the* uh-oh, I can't demember.

J: You can't re-mem-ber? The word is ca-bi-net.

N: Ca-bi-net. Look in the cabinet for some money.

J: Sounds good to me. No, you can't look yet. I was hoping you'd write the words on the blanks. You can do that, then look in the cabinet.

N: How you spell look? L—

J: Think about it. That was one of your spelling words.

N: I denember. L-O-O-K! (He writes it and then continues to do the task carefully until he gets to the unfamiliar word.) I don't know how spell cabinet. I don't know.

J: What should you ask me? How — do —

N: How do you spell cabinet? It easy?

J: Sure. There are seven letters. Listen to four. C— hold it. Don't write until I give you four letters. C-A-B-I. (Nicholas writes those letters, repeating them softly to himself as he does so.) Ready? C-A-B-I-N-E-T.

(Nicholas finishes writing the new word and continues writing the sentence, saying each word until he gets to *money*.)

N: Money — M-O... What's next?

J: M-O-N-E-Y. There are five letters. M-O-N-E-Y.

N: I finish it. *Look in the cabinet for some money.*

J: Okay. Follow the direction. (To Mom) It's important for Nicholas to understand that what's in writing is real, with a message and consequences. How do you think you could carry this over to home or some other situation?

Mom: Maybe his brother could make a message for him. Or, Nicholas could make messages for Ryan or his Dad to listen to.

J: The nice part about that is that Nicholas could see how someone else puts his speech into print. It should be something that would be important and enjoyable to him.

N: See. I got some nickel, dime, quarters. No dollars. That's too bad. I like dollars.

J: So I see. Did the tooth fairy ever bring you any money?

N: I got some unner my pillow. Two dollars. Denember, Mom in 1995, no 1996. I got money unner my pillow.

J: *Under,* right?

N: Under, see how many nickels — one, two; quarters, that's 25 cents. And one dime, that's 10.

J: Let's put the money in the play cash register as we count it.

(To Mom) Well, you can see that took some time. But he'll soon get the idea of what we want, and he's already becoming aware of the connection between speaking and writing. We can let him know there's always a way to figure out the connection between speech and writing.

(The activity continues. Another direction is presented on the language master card, *Listen to the Song*. This provides practice with the /l/ and /t/ in another sentence. It also directs him to listen to the song we practiced last week on the tape recorder.)

Parent Guidance

✔ This week, help Nicholas think up messages for Daddy to hear and copy from the tape recorder.

✔ Clue Daddy into the process of thinking out loud as he writes the messages.

✔ Let Nicholas watch Daddy go through the process, so he can see that grown-ups don't automatically know everything.

✔ Be sure to show Nicholas that there are times that you don't recognize some words.

Twenty Questions

This activity is an adaptation of the verbal Twenty Questions game. Initially, we use objects such as those found in the Getting Ready to Read Kit™ (Houghton Mifflin). Using category names, such as *animal, vehicle, furniture,* and attributes, such as *size, color, function,* Nicholas, his mom, and I try to identify the hidden object. Twenty Questions requires careful thinking about the intention of a question. It teaches a way of making questions that is different from the "wh" questions. It also teaches Nicholas to use questions that start with auxiliary verbs.

Jan: Take a look in this box, Nicholas. What do you see?

Nicholas: I see a racing car, a zebra, a pie, a bear, ahh, I don't know —

Mom: That's called a bulldozer. You've seen one by the school where they're going to build some new houses.

N: Oh yea. They're loud.

J: Yes, it's a noisy machine.

N: A top, and a baseball bat. They little.

J: Yes, they are not real, but we'll pretend they are real. Here are some things you can ask me about.

(I show Nicholas and his mother a list of characteristics: color, shape, size, what it's used for, who uses it, what you do with it, where you see it. I model a few questions for them that can be answered only with "yes" or "no": Is it an animal? Is it bigger than a backpack?)

J: Both of you close your eyes while I hide one. (I put the bulldozer into the cup and invert it on the table.) I am ready. You've only got 20 questions. If you use more, I win.

Mom: Is it something I have in the house?

J: No, it is not.

Mom: Can I pick it up?

J: No. You cannot pick it up.

N: Oh, I know. It's a baseball bat.

J: You have to start with *is*. Is it _____?

N: Is it baseball bat?

J: No, it is not a baseball bat. That's three questions gone. First try to figure out about the object, before guessing.

Mom: Can it move heavy things?

J: Yes. It can move very heavy things.

N: Oh, I know, I know. It a — ah, ah Mom, I can't denember. Help me.

Mom: (In a soft voice) A bulldozer.

N: A bull*doner?*

Mom: (Whispering) A bull-*doze*-er

N: That it. A bulldoner

J: Hmmm. I don't think I have one of those here.

N: It move things.

Mom: (Whispering) a bull-*doze*-er

N: That it! A bull*doze*-er.

J: (Prompting) Is it _____?

N: Is it bulldon — ah — bull-doze-er? It move dirt 'n rocks.

J: You're exactly right. It moves heavy things; it's not in the house; and you can't pick it up with your hands. Let's see, you used five questions. How many questions do you have left? 20 − 5 = 15. It's your turn now. I won't look until you tell me you're ready.

(Nicholas takes a turn as the game continues.)

Parent Guidance

✔ When you play this game, try to focus on *one language target:* Make sure Nicholas starts each question with an auxiliary verb. Don't take away points if he doesn't think to do it spontaneously at this time. The game can, however, become that specific, depending on what your goals are.

✔ Play tic-tac-toe using a grid with auxiliary verbs. You must ask a question starting with the verb before putting on the "x" or "o."

is	are	can
do	will	does
was	were	did

✔ Play the I Spy game using characteristics for descriptions (e.g., I spy a vehicle that has two wheels and you ride it to school).

✔ Play Brainquest™ or one of the trivia games that are available at various age levels.

Brown Bear, Brown Bear

Portions of the lesson, Brown Bear, Brown Bear, What Do You See? are selected and incorporated into this session. (See pages 246–256.)

Summary

At the end of the session, Nicholas chooses books from the children's book shelf while his mother and I discuss the session. We discuss the improvement in Nicholas's auditory memory of letter names when spelling. He is more confident when listening to tape-recorded speech. Production of /l/ is improving. He understands and hears the differences in words that rhyme. He is learning strategies for filling in words he does not know. He is using questions to gather information and to seek help.

We discuss specific carryover activities related to therapy goals. Nicholas's mom writes down the weekly home plan. I assure her that things are going well.

Lesson Plan for Chase

K. Todd Houston, MSP, CCC-SLP, Cert. AVT

In August 1995, I met Chase, a handsome little boy who had just celebrated his third birthday. One month earlier, he had received a Nucleus 22 cochlear implant. The initial MAPping of his speech processor had just been completed, and he was eager to show off his new toy when his mother came to obtain a comprehensive speech and language evaluation and to enroll him in therapy.

Chase's parents first suspected he was not hearing when he was six months old. After visits to his pediatrician and finally to an audiologist, Chase was diagnosed with a profound hearing loss in the right ear and a severe-to-profound hearing loss in the left. The detailed case history revealed that Chase's hearing loss was attributed to cytomegalovirus (CMV).

He was immediately given bilateral behind-the-ear (BTE) hearing aids, but his aided responses were not within the speech range on the audiogram. At 11 months, after a second opinion from another audiologist, Chase was given more powerful aids. His aided responses were just within the speech range at 500, 1000, and 2000 Hz but outside the speech range above 2000 Hz.

Chase's parents were pleased that his vocalizations increased after acquiring the new hearing aids and wanted him to use spoken language, so they looked for local professionals to help them. To their surprise, however, the only approach available was total communication. This forced them to look outside their area. They finally enrolled Chase in an auditory-verbal practice and traveled the long drive from home twice a month.

After a year of therapy, formal evaluations revealed that Chase had made limited progress in communication development. The therapist discussed the limited amount of auditory information available through Chase's current amplification and suggested that cochlear implantation be considered. Following many discussions with parents of children who had received implants and with other professionals, Chase's parents decided to investigate this option.

In the spring of 1995, Chase was evaluated by the implant team and determined to be a candidate. Two months later, he received his cochlear implant with a full insertion of 22 electrodes. His aided responses with the implant are between 30–35 dB HL across all frequencies of the audiogram.

One month following surgery and a few days after the initial MAPping of his speech processor, Chase arrived for a speech and language evaluation to establish baseline skills in speech, language, cognition, and listening. Chase had just celebrated his third birthday and was eligible to receive services from his local school district, which had decided to contract with my center for auditory-verbal services.

The assessments revealed that Chase had auditory pattern perception and some word recognition. That is, he could discriminate between one-, two-, and three-syllable words containing a variety of stress patterns and recognize familiar words in a known context through audition alone. Spontaneous speech was limited to a few early developing consonants (b, m) and vowels such as (a, u). He repeated and alternated syllables to approximate one- and two-word utterances, and occasionally, he approximated some three-word combinations.

Two weeks after the initial evaluation, the family enrolled in therapy for three 45-minute sessions per week. Chase also continued to have sessions with his first auditory-verbal therapist once a month.

Over the past two years, Chase has made remarkable progress in communication development due to a number of variables, including excellent family support and consistent intervention. In fact, nine months after receiving his implant, Chase was evaluated using a variety of assessments normed on children with typical hearing. Results indicated consistent word recognition, auditory processing of four critical elements (e.g., Put the *yellow car in* the *box*), ability to follow two-step directions, age-appropriate receptive language, and only a six-month delay in expressive language. In conversational speech, however, Chase did exhibit numerous substitutions, omissions, and distortions.

Chase is now four-and-a-half years old and is approaching his second anniversary with his cochlear implant. He currently has two therapy sessions per week and attends a self-contained auditory-oral preschool program two days per week and a church-based preschool during the remaining three days. In this lesson plan, I focus primarily on fine-tuning Chase's listening skills, expanding expressive language, and improving speech intelligibility.

Introduction to the Lesson

The center consists of a main building and an annex, where my office and therapy rooms are located. Therapy sessions begin in the parking lot, where I usually meet the family getting out of their car.

As Chase walks ahead, Mom and I discuss what has occurred since the last session. Interesting events such as a birthday party, trips to the zoo or a football game could be used as topics of conversation.

The therapy room is small, containing a child-sized, rectangular table and toddler chairs. I share the therapy rooms with six speech-language pathologists and currently do not have one room designated just for auditory-verbal therapy. I keep all therapy materials in my office and transport required items to the therapy room prior to each session.

After nearly two years in therapy, the interesting-toy-on-the-table strategy is no longer necessary with Chase, and he comfortably follows the *rules of therapy:*

- We listen to each other.
- When we talk, we use our *quiet* voice.
- We cooperate and help each other.
- We have fun!

Chase readily enters the therapy room and goes straight to his seat. I sit beside him on his right in order to speak closely to the microphone of his cochlear implant. Mom sits across the table from Chase, ready to record the important points of the session, and a graduate clinician sits across the table from me.

The session begins with a conversation that engages everyone in the room, especially Chase. This seems very informal, but conversation is actually the most natural way to target developmentally appropriate vocabulary.

The Initial Conversation

GOALS

Listening:
- to follow a conversation about a known context through listening only.

Speech:
- to generalize emerging speech sounds to connected speech.

Language:
- to increase utterance length using correct grammar and syntax.

Cognition:

- to learn developmentally appropriate vocabulary, concepts, and figurative language during natural discourse.

Communication:

- to develop the conversation skills of initiating, maintaining, topic transition, and closure.

DISCUSSION

Chase's conversational language is above average compared to other children with similar case histories. He is able to initiate a discussion and respond to the comments of others, but he experiences difficulty maintaining a conversation. In order to help him, I ask Mom or the graduate student to model the correct response. If I ask a question and pause expectantly for Chase to answer and he doesn't, Mom or the graduate student will model the correct response. Chase will usually repeat it, and we continue the conversation. I introduce new vocabulary such as *grandparent, grandmother, grandfather, aunt, uncle,* and *cousin* throughout the conversation.

ACTIVITY

Todd: "So, Chase, Mom said you are going on a trip this weekend."
Chase: "Yes! I'm going on a trip."
T: "Where are you going?"
C: "I'm going to see G-Pop in Georgia."
T: "Oh, yes, G-Pop. He's your *grandfather,* right?"
C: "What?"
T: "G-Pop is your *grandfather* and Grandy is your *grandmother.*"
C: "Yes, grandfather and grandmother."
T: "G-Pop and Grandy are your *grandparents.* You will visit your grandparents in Georgia."
C: "My grandparents wive in Georgia."
T: "That's right, Chase. They do *live* in Georgia. How *long* a drive is it?"
C: "We drive for a *wong, wong,* time. Two hours!"
T: "That is a *long, long* drive! What do you do while Mommy and Daddy drive?"
C: "I watch movies in the van."
T: "You watch movies in the van?"
C: "Yes! The Wion King. I watch the Wion King."
T: "Wion King.... what's that? I've never heard of the Wion King."

C: "No, it's not WION King... it's Wion King."

T: "Oh, you mean the Lion King... Simba!

C: "Yes...Simba in the Wion King."

T: "Chase, *you're pulling my leg*. You can't watch The *Lion* King in the van."

C: "What?" (Chase looks under the table at my legs.)

T: "You're *pulling my leg*. I think you're *teasing* me."

C: "No, I'm not!"

T: "You really have TV and VCR in your van?"

C: "Yes!"

ANALYSIS

In addition to conversational skills, I carefully monitor speech production. Chase substitutes /w/ for /l/ and /d/ for /g/, which are current targets. I model correct production of these phonemes and use acoustic highlighting when necessary. This conversation provided an opportunity to introduce a new idiom — *you're pulling my leg*.

Chase used individual nicknames to refer to his grandparents, so the terms *grandfather, grandmother,* and *grandparents* were new. This new vocabulary was introduced naturally in the conversation.

Although Chase has made tremendous progress in receptive and expressive language, more abstract language forms, such as idioms (*you're pulling my leg*), words with double meanings, and homonyms, are challenging. Even though he did not initially understand the idiom, I repeated it, provided a definition (*you're teasing me*), and Chase was able to grasp the idea. This is learning from the known to the unknown, the easy to the complex, and the concrete to the abstract.

I carefully monitor his speech production of /l/ and /g/. If Chase misarticulates or omits these phonemes, I provide the correct model using acoustically highlighted sounds. I also repeat exactly what he has said and ask him if the statement or word was correct (e.g., when he mentioned the Wion King). Through my puzzled expression, Chase was able to discriminate what was wrong, but when *he* corrected *me*, he still made the error. This diagnostic information tells me that he can discriminate between the /w/ and /l/ sounds when he hears them but cannot self-correct this speech error. The /l/ is emerging. He can discriminate the sound through listening and must now learn its production. If Chase is not able to acquire this sound through listening alone, I will provide more acoustic information, using a variety of techniques before presenting visual cues. If visual cues are required, the final therapeutic step is to *put the sound back into listening*.

New vocabulary was introduced, and pragmatic skills were reinforced. Chase was able to maintain the conversation by providing relevant information and introducing new topics.

Parent Guidance

When developing conversational competence:

✔ Capitalize on *natural* interactions, especially at the dinner table or when Chase wants to share something important, such as what he did at school that day.

✔ Use vocabulary and language introduced during this session such as *grandfather, grandmother, grandparents,* and *you're pulling my leg* in conversation at home.

✔ Find books and stories containing the same vocabulary and expressions in other contexts. In the library you might find interesting stories about relatives or books of idioms.

✔ Draw pictures of some simple idioms *such as you're pulling my leg, a green thumb,* and *it's raining cats and dogs.* You can talk about each picture and what the expression really means. You will extend Chase's comprehension from the literal meaning of the phrase to the abstract.

Speech Babble

GOALS

Listening:
- to detect and identify misarticulated phonemes and to develop correct production through audition.
- to continue development of auditory self-monitoring of speech.

Speech:
- to improve speech intelligibility by repeating and alternating targeted phonemes at the syllable level.

DISCUSSION

Even though Chase has intelligible speech, he still misarticulates a few current targets, /k/ and /l/. Chase enjoys reinforcement for correct productions by writing steeples (+'s) on the data sheet developed for tracking progress.

I usually start speech babble with the Ling Six-Sound Test, and I know immediately if his implant is functioning correctly by the *quality* of Chase's responses. I say each of the six sounds /sh/, /m/, /i/, /u/, /s/, and /a/, and vary my pitch with each one. Chase repeats all sounds correctly and quickly writes six steeples on the data sheet. This takes less than two minutes!

ACTIVITY
I begin speech babble by saying, "gagagaga." Chase responds "dadada-da," and writes more steeples on the data sheet.

Todd: "Chase, I want you to try *gagagaga* once again."
Chase: "Dadadada."

(I try to use an anticipatory set of phonemes to elicit correct production of /g/.)

T: "Chase, let's try *babababa*."
C: "Babababa."
T: "Very good! Now try *dadadada*."
C: "Dadadada."
T: "Great Chase. Let's do *gagagaga*."
C: "Dadadada."

(I double-check to see if he can discriminate the sounds through listening.)

T: "Chase, are these sounds the same or different — *dada... gaga?*"
C: "Different!"
T: "Yes. Now, let's listen again — *gagaga*." (I lean over to within six inches of the microphone and repeat the stimulus.)
C: "Dadada."
T: "Good try. Listen for this sound... *kakaka*. Can you say kakaka?"
C: "Kakaka. Like cat, right?"
T: "Yes, like the word cat. Can you feel where the kakaka sound is made — way back, right?"
C: "Kaka — yep."
T: "That's the same place for gagaga. Try it again, *gagaga*."
C: "Dada.... gagaga!"
T: "Excellent, Chase. Now, let's try *gugugu*."
C: "Du... gugu... du... gugu."
T: "Good. You are doing fine. Let's try a different sound — *lalala*."
C: "Wawawa."

T: "Try it again... lalala." (I again move to approximately six inches from the microphone.)

C: "Wawawa."

T: "Wawawa... is that the same as lalala?"

C: "No!"

T: "You're right. These are different, too. Let's try a l-l-l." (I place the /l/ in the final position of the syllable and lengthen its duration.)

C: "Ah... all!"

T: "Great, Chase. That's right, *all*. Try it again, a l-l-l."

C: "Ah... ah... all." (Chase noticeably pauses between productions before he correctly says *all*.)

T: "Here's a harder one. Try, a l-l-l a." (I purposefully lengthen the /l/ again and release it into the same initial vowel, /a/.)

C: "All... ah."

T: "Good, Chase, but listen for my long sound and say /a/... a l-l-l a."

C: "All-la."

T: "Right, Chase! Now, try *alalala*. Remember where we make that *long* sound." (When I say the word *long,* I use acoustic highlighting to emphasize the /l/.)

C: "Ahlalala!'

T: "Perfect, Chase. That's it! You got it!"

With the correct productions, speech babble ends as Chase records more steeples.

ANALYSIS

Short sessions of speech babble give Chase specific cues about correct production of these phonemes at the syllabic level. He was able to produce each successfully after specific strategies were used. I began by using an anticipatory set to reinforce the correct manner and voicing of the phoneme /g/, but Chase was still unable to produce /gagaga/ accurately. I moved closer to the implant's microphone to provide a more audible speech signal. Unfortunately, this still did not work. Lastly, building on his responses and knowing that he knew the correct manner and voicing characteristics for the /g/, I gave him a place-of-production cue with the /k/. Since he has mastered the /k/, it was easier to remember the tongue placement and correctly produce the voiced correlate, /g/.

Chase substituted /w/ for /l/. He did not have the correct tongue placement. I moved closer to the microphone of the implant, but Chase still could not produce the /l/. I determined he could hear the difference between the /l/ and /w/, so I continued to target the /l/ by placing it in the final position of the syllable. Using the /a/, I modeled the production, releasing the /a/ into a sustained /l/ which can be an easier context in which to learn it. During his first successful production of the /l/, Chase noticeably paused to check his tongue placement before saying *all*. This indicated that he was self-monitoring his own speech. I quickly tried to elicit /l/ in the medial position by saying *alla*. Essentially, /l/ is moved to the medial position, lengthened, and released into the /a/ and then moved to the initial position.

Parent Guidance

✔ Continue to work on these sounds by selecting books and other materials that contain them.

✔ Do not correct Chase's misarticulations or approximations of /g/ or /l/.

✔ Reinforce correct production of the sounds through modeling and acoustic highlighting.

✔ Reduce visual cues and encourage Chase to *listen* to the sounds.

Story Time

GOALS

Listening:
- to increase auditory memory.
- to sequence events in a story with and without the use of pictures.
- to develop the ability to retell a story by including its critical elements.

Speech:
- to develop appropriate suprasegmental features (pitch, loudness, duration, and intonation).
- to emphasize targets speech sounds such as /g/ and /l/ through acoustic highlighting.

Language:
- to increase length of utterance using correct grammar and syntax.
- to introduce new vocabulary, such as *huge* and *gigantic,* and idioms in story context.
- to reinforce the question form: *Which one?*

Cognition:
- to reinforce the concept that a story has a *beginning, middle,* and *end.*
- to reinforce the concepts of *first* through *fifth,* and *last.*
- to reinforce the concept of *left* and *right.*

DISCUSSION
In each activity, I try to incorporate goals in listening, speech, language, and cognition as often as I can. The primary goal of Story Time is to develop Chase's auditory memory so that he can retell the story by correctly sequencing the events. I use a variety of clinician-made and commercial sequence cards, which complete a story, instead of the somewhat limiting single-event cards. I can illustrate a complete story and embellish it as much as I wish. I often create silly character names that contain the targeted speech sounds. Chase loves to listen to these!

ACTIVITY
I hold the set of cards for a story titled, *Gus Goes Fishing.* I hold each card and tell the story, using targeted vocabulary and/or concepts. Chase listens to the story through all five pictures. He listens as I begin:

"One day, Gus decided to go fishing. He went to the pond and fished off of the pier. Suddenly, his fishing pole starts to bend. Gus thinks he has finally caught a huge, gigantic fish. He lifts his pole out of the water and there is something on his fishing line. What do you think it is, Chase?"

Chase: "It's a huge fish!"
Todd: "A big, huge fish? Do you think it is a GIGANTIC fish?"
C: "Yeah!"
T: "Sorry, it's not a fish! It's an old, stinky, soggy boot! Let's find out what Gus does next. Maybe he'll catch a fish now."
C: "Yeah... a huge fish."

I present the fourth card.

"Gus's fishing pole was bent over again. He has something very, very heavy on his fishing pole. He pulls it out of the water and guess what?"

C: "What... what?"
T: "It's another boot. He caught another old..."
C: "He got another stinky, soggy boot!"
T: "That's right... another stinky, soggy boot. Now he has two boots to wear. This time a fish was in the boot, and it jumped back in the water."
C: "Why did the fish jump in the water?"

"Fish live in water. If he stayed out of the water, he'd die. After Gus pulled the second boot out of the water, he dried them both off. Gus decided that catching a pair of boots was better than nothing at all. He decided to keep his boots, and he wore them home to show his Mom."

After finishing the story, I turn the cards face down on the table and mix them up. I tell Chase to turn over one card at a time and tell me what is happening in the picture. He must also decide if the scene occurred at the beginning, middle, or end of the story. He turns over the first card.

T: "What's happening here, Chase?"
C: "He has a boot on the pole."
T: "Who has a boot? What's the boy's name?"
C: "His name is Dus."
T: "Dus or Gus?" (I again move to approximately six inches from the implant microphone and acoustically highlight the /g/ in *Gus*.)
C: "Dus."

I instruct Chase to remember the cat sound, *meow*, as a cue for correct tongue placement and ask him again, "Was it Dus or Gus?"

C: "Um... Du... Gus!"
T: "Right! So, Gus has one boot. Was that at the beginning, middle, or end of the story?"
C: "Uhhh... beginning."
T: "That's right, Chase. This happened at the beginning."

I place the card face up on the far left side of the table. As Chase turns over each card and describes the scene, he decides where each will go on the table (far left, in the middle of the table, or on the far right, depending on *where* the scene occurred). He carefully sequences the story cards.

T: "Chase, what happened *first?* Look at the cards on the *left*. They happened in the beginning of the story. Which one happened *first?*"
C: "Uhhh… This one. Du… Gus is fishing on the pier."
T: "That's right. Gus is fishing on the pier, and his pole is really bent over! What happened *next?* What was the second thing that Gus did?"

We continue until he has correctly sequenced all the cards. Chase pauses, looking at all the cards, and retells the story:

"This boy… his name is Dus. He does pishing and he caught a boot. Then, he catches another boot. He cweans the boots, because they stink and they are wet and soddy. He puts them on his feet and does home to show his Mommy."

I compliment Chase on his story and then ask Mom and the graduate student to take turns randomly describing one card, while expanding the story. Chase listens in order to select which scene is being described. I encourage at least two or three sentences in each description. Chase pauses, thinks, and selects the appropriate card. We continue until all the cards are put away. Then, *without looking at the pictures,* I tell Chase another story called *Leo the Pig.*

"One day Leo decided to go for a walk in the forest. It was a beautiful spring day. It was warm, the flowers were blooming, and the birds were singing. Leo was very happy. As he walked, he met his friend, Mr. Duck. Mr. Duck told Leo that his foot was hurting and asked if he could ride on Leo's back. Because Leo was such a good friend and was in a very cheerful mood, he allowed Mr. Duck to ride on his back. Leo and Mr. Duck continued walking through the forest. Then, suddenly, they met another friend, Mr. Kackle, a chicken. Mr. Kackle saw Mr. Duck sitting on Leo's back. Because he, too, had recently injured his foot, he asked if could join Mr. Duck. Leo, a true friend, said 'Sure, the more, the merrier,' and the three friends continued walking through the forest, enjoying the beautiful spring day."

Chase retells the story:

"Weo was this pig and he was walking in the forest and saw a duck. The duck hurt his foot and climbed on Weo's back. Then, Weo saw a chicken. He hurt his foot, too. He wanted to sit on Weo's back… like the duck. The chicken and the duck sat on Weo's back and they walked in the forest."

Mom asks, "Chase, how was the weather when Leo went on his walk?"

C: "It was warm outside."
M: "Which season of the year was it... spring or summer?"
C: "Uhhh... summer."

Mom replies, "No, think again. Remember, the birds were singing and the flowers were blooming. When does that happen?"

C: "Spring!!"

Mom replies, "That's right!"
Then, the graduate student asks, "Chase, who did Leo meet *first?*"

C: "He met the duck, then the chicken."
GS: "Good, Chase!"

ANALYSIS

Chase had the benefit of the pictures for the first story, which made it easier to retell. Chase was successful retelling the story *without* the pictures. The ultimate goal is to listen to a long, detailed story and to *retell the story from memory.*

Sequencing a story is an important task because it reinforces that stories have a beginning, middle, and end. As Chase develops conversational competence, he will learn that his own stories must have the same components. Within these components, there are critical details that he should remember and retell. This is important diagnostic information about his auditory memory.

Throughout both stories, I expanded vocabulary and concepts such as *huge, gigantic, beginning, middle, end, left, right,* and *first* through *last.*

I often stopped to evaluate his comprehension and used auditory closure to help him ("He caught another old..." I paused to check his understanding of specific vocabulary in this sentence, *stinky* and *soggy*). Chase was primed for this vocabulary, and he answered correctly.

Chase substituted /d/ for /g/, especially in the word *Gus.* I moved closer to his microphone and asked him to discriminate between these two sounds. This was ineffective, so I reminded him of the placement cue (the "cat" sound). He remembered the correct tongue position and accurately repeated *Gus.* When he retold the story, however, he was unable to produce the /g/ correctly in *Gus, goes,* or *soggy.* Chase also continued to substitute /w/ for /l/ in the second story. Both phonemes are emerging. He is stimulable for each at the word level, but needs more practice at the phrase, sentence, and conversation levels. Because he has acquired these sounds through listening and verbal cues (the "cat" sound), I will speak closer to the microphone and use acoustic highlighting to encourage correct production. He demonstrated some ability to self-correct both sounds, a vital step in building his auditory feedback loop!

When Chase's mom asked him about the season of the year, he answered incorrectly. She immediately offered a closed set of two choices, *spring* or *summer.* Chase, who was probably *not really listening,* answered with the last word he heard, *summer.* She then described exactly what happens in the spring of the year, using *another closed set* of choices. Chase easily responded correctly. Although reducing choices to a closed set is a good strategy to use in some situations, it was not the best here. Instead, when Chase could not remember the season, she could have asked him an *open-set question* such as, "What do you remember about the story?" Or, "What did Leo see on his walk?" As he remembered the things Leo saw on his walk (birds singing and flowers blooming), he might have reasoned that the season was spring.

Parent Guidance

✔ Read and tell stories to Chase that have a clear *beginning, middle,* and *end.*

✔ Use the vocabulary *first, second, third, fourth, last,* and *next.*

✔ Encourage him to make choices by using the question, *Which one?*

✔ Use puppets or other props to practice retelling stories.

✔ Common children's stories such as *The Three Little Pigs* or *Jack and the Beanstalk* are excellent to use because they contain repetitive vocabulary and build shared knowledge with Chase's peers. These are important readiness skills for inclusion in the regular school.

✔ Develop conversations by sharing what *you* did that day while Chase was at school.

✔ Encourage him to tell the events of his day in sequence.

✔ Use *open-set* questions to challenge Chase's auditory memory.

What's Wrong?

GOALS

Listening:
- to process various question forms.

Speech:
- to reinforce speech intelligibility by developing emerging phonemes, especially /g/ and /l/ at the word and phrase levels.

Language:
- to respond appropriately to *What's wrong? How?* and *Why?* questions.
- to increase expressive language using appropriate grammar and syntax.

Cognition:
- to reinforce reasoning, abstract thinking, and problem-solving skills.

DISCUSSION

One of Chase's favorite activities is talking about *What's wrong?* picture cards. This set of cartoon-like cards consists of scenes which portray events that are obviously wrong or illogical (such as a person driving a car on water). Chase refers to them as the *sil-we* (silly) pictures. Chase looks at one card at a time and must describe what's happening to his mom and the graduate student without letting them see it. They must try to figure out what's happening and then ask Chase questions about it. If there are obvious errors in his speech production, grammar, or syntax, Chase's mom, the graduate student, or I will provide correct models.

ACTIVITY

Chase starts with a card involving a woman driving a car on water.

C: "There's this woman. She is driving a car. It's on a wake (lake)."

Chase's mom says, "Oh, that's silly. What's wrong with that? Why can't she drive on a lake?"

C: "She can't drive on water. The car will sink."

His mom continues, "You're right, Chase. The car will sink. It can't...."

C: "Fwoat (float)!"

M: "Right, the car can't float. It will sink and go to the bottom of the lake," (Mom replies as she acoustically highlights the fl-blend in the word *float*.)

C: "She can drive on the road, not on the water. That's a silwy picture."

Chase hands me the first card and quickly asks for another.

C: "There's this chair and a girl is sitting on it... but it doesn't have any wegs (legs)."

The graduate student replies, *"Legs,"* as she moves closer to him and slightly emphasizes the /l/.

C: "Yes... la... legs."

GS: "No legs? What do you mean... the girl had no legs?"

C: "No, silwy... the chair. The chair doesn't have wegs."

GS: "Oh, the chair doesn't have legs. Then, how does the girl sit in the chair without falling down?"

C: "I don't know. That's very silwy. She might fall down!"

GS: "It is silly. If the chair doesn't have legs, she should fall down. It can't hold her up."

C: "Yes, very silwy picture.

We continue until we have worked through approximately 10 cards. This game is highly motivating for Chase.

ANALYSIS

The silly pictures are useful in developing a variety of skills. Abstract thinking, reasoning, problem solving, vocabulary building, expansion of expressive language, speech production, and conversational competence were all targeted and/or reinforced.

Chase is stimulable for the /l/ at the word level, so the graduate student simply repeated the word *legs* with a slightly highlighted /l/, moving the sound from a known context (single word) to an unknown context (connected speech).

The graduate student asked Chase if the girl was missing legs, but Chase had already used the pronoun *it* to refer to the legless chair. It was not the best question and interrupted the natural flow of the conversation.

The silliness, comedy, and light-heartedness of each situation portrayed by these cards is very motivating. Chase loves the idea that only he and I see the cards at first and feels that *he* is the authority and can share information that the others do not know.

Parent Guidance

✔ Use home situations to develop abstract thinking, reasoning, and problem solving, such as telling Chase to cut his sandwich with a spoon, cut paper with a ruler, or paint a picture with a hair brush.

✔ *Sabotage* of a situation can also be effective for reinforcing problem-solving skills such as coloring a picture with an empty box of crayons or cutting paper without scissors.

✔ Predictable books and stories also reinforce abstract thinking. Books such as *Brown Bear, Brown Bear* and *Hattie and the Fox* will encourage Chase to predict what might happen next.

Rhyming Bingo

GOALS

Listening:
* to discriminate between rhyming words having sounds that differ in manner, place, and voicing.

Speech:
* to use targeted speech sounds correctly at the word level and in conversation during a game activity.

Language:
* to increase understanding and use of synonyms and homonyms.
* to develop rhyming words.

Cognition:
* to begin to develop sound–letter associations.

DISCUSSION
Discrimination skills at the word level help with understanding and perceiving rhyme. The ability to understand rhyming words demonstrates

that Chase can recognize both similarities and differences in speech sounds. He needs to develop this reading readiness skill as he prepares to enter kindergarten.

To play this clinician-made game, each player chooses a game card that has eight monosyllabic (one-syllable) words illustrated on it. The game also contains single-picture cards, which players select and label. The object is to listen to a player name a card and then try to find an object that rhymes with it among the eight pictures on one's game card. For example, a player may select a card that is a picture of a cat. The player says, "Cat." The remaining players look at their cards and try to find something that *rhymes* with cat.

ACTIVITY

The activity begins by passing out a game card to each player, and the single cards are stacked in the middle of the table. I turn over the first card and begin by calling out the word *coat*.

Todd: "Coat. Who has something that rhymes with coat?"

Mom: "I do… I do," Mom replies as she quickly covers a picture on her card with a chip.

T: "Chase, what do you think Mom has on her card?"

C: "I don't know."

T: "What's something that sounds like *coat?*"

C: "I forgot!"

T: "Well, I can think of an animal… the word sounds like *coat…*"

C: "Oh, a doat (goat)!!!"

T: "Yes, a *goat*. Goat and coat rhyme, don't they? (I acoustically highlight the /g/ in *goat*.) OK, Mom. Let's see what's on your card."

(His mom moves the chip to reveal a picture of a goat.)

T: "Chase, our first word was *coat*. What's another word for *coat?*"

(I pause to wait for Chase to answer.)

C: "Uhhh… I don't know.'

T: "If it is cold outside, you could wear your coat or you might wear your…"

C: "Jacket!"

T: "Right, your jacket or parka. Those words *basically* mean the same thing as coat. Let's see… who's next?"

The graduate student says, "OK the next card is a *shell*. Who has something that rhymes with *shell?*"

"I do," Chase replies as he covers the item on the game card.

GS: "Well, Chase, what could it be? I guess we'll need to guess."

We each take turns asking Chase what the item is.

T: "Is it a *pail?*"
C: "No."

His mom says, "It must be *mail* like a letter or envelope."

C: "Nope."

"I know. I think you have a *bell* on your card, " the graduate student says.
"Yeah...I have a *bell,*" Chase replies.
We continue the game in this manner until someone has acquired at least four covered pictures in a row and yells "Bingo."

ANALYSIS

At first, Chase had real difficulty discriminating between these words. Often, as illustrated with the word coat, I extend the game by asking if he knows another word that also rhymes. This reinforces the concept of rhyme and encourages him to *think*. This is an open-set task that fine-tunes his listening skills at the word level.

I extended the activity by asking for a homophone of coat to expand vocabulary. Being from the warm South, I doubt if Chase is familiar with term *parka*.

I reinforced correct production of /g/ by moving closer to Chase and emphasizing the target sound while repeating the word. He subsequently misarticulated the sound again during connected speech, illustrating the need for continued work at the word level.

Rhyming Bingo is a *word discrimination through listening* task, but many other speech, language, and cognitive goals can easily be incorporated. Generalizing Chase's discrimination skills to as many contexts as possible helps expand his receptive and expressive language and encourages auditory self-monitoring of speech.

I may use auditory closure activities to help Chase understand rhyme. For example, I could give him an open-ended statement such as, "Jack and Jill went up the..." He will *close* the sentence with the correct rhyming word. Card games such as Go Fish with rhyming words are also motivating.

Parent Guidance

✔   Highlight rhyming words found in children's poems and songs. Dr. Suess books such as *The Cat in the Hat, Hop on Pop,* and *There's a Wocket in my Pocket* are ideal.

✔   Make games to target auditory closure.

✔   Practice a poem or nursery rhyme; take turns saying each line.

✔   Cut homonym and synonym picture cards from magazines, catalogs, or sale flyers.

Listening in Noise

GOALS

Listening:

• to comprehend sentence-length information and instructions in the presence of noise.

DISCUSSION

Recently, his mom has noticed that Chase has difficulty playing a board game while the radio is on. He also has difficulty responding to her when his grandparents are engaged in a conversation only a few feet away. It is time to introduce noise into the therapy sessions.

I introduce a portable radio placed slightly behind Chase approximately three feet from his chair. It is tuned between two radio stations, which produces *white noise* or static. I begin with white noise, because it is easier to understand spoken information in white noise than in speech. Chase is required to follow relatively simple directions that will become progressively more complex. I use drawing as the reinforcement for this activity.

ACTIVITY

Todd: "Chase, draw a picture of a *boy with a red hat.*"

As the noise plays, Chase listens and successfully completes the picture. I am careful not to increase the volume of my voice and try to keep it a normal, conversational level. After each successful drawing, I add a little more information, using the carrier phrase, *Draw a picture of...*

A boy with a red hat.
A big flower next to the boy.
A girl with long, blond hair next to the flower.

The instructions become more difficult and more complex. Chase begins to have some difficulty.

T: "Draw a picture of a red ball next to the tree."

(Chase pauses and does not start to draw.)

C: "What ya say?"
T: "What did you *hear?*"
C: "Draw a picture of a ball..."
T: "Right. Draw the ball where... (pausing)... next to the..." (I pause again.)
C: "Draw the ball next to the tree!"
T: "Very good, Chase. What color is the ball?"
C: "Uhh... blue!"
T: "No. Listen as I repeat the entire sentence again. Draw a picture of a red ball next to the tree."
C: "Oh... red!"

ANALYSIS

Chase demonstrates improved listening skills in white noise. In this session, he had difficulty hearing all the words in the sentence, "Draw a picture of a red ball next to the tree." I used the carrier phrase *Draw a picture of...* for each presentation to reduce the level of difficulty. When he had difficulty, I did not repeat the entire sentence. I encouraged him to recall as much information as he could. He was able to recall only a little, so several adaptive strategies for listening were required.

The ultimate goal is that Chase will understand spoken language when competing conversations are occurring around him (listening to the teacher's voice while classmates are chatting or to conversations while the radio and television are playing). I will eventually move from white noise to single-talker to multitalker taped stimuli.

Conclusion

This therapy session targeted three major areas: listening, expressive language, and speech intelligibility. Listening skills were addressed in three different ways: by encouraging development of auditory memory and sequencing with story retelling, enhancing discrimination skills

---

Parent Guidance

✔ Situations such as listening with the radio or television on or with a competing conversation are challenging! We want Chase to be able to communicate effectively in these situations.

✔ Think about how situations can be altered to *help him hear optimally.*

✔ Listening during noise develops in a hierarchy. Chase needs experiences listening in white noise as the information increases in complexity. After he refines his listening in white noise, we will introduce cafeteria-type noise that contains a mixture of environmental sounds and speech. *Tuning out* competing linguistic information is a much more difficult task than simply listening in white noise.

✔ As his listening skills develop in the presence of various kinds of noise in the sessions, he will have more successful listening experiences with competing stimuli in various settings.

✔ In school, make sure Chase has an appropriate FM system.

---

through rhyming words, and challenging Chase's listening skills in the presence of noise. Expressive language and speech production were targeted throughout the session.

Chase is making good progress in receptive and expressive language. He demonstrates the ability to discriminate between rhyming words that differ in manner, place, and voicing of the initial consonant, which is an important readiness skill for reading. He comprehends increasingly longer and more difficult *strings of information* in the presence of noise. His speech intelligibility is improving, and I expect him to master /g/ and /l/ soon.

In August 1997, exactly two years and one month after receiving his cochlear implant, Chase will enter a mainstream kindergarten for five-year-olds at his local public school. He is a highly motivated child and, with the support of his family, friends, and the professionals on "Chase's team," this kid is on a roll!

Lesson Plan for Jason

Nancy S. Caleffe-Schenck, M.Ed., CED, CCC-A, Cert. AVT

One of the most powerful tools used to enrich Jason's development is children's literature. This lesson plan shows how to integrate specific goals for Jason by using one book. This may stand as one full lesson or be abbreviated and included as part of another.

Learning through Literature: *Brown Bear, Brown Bear, What Do You See?*

Brown Bear, Brown Bear, What Do You See? by Bill Martin, Jr., with illustrations by Eric Carle, is a popular book found in many classrooms and homes around the world. The text of the book is repetitive in that the same question is asked throughout: *What do you see?* The response is: *I see a _____ looking at me.* Examples of animals seen in the book are: a red bird, a yellow duck, a white dog. This book may be adapted for use with children with cochlear implants at various stages of development. For younger children, toy props representing the animals in the book are very useful. These props assist in maintaining a child's interest and promote the integration of audition, speech, language, cognition, and communication. For example, a stuffed yellow duck can be related to a plastic duck and to pictures and puzzle pieces. For an older preschooler, an abstract item such as a bottle cap can represent the duck. The goal is that language such as *yellow duck,* learned through listening, represents to Jason a wide array of impressions, ranging from something he sees on a pond to something he talks about in a conversation with a peer or adult.

PREREQUISITE SKILLS

Brown Bear, Brown Bear may be used to develop the foundations of listening, language, speech, or cognition. Jason has had experience and exposure to children's books as a pleasant and successful way of interacting with his parents, teachers, and therapist. He has been reading *Brown Bear* by memorizing the repetitive phrases and using the pictures as cues. He has learned to attend to, discriminate, imitate, and identify the *learning to listen* sounds and the words associated with these sounds. For example, when he hears a *bark* like a dog, Jason imitates the sound that he hears and associates the sound and word with the family dog, the neighbor's dog, toy dogs, and pictures of dogs. He spontaneously says *dog*. He monitors his speech by listening, *so that it sounds like the speech he hears*. For example, if Jason substitutes /g/ for /d/ when saying the word *dog,* he changes his speech from /gog/ to /dog/ after an adult models the target sound by babbling /da da dog/ while Jason listens. If Jason does not correctly self-monitor his speech for sounds that he previously used, it may indicate that his speech processor needs to be reprogrammed. Jason has developed an auditory memory for three items and shows what he remembers by picking up three toys in correct order. He participates in barrier games by putting the correct toy *in the water* or *under the blanket*. He knows the vocabulary for the color words used in *Brown Bear.* He enjoys coming to therapy and going to school.

MATERIALS
- animal stamps and stamp pad.
- a colorful gift bag.
- the book, *Brown Bear, Brown Bear, What Do You See?*
- small toys to represent animals in the story: a brown bear, a red bird, a yellow duck, a blue horse, a green frog, a purple cat, a white dog, a black sheep, a goldfish, a mother, and children. (You may paint, color with magic marker, or dye the toys if you cannot find them in the right color, such as a purple cat or blue horse.)
- flannel board figures or colored pictures pasted on popsicle sticks may be substituted or used in addition to the props.
- construction paper (blue to represent the pond and green for the pasture), green tissue paper and/or play dough for the forest; popsicle sticks to use as tree trunks, fences for the pasture and puppet handles; a cardboard box decorated as a house; and a pair of scissors.
- a tape recorder and/or language master.
- the book, *Good Dog Carl.*
- pictures of real animals (from nature and animal magazines).
- baby animal books and/or "go together" cards.
- a stuffed teddy bear.
- markers and 8 1/2" x 11" paper (folded in half to make a book).
- 3" x 5" index cards.

GOALS

Audition:
- to self-monitor speech through listening.
- to process descriptions and directions.
- to listen through an electronic sound source (tape recorder and language master).
- to increase distance hearing.
- to extend auditory sequential memory (remember items in correct order) to four items.
- to use auditory closure to complete a repetitive sentence, such as, *I see a _____ looking at me* or *Sheep, horse, and cow are all farm animals.*
- to remember the song, *Teddy Bear, Teddy Bear, Turn Around.*

Speech:
- to integrate speech targets /l/ and /t/ into conversation.
- to improve pitch in singing.

Language:
- to understand and verbalize descriptions.
- to use the question form, *What do you [verb]?* (verb= see, hear, eat, wear, etc.).
- to use final /s/ for third-person singular verb tense.
- to follow various directions.
- to understand the question forms, *What do you [verb] with?* and *What [verb]s?*
- to understand and remember a made-up story.
- to create and to tell a story using props or pictures.
- to integrate reading, writing, and spoken communication.
- to rhyme words and phrases.
- to expand vocabulary (*in front of, pond, pasture, graze, quickly, safe, stripe, carton, cub, duckling, foal, tadpole, lamb*).

Cognition:
- to visualize a story.
- to use props to put on a play.
- to discuss how things are the same or different.
- to understand *real* versus *pretend*.
- to categorize animals by labels (*pets, wild, or farm animals*) and by where they live (*house, forest, pasture, pond*).

Conversation:
- to request assistance.
- to inquire or to ask for additional information.

Introduction to the Lesson

Jason, his mother and I greet each other and have a short, friendly discussion. I inquire about the week and the carryover of last week's goals and jot notes from this parent report. I glance quickly through the back-and-forth book from his classroom teacher. I present the six Ling sounds and a variety of others (e.g., /h/, /p/, /w/, /f/, /ou/, /n/, /l/, /t/) close to him and at a distance. Jason identifies these sounds. I feel that he is hearing appropriately, and we are ready to begin the lesson.

All activities are presented first through listening only.

Speech Stamps

We practice speech babbling from auditory cues for the sounds /l/ and /t/. Jason stamps an animal onto paper after each imitation. First I provide the model, then his mother presents a model, so that she develops confidence and a good ear for judging his productions. The phoneme /l/ is repeated in the final position in syllables using different vowels (e.g., ululul, alalal), next in the middle (e.g., ala, alee, ula), then in the beginning (e.g., la, lu , lee, lay). Words with /l/ from the lesson are practiced (e.g., pull, yellow, looking, listen, purple) and put into sentences (e.g., I see a yellow duck looking at me). When his production of /l/ is not correct, I put it back into babble through listening as we did at the start of this activity. We continue in a similar way with /t/. This time, we start the babble with /t/ in the beginning position of syllables, next in the middle, then at the end. Again, we practice the sound in words (e.g., purple cat) and sentences/questions (e.g., Purple cat, purple cat, what do you see?). Before finishing this activity, Jason imitates syllables with alternating consonants (e.g., talu, latee). The stamps are put away and his stamped picture is put beside his backpack.

Colorful Bag

I pull out a colorful gift bag containing the toy props for the story. I describe the toy before I reveal what it is. "It's an animal that lives on a farm. We get wool from him."

Jason responds. "Horse?"

I continue, "No, we don't get wool from a horse. The baby is called a lamb and it says baa."

He guesses, "Sheep?"

Jason's mom models for him to repeat, "Is it a sheep?" She takes a turn describing a toy, then Jason takes a turn. We put the props on the table.

I get out the book, *Brown Bear.* We take turns reading from the book. We put each question/sentence on a language master card: *Brown bear, brown bear, what do you see?* After we finish the book, I shuffle the language master cards. Jason plays back a card, matches it to the page in the book, and lines up the toys in an animal parade. After all the cards are put back in order, we play them again and verify what we hear by the order of the animal parade. Jason completes this activity with ease.

I ask his mother to move away from the table and even out of the room and say, "What does the yellow duck see?"

Jason practices distance hearing and responds, "The yellow duck see the blue horse."

I ask Jason to listen as I acoustically highlight the final /s/ for the present verb tense. *"Sees.* The yellow duck *sees* the blue horse."

Jason listens and corrects himself. His /l/ in *yellow* was a good production, and I comment on this. We continue with a few more questions from a distance.

Changing the Scene

Now it is time to change the scene. I take out blue and green construction paper. I ask Jason, "What do you cut with?" He relies on the context and answers correctly. I continue with, "What cuts?" He's not sure how to answer, so I refer to his mother.

She replies, "Scissors." I encourage her to continue to name something else that cuts.

At that point Jason understands and adds, "knife."

I model, "A knife cuts" (third person /s/). I direct him to cut the blue paper into a big circle to make a pond. I explain that a pond has water in it. The green paper is the grass, or pasture, where the farm animals *graze.* Jason is learning new vocabulary in the context of play related to the book. I direct Mom to *put the goldfish in front of the purple cat.* I ask Jason to *put the red bird in front of the dog.* He does this. I then encourage auditory memory development and tell him to *put the yellow duck and green frog on the pond and the blue horse in the pasture.* He places the duck and frog and picks up the blue horse, but doesn't remember what to do with the horse. I put the toys in the line again and repeat the entire sentence, but this time I add, "The pasture has green grass." He then puts all the toys where they belong. His mother gives a direction, then Jason gives a direction.

A New Story

I move the red bird and white dog in front of Jason and push the other toys to the far end of the table. I ask him to listen to a new story that I made up about the red bird and white dog:

"The red bird was enjoying the spring day. She was looking for worms for her baby bird. The white dog started barking, then chased the red bird. The red bird flew away quickly. She was safe, but the white dog was hungry!"

Jason's mom repeats the story and acts it out, using the toys. Jason takes a turn. He forgets a part of the story. I encourage his mother to wait for him to ask for our help instead of coming to his rescue. He looks at us and shrugs. I model for him to ask his mother, "What's the next part? I forget."

He repeats, "Whas nek? I forget."

I do not correct his speech when he omits /t/ in the words *what's* and *next*. These are consonant blends and a challenging target for him. At this moment I want him to ask for help. We don't want to discourage him by working on several new targets within one interaction. I reinforce by repeating the model and encouraging him to ask if he needs help. "What's the next part? I forget. That's great that you asked us for help when you needed it."

I ask him to record his story on the tape recorder while using the microphone. He enjoys talking into the microphone. His mother tapes the same story right after his recording. We listen to the two recordings of the story. I explain to him and Mom that he can make up a story at home using a few of his toys.

Auditory Pick-Me-Up

It is time to put these toys away and go on to a different activity. This is a wonderful opportunity for Jason to remember single items. Using auditory-only cues, I ask him to put four of the many toys on the table into the gift bag. He picks up all the right toys and in the correct order. Next, I ask him for five toys. He needs some coaching for this.

Extension Activities

For the remainder of the session, I demonstrate for Jason and his mother some extension activities they can try during the week. *Good Dog Carl* by Alexandra Day is a picture story without words and continues the dog theme. I turn to a picture, but do not show it to Jason or his mom. It is a colored illustration of a big, black dog named Carl who is sitting down with a carton of milk in his mouth. A baby with blue-and-white striped pajamas is sitting under Carl's mouth holding a cup. The milk is spilling right into the baby's cup. I tell Jason that I am going to describe the picture to him. I ask him to *take a picture in his mind* of the picture I am describing. If he closes his eyes, it is easier for him to take the picture. I explain in detail what I see. I describe the characters, what they look like, what they are wearing, their expressions, the colors in the picture, the action, and so on. Jason and Mom visualize what the picture looks like. They ask me questions to get a better picture, such as *What color is the baby's eyes?* I show them the picture and we discuss how it is the same or different from what they saw in their mind. This strategy will help Jason remember stories and recall details.

Photographs

Since we are looking at pictures, I take out the photographs I have collected of *real* animals. We compare these with *pretend* animals such as illustrations from *Brown Bear,* toy props, and stuffed animals.

Go-Together Puzzle

I get out my baby animal go-together puzzle. As Jason matches the puzzle-piece pairs, his mother and I provide the new vocabulary, such as: *tadpole, foal, duckling,* and *cub.*

Let's Move Away

Jason has been sitting for a long session, so we move away from the table. We set up a forest in one corner of the room using green tissue paper or play dough and popsicle sticks for tree trunks. The blue construction paper pond and green paper pasture are set up in other corners. The cardboard house is *built on a hill* (a chair). Jason sorts the props from *Brown Bear* according to where the animals live. I then sit down beside him and say, "Dogs, cats, and goldfish are all _____" (pets). "They live in a _____" (house). I encourage Jason to use the context to complete the auditory closure activity. We continue with additional incomplete sentences.

Teddy Bear, Teddy Bear

I bring out the teddy bear. Jason's mom and I sing the song as Jason helps the teddy bear act out the song:

"Teddy bear, teddy bear, turn around. Teddy bear, teddy bear, touch the ground.

Teddy bear, teddy bear, tie your shoe. Teddy bear, teddy bear, I love you.

Teddy bear, teddy bear, go upstairs. Teddy bear, teddy bear, say your prayers.

Teddy bear, teddy bear, turn out the lights. Teddy bear, teddy bear, say good-night."

I return to the question form, *What does he [verb] with?* (walk, kiss, touch). This is an opportunity to reinforce the third-person singular tense: *He kisses with his lips. He touches with his hand (or paw).* The *-es* in *touches* is easier for Jason than the /s/ in *walks,* because it is the /z/ sound within an extra syllable.

Back to the Drawing Board

It is important that Jason understand the relationships among reading, writing, and spoken communication. We return to the table and I show him how to write a book by folding several sheets of paper in half, deciding on a title and repetitive phrases, and using one illustration per page. I give him a few examples for titles, such as *Furniture, Furniture, What Do You See?* He decides on *Children, Children, What Do You Eat?* He initially uses the repetitive answer *I eat color + food* (red apples). I suggest that his mom encourage more descriptive adjectives, such as *crunchy* carrots, *shiny* apples, *creamy* yogurt.

Rhyme Time

We finish the session with a game to reinforce a rhyming word unit from school. On 3"x5" cards I have written selected words from *Brown Bear:* cat, frog, sheep, fish, bear, mother. Jason, with assistance from his mother, writes words or phrases that rhyme: fat, log, keep, dish, wear, brother. We play a quick game of Concentration using the rhyme pairs. I give Jason the cards for playing Concentration while his mother and I talk, and he takes them home.

Parent Guidance

Jason's mother and I review the goals and activities of the session. I rate his *glows* (what he did well on) and *grows* (what he needs to work on). She writes in her notebook as we talk. His mom will share this information with Jason's classroom teacher.

I suggest activities related to the goals and remind Jason's mom to proceed from simple to complex, known to unknown, and concrete to abstract.

✔ Look at the *I Spy* books by Walter Wick and Jean Marzollo. Describe things to look for.

✔ Play I Spy with descriptions and rhyme words.

✔ Set up scenes with toys or complete household routines, such as setting the table or grocery shopping, by following four- or five-item auditory directions.

✔ Play Simon Says using four or five directions together.

✔ Play a scavenger-hunt game where Jason finds objects for the question forms *What do you [verb] with?* (pound, peel, sweep) and *What [verb]s?* (rings, scrapes, twists).

✔ Dictate, write, and act out home-made stories.

✔ Describe an image, ask Jason to *take a picture in your mind,* then have him draw a simple picture to match the description. Compare this with the stimulus picture.

✔ Discuss whether pictures, stories, movies are *real* or *pretend.*

✔ Sing and act out the song, *Teddy Bear, Teddy Bear Turn Around.*

✔ Finish his *Children, Children, What Do You Eat?* as a home-made book. The activity will be fun if Jason can taste the foods he mentions in his book.

✔ Take a walk through the neighborhood or a zoo, or visit a farm. Discuss what you observe. For example, if you see a dog limping, talk about how he may have gotten hurt. Relate this to other dogs you have read about. Talk about how the dog is the same or different from the dogs in the Walt Disney movie *Homeward Bound.*

✔ Discuss the diversity of the children pictured at the end of *Brown Bear* (race, color, sex, age, and size). Explain that everyone is different and wonderfully special.

(cont'd on next page)

Parent Guidance *(cont'd)*

✔ Listen for carryover of the speech targets /l/ and /t/. Model correct speech without interrupting communication.

✔ Review new vocabulary presented this week by *mailing* the word into a box with a slot in it. Keep a list of words that crop up that he does not know.

✔ Visit the local library to find books that extend the ideas in *Brown Bear.*

Summary

The success of using children's literature as the basis for Jason's auditory development depends on:

- following appropriate stages of development which provide successful auditory experiences for Jason.
- being clear about the goals.
- incorporating several different auditory levels within the same activity (e.g., self-monitoring, memory, processing, and understanding).
- integrating audition, speech, language, cognition, and communication at all levels.
- utilizing books and materials in creative and satisfying experiences that are meaningful to Jason.
- empowering Jason's parents and teachers to incorporate meaningful auditory interactions throughout the day.

Related Books

• *Sam's Teddy Bear* by B. Lindgren is a simple book to read with one picture per page. It is clever to act out. The only props needed are a teddy bear and stuffed dog. Jason can be Sam.

• *The Boy with a Drum,* a Little Golden Book, has language that is repetitive with many of the same characters as *Brown Bear:* cat, frog, dog, horse. The lyrics rhyme and the drum says *rat-a-tat-tat,* which allows for carryover of the /t/ speech target.

• *Go, Dog, Go!* by P.D. Eastman has a 75-word vocabulary. Different colored dogs (red, blue, and green) play and work together in silly ways.

(cont'd on next page)

Related Books *(cont'd)*

• *Polar Bear, Polar Bear, What Do You Hear?* by Bill Martin, Jr. and Eric Carle is a logical follow-up to *Brown Bear*. Zoo animals hear interesting sounds made by other animals (hissing, trumpeting, snarling). The repetitive phrases and illustrations resemble those in *Brown Bear*.

• *The Very Hungry Caterpillar* by Eric Carle continues the study of books by the same author. It shows a vivid and colorful transformation of the caterpillar into a butterfly.

• *The Greedy Python* by Richard Buckley and Eric Carle is a story with animals as characters. There are complex sentences, using the relative clause *that*. We do not expect Jason to be using this language yet, but the exposure is appropriate for his age.

• *Baby Animals, A Change-a-Picture Book* by Larry Shapiro, distributed through Discovery Toys, is an interactive book that provides general information about baby animals. Jason can turn a ribbon for each page and watch the transformations: caterpillar → butterfly; tadpole → frog, and egg → fish.

• *Alphabears* by Kathleen and Michael Hague fits in well with the teddy bear theme. There are rhyming phrases and letter-to-word associations (e.g., *A is for Amanda*). This book can serve as an introduction to the other excellent books by the Hagues.

• *Quick as a Cricket* by Audrey and Don Wood provides adjectives associated with animals (e.g., *weak as a kitten, gentle as a lamb*). It is a child-centered introduction to analogies and similes (e.g., *I'm as brave as a tiger*).

• *Berenstain Bears First Time Books* (e.g., *Too Much TV, Learn About Strangers*) by Stan and Jan Berenstain are thoughtful and practical stories about challenges faced by a pretend bear family.

• *Berenstain Bears Chapter Books* (e.g., *Gotta Dance*) by Stan and Jan Berenstain are enjoyable books for children who know the family and are ready to read chapter books.

• Nonfiction books such as *How Animals Sleep* by Millicent Selsam include general information and facts about the animals in *Brown Bear* (e.g., *Does a goldfish sleep?*). The answers can be read to Jason to develop his memory, processing, and understanding of general information.

• *Ranger Rick*, a monthly magazine from the National Wildlife Federation, is an entertaining and informative periodical about wildlife. Jason would appreciate receiving these at home each month or looking at them at the library.

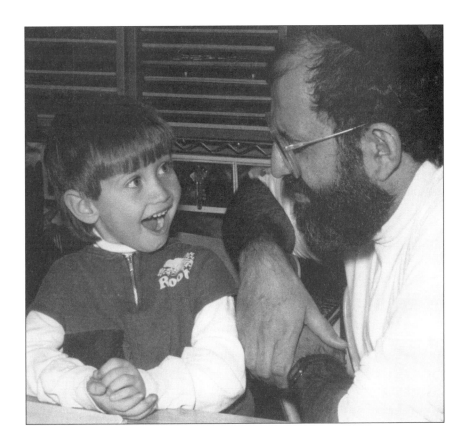

PART IV

Family Stories from Around the World

Lewis

Dianne Blair

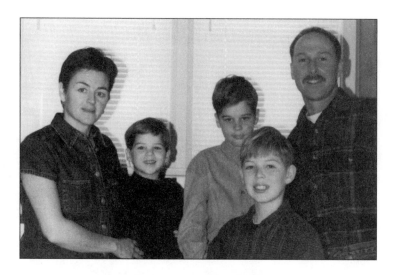

Lewis Blair (centre left) and family

The other night I watched the movie *Before and After*, starring Meryl Streep and Liam Neeson. Although this movie has absolutely nothing to do with deafness or my son Lewis's story, I was struck by the opening narration.

> Your whole life can change in a second and you never even know when it's coming. Before, you think you know what kind of world this is and after, everything is different for you. Not bad maybe, not always, but different, forever. I didn't used to know that till the day it happened for my family. I didn't even know there could be such a thing as "after." I didn't know that for us, "before" was already over.

Our "after" began on a Saturday morning in July four years ago, when Lewis, at seven months, woke up with a fever. Lewis is the youngest of our sons, and we'd been through enough childhood illnesses not to be particularly concerned. He was irritable that day and not interested in his favorite mashed bananas. I was still nursing him, and he continued to nurse well throughout the afternoon and evening.

The following day, even though his fever was down, I called our local hospital emergency department. They said to bring him in if I was concerned.

At the hospital, Lewis's temperature was slightly elevated. The doctor told us he probably had the flu, and sent us home with a prescription for an antibiotic. As Sunday wore on, I became anxious: Lewis didn't seem like himself, appearing agitated and irritable. His cry was unusual, and he practically slept through his evening bath. I had planned to wait until the next morning to take him to our family doctor, but as I got ready for bed around 11 o'clock, my husband Kelly gave me the push I needed to take Lewis back to emergency, saying that I would feel reassured having him examined again.

Another doctor examined Lewis this time, and it soon became clear from her questions that this was something more than flu. The doctor wanted to send him to the Children's Hospital in London, Ontario by ambulance. She thought it was meningitis. I asked no questions, but called Kelly and told him to meet us in London. Lewis cried all the way in the ambulance.

At the hospital in London, a lumbar puncture confirmed that Lewis indeed had meningitis. Kelly and I sat in the waiting room, stunned and silent, while many people came and went from Lewis's examining room.

We had sat in a hospital waiting room like this before. Seven years before Lewis was born we lost our first child, a little girl. She was stillborn at full term, and the cause was never known. Now, those same feelings — shock, disbelief, pounding heart, agitation, nausea, shaking — were all too familiar. But as the examining room door opened and we rose from our chairs, we were both calm. Yes, it was meningitis. They would start an antibiotic immediately... at least a 10-day hospital stay... complications... side effects. I didn't hear too much after that.

Lewis was taken to a private room and an IV was started. He was put on a heart monitor. Kelly went home around 3 a.m. I held Lewis a lot that night, rocked him in a rocking chair, sang to him, nursed him, and tried to comfort him.

Kelly, who is a teacher, was then on summer holidays and so was able to be at home to look after our two older boys, Sam, who was 6, and Liam, who was 5. When he arrived at the hospital the next day, I drove home, relieved the babysitter, and packed some clothes for a 10-day hospital stay. I took Sam and Liam back to the hospital with me, where Kelly was waiting for us near the entrance. Lewis was having difficulty breathing and had been moved to the Critical Care Unit.

Capped and gowned, we walked into the CCU, where Lewis was in an oxygen tent. Part of his head had been shaved and he was on an IV. His eyes were closed, he was hooked up to monitors, and a nurse was watching his vital signs.

I slept on and off during that night and frequently went in to see Lewis, but I couldn't hold or nurse him.

The following day the doctors felt that Lewis was stable enough to move back to the floor. Once he was out of the CCU, I felt that everything would be fine. Although Lewis seemed weak and lethargic, he was nursing again and didn't seem to be as agitated. There were many tests, many groups of residents to examine Lewis, and many questions asked. It was confirmed that Lewis had pneumococcal meningitis, the second most common type of meningitis in children under the age of two, stemming from a very common bacterium that causes illnesses such as strep throat.

Friday of that week I sat nursing Lewis in a rocking chair when I felt his legs suddenly stiffen. His eyes rolled backwards, and his left arm and leg began to twitch. He was having a seizure. I shouted to a passing nurse, who came on the run. The seizure lasted less than a minute, and within the hour Lewis was sedated and having a CT scan. The doctor told us there were some irregularities, some dark areas on Lewis's scan, but they couldn't say what that meant. They started an antiseizure medication, and the pediatric neurologist arrived. Reassuringly, she told us that further CT scans would be done and that most infants recovered, or made adjustments to the damaged areas of the brain.

Ten days after hospital admission, we were feeling that maybe we were in the clear. Lewis could probably go home in a few days. Subsequent scans were clear, and the IV antibiotic was finished. An audiologist came to do an auditory brainstem response (ABR) test. Lewis was sedated. I was certain that there was nothing wrong with his hearing!

When we returned from lunch, Lewis was still asleep and the audiologist said, "I didn't get the results I wanted. There was no response to the limits of the equipment. More tests are required. We suspect at least a severe hearing loss." We were stunned. The otolaryngologist came later and briskly sketched an audiogram on the back of a piece of paper. Then he was gone.

A World without Sound

Although the doctors had mentioned the possibility, deafness was the farthest thing from our minds. Instead, we had feared physical handicaps, brain damage, seizures. That day I stared out the window of the hospital room at the cars moving silently along the road and wondered what a world without sound would be like. I thought of Lewis, no longer able to hear familiar sounds, the sound of my voice, the squeak of his favorite toy. I had seen the movie *Children of a Lesser God*. I recalled many years earlier being in a coffee shop when a man approached and handed me a card stating that he was deaf and asking if I would buy something from him. That was my total experience with deafness.

Lewis was examined by a pediatric ophthalmologist because his eye muscles had been weakened by the meningitis. His eyes needed patching alternately for three hours a day over six weeks, when he would be reexamined. We left the hospital two days later with prescriptions, instructions, follow-up appointments, and Lewis.

I wish now that I had kept a journal of my thoughts and feelings at that time. It's difficult to remember everything. But I do recall feeling sad coming home... as though someone had died.

Home Again

We were back in our familiar surroundings, yet everything had changed. In Lewis's room there was a favorite mobile hanging over his crib that played Brahms's lullaby; it had hung over all our children's cribs. I was sad to think that he couldn't hear it now. I wanted to take it down, but left it up — just in case the hearing tests had been wrong.

Lewis had been admitted to hospital on July 26 and discharged August 6. He was to return for further hearing tests on September 1. The wait seemed interminable.

Kelly brought home books about deafness from the library. One was *Choices in Deafness*. We began to inform ourselves about the different approaches to educating children who are deaf. We read encouraging stories about children learning to listen and speak, even those with profound hearing losses. We were heartened, but we still hoped the first hearing test was wrong.

Hearing Aids

When we returned to the hospital in September, Lewis had made a good physical recovery. He was sitting up by himself again; there had been no further seizures, and he was eating and sleeping well. We had repeatedly conducted our own hearing tests — loud music, pots and pans, shouting, banging on doors. Lewis had not responded. I sat with him in the audiology booth that morning as the sounds became louder and louder. Lewis didn't respond. The audiologist said little. She sent us for another ABR and referred us to a hearing-aid dispenser. Lewis was tired and irritable, fell asleep during the ABR, and continued to sleep right through the making of his earmold impressions. The degree of his hearing loss was not confirmed. He was young and would require further testing with his hearing aids.

A month later, the audiologist put the hearing aids on and did some tests, but Lewis still didn't show any reliable responses. She assured me that it would take a while for him to adjust to the hearing aids and begin to respond to sound.

We began a program with a teacher of the deaf, from our provincial Ministry of Education, who came to our home once a week. She was an important source of support and information during those early days. We were confused by the conflicting information and uncertain about which communication approach to follow. Subsequent tests showed that Lewis had very little hearing in the speech range. As he was only nine months old, we didn't feel pressured to choose a method of communication. Looking back now, I know that we wasted valuable time in that first year. We struggled with Lewis to keep the hearing aids in; the feedback from them drove me crazy! When I complained to the audiologist, she said, "Just turn them down." We soon found a compassionate, knowledgeable, and skilled audiologist who was highly recommended by many parents. He spent two hours with us at the first appointment, explaining the testing, talking about the results, and answering all our questions.

Lewis's hearing loss was confirmed: a left-corner audiogram. More powerful hearing aids were prescribed; earmolds were made of a material to provide a better seal, so the appropriate volume could be used. There was still little benefit.

Like most parents of children who are deaf, we wanted Lewis to be able to speak intelligibly and function in a hearing world, but his hearing loss was very profound. I felt we would probably need a total communication (TC) approach. We wanted to be able to communicate with Lewis as effectively and efficiently as possible. The stories I had read about the auditory-verbal approach felt intimidating: it seemed to require extraordinary efforts from the families, especially the mothers. I felt very much like an average mom, and I questioned my ability. We did, however, investigate this approach, and finally decided to give it a go.

Auditory-Verbal Therapy

Kelly and I drove two hours to a Toronto hospital to talk about auditory-verbal therapy with the staff there. I still remember the five children I saw that first day at the clinic. The little three- and four-year-olds listened intently and worked hard. Their committed parents scribbled down notes and actively participated. The last child that day was a seven-year-old girl with a profound hearing loss. I played a game of "Guess Who" with her; her speech was excellent. Driving home that night, I thought, "I can probably do this."

We began the program in September 1993, when Lewis was 20 months old. The therapist helped us to gain confidence and direction, by listening to our story and our concerns.

We have kept almost all our auditory-verbal sessions on videotape. When I look back at Lewis's first therapy session now, I am struck by how small he was and how little he heard! Yet, in our first session, I was amazed at how quickly Lewis learned the routines and expectations. The therapist engaged him for 50 minutes with the *learning to listen* sounds, musical clowns and clocks, chimes, clickers, songs, and games. Lewis was attentive and willing to participate, and I went home with notes, ideas, and instructions! We attended weekly therapy sessions for several months and followed up with daily lessons at home. During this time, however, we saw no real responses to sound and no changes in Lewis's auditory or verbal behavior. We began to feel discouraged.

After several months, Lewis's therapist expressed concern about his lack of auditory responses and language development, and questioned his suitability to the auditory-verbal approach. He suggested that Lewis might benefit from a cochlear implant.

The Cochlear Implant

We had heard about cochlear implants and had even seen a story about them on the TV program *60 Minutes*. But that was New York City! The operation seemed inaccessible and unattainable. However, we soon learned that the surgery was being done at three hospitals in Ontario, two of which were fairly close to our home.

We read everything we could, including research studies published in current journals. We scheduled an appointment with the audiologist from the nearest implant team to discuss the assessment process.

Although the implant was FDA approved for children over the age of two, the nearest hospital was not a pediatric hospital, and children's programs there began at three years of age. Lewis was not yet two, so we had an entire year in which to consider the decision of surgery. However, we felt that Lewis could not continue without language, so we began to introduce him to some sign language.

In November 1993, we completed a questionnaire and were introduced to the candidate selection process. We had many questions; most had to do with the risk of surgery, the reliability of the device, and the long-term effects of implant use. The assessment process seemed very long: there were many hearing tests, a hearing-aid evaluation, a medical evaluation, a speech and language assessment, and a three-month trial with different amplification devices. There would be a CT scan, perhaps another ABR, and evaluations by a psychologist and a social worker.

We also attended a parent workshop, where we heard encouraging stories from a panel of parents whose children had cochlear implants, and one adult who has a implant. These accounts were more affirming than all our reading of articles and information from the professionals. It was exciting to learn about these children's progress in hearing, listening, and talking. The adult user spoke of how the implant had brought her "back into the world of the truly living" after years of social isolation resulting from her deafness. We were inspired.

At our next appointment we asked the audiologist about an earlier surgery date. She explained that that decision would be made by the surgeon. We presented our arguments to the doctor: this was a critical period for Lewis's language development; we would have to introduce sign language if surgery was a year away, and we preferred him to have access to spoken language as quickly as possible. The surgeon agreed.

Before Lewis's second birthday in December 1993, we had a commitment from the implant team that Lewis's surgery could be done when his assessment was completed. We were able to forgo the three-month trial with other amplification, as Lewis had been wearing hearing aids for more than a year and had had months of auditory-verbal therapy. The CT scan showed that his cochleae were clear of ossification, and we made it through the psychological evaluation. Lewis's candidacy for the implant was approved, and his surgery was scheduled for Tuesday, March 15, 1994. School was in recess that week, so Kelly could be at home while I stayed at the hospital with Lewis.

As with most parents, our biggest concern was, of course, the surgery. Our child had already been critically ill; why put him at risk again? We knew that the risks of the surgery were statistically low, but we had been beaten by the odds three times before: first in losing a child, second in having a child develop meningitis, and third in having that child lose his hearing. After such experiences, risk factors and statistics have little meaning.

Surgery

We couldn't sleep the night before the surgery. The next day, we awoke to a world covered in ice: freezing rain had fallen all night. Our babysitter's garage door was frozen shut, so Kelly scraped the ice off our car and went to pick her up. We were supposed to be in the hospital admitting room at 7:30 a.m. We didn't leave home until 7:00, and the hospital was an hour away. The roads were treacherous, with cars slipping and sliding off the road. We drove slowly and silently to the hospital, arriving at almost 8:30. Lewis's surgery was scheduled for 9:00. We went directly to the lab for blood and urine tests, and then quickly ran to surgery. Maybe the rushing was a good thing: we didn't have much time to worry about the day's events. The surgeon spoke reassuringly to us, and the anesthesiologist carried our unconcerned and unaware Lewis into surgery.

I felt quite calm, but Kelly was upset as we sat down for the long wait. The surgeon came out about 11:45. Everything had gone well. There was some ossification, but all 22 electrodes had been inserted, and Lewis was in the recovery room. About an hour later Lewis came out of the anesthetic. He had a huge gauze bandage wrapped around the right side of his head and across his right eye. He received an injection for pain and nausea, and he slept on and off most of that day. I stayed with him as he slept comfortably through the night.

Lewis recovered quickly. As we all drove home two days later, his hat came off taking his bandage with it, revealing his incision for all to see. For once in their lives, Sam and Liam were speechless. Lewis won a new respect from his two older brothers that day!

Turning On the Implant

Seven weeks later, Lewis's implant was switched on. His stitches had been removed, his incision had healed well, and his hair was growing back. The programming went slowly, and Lewis's responses were inconsistent. The initial stimulation was unremarkable, with Lewis showing little response to the sounds he was receiving. Why did I expect him to turn in response to his name on that first day? We went frequently for MAPping over the next six months. Lewis eventually learned the routine, although he was not always cooperative.

Return to Therapy

We started back to auditory-verbal therapy in June 1994. Looking back, I am amazed at the difference the implant made in such a short time. In his first therapy session Lewis responded consistently to play audiometry at the sound of a drum, a horn, a clacker, and speech. In the second lesson he was vocalizing "ahh" for the airplane, clicking his teeth for the sound of the horse, and waving at the words "bye-bye." This was amazing because, in four months of therapy with his hearing aids, Lewis had never vocalized for any of the *learning to listen* sounds, and most of his responses in play audiometry had been inconsistent. He quickly learned the expectations of play audiometry, began to say some sounds, and relearned the rules of therapy. We played with many noise-making activities, always alerting Lewis to sounds by pointing to our ears; we made *learning to listen* games and overall, had an exciting summer. Lewis was now spontaneously responding to many sounds: the lawn mower, the ringing of the telephone, the beeping of the microwave and, most rewardingly, the sound of his name!

By September, he was saying "bye-bye," "up," "no," and "mum," and making approximations for other words. We have never looked back. When I look through my notes and Lewis's Experience Book from that first year of therapy, I am astonished at how much he accomplished. In four months, Lewis went from hearing and saying nothing to speaking in three-word phrases.

Lewis was three-and-a-half years old when we began to consider the next step: a preschool program for the coming year. We looked at mainstream day-care centers and preschool programs for children who are hearing impaired, and after much consideration, chose a preschool in a school board outside our own, as ours provided few services for children who are deaf. Further, our local day-care centers had little or no experience with deafness or with children with cochlear implants, and they seemed busy and loud places. I wondered if Lewis would hear anything in that environment compared to a program with strong emphasis on speech and language development and a ratio of one teacher and an assistant to three children. Our choice meant that Lewis had a 50-minute taxi ride twice a day; he went to school four mornings a week, and we continued with auditory-verbal therapy.

Throughout the second year post implant, Lewis's speech improved, his vocabulary increased, and his grasp of language steadily expanded. As Lewis grew and became more independent, his therapy sessions were becoming more difficult. His therapist has always referred to Lewis as "a little challenge and a gift!" At this time, although Lewis seldom became angry or defiant, he would often lose interest, look around the room, or pretend he was tired. He needed much encouragement and refocusing to complete a task. When sessions at home also became difficult, I turned the job over to my husband, who has more patience and was usually able to obtain Lewis's cooperation.

At school the first year, Lewis needed much more direction than the other children simply to attend and to complete an activity, especially if it was something he didn't want to do. These behaviors have become more pronounced as demands on him have increased, and I'm now convinced that he has been affected with yet another "handicapping condition" — Attention Deficit Disorder (ADD), which seems to be prevalent in the males in our family. We have not had him officially diagnosed, but I don't know that I need to have anyone tell me! This condition will probably be more challenging than his deafness.

Lewis is now attending a typical kindergarten program in the mornings and a program for children who are hearing impaired in the afternoons, and we continue weekly auditory-verbal therapy. The therapist and I are constantly looking for new ways to keep his attention and meet therapy goals. Lewis's articulation and speech are now quite good, and his auditory perception is excellent. Last night I called to him in the neighbors' yard, where he was playing behind a big cedar hedge and couldn't see me.

"Lewis," I called.

"What?" came the reply.

"Time for dinner."

Silence — had he heard me?

"I don't want any dinner."

I marveled at the cochlear implant technology, and then walked over to the neighbors' yard to engage in a five-minute argument, finally bribing Lewis home for dinner!

Life Goes On

The cochlear implant is a miraculous device, but most of the time we take it for granted when we put it on Lewis every morning. We didn't take it for granted, however, the day he fell out of a canoe at a friend's cottage. (We have since purchased a waterproof fanny pack.) Nor did we take it for granted on the Saturday evening (why is it always a weekend?) when the device stopped working because the speech processor had lost the MAP. Had the internal device failed? Would Lewis need more surgery? Could his device be reimplanted? Although I hope we never have to make that decision, I would not hesitate if reimplantation were necessary.

Of course, the cochlear implant is not a cure for deafness. At times, I think I tend to overemphasize my child's progress and understate the amount of work we've done to get there, complete with all the doubts, guilt, worry, and frustration. I'd like to believe that Lewis is going to hear and speak like the four-year old around the corner, that he'll go to the neighborhood school next year and, although he might not be an "A" student, that he'll struggle by. But this may not happen. It is a continuing process; we will be flexible and do what we think is best for Lewis and our family, just as we have in the past.

The Family

Lewis's deafness has been an experience for our entire family. Sam and Liam have been, and will continue to be, influenced — both for good and for ill — by this event. Time and patience have often been in short supply. Liam is now nine, and after listening to three years of Lewis's lessons, he has become an accomplished auditory-verbal therapist himself (though not yet certified). Although he pictures his future in the Canadian Coast Guard, I truly believe that Liam will in some way enter a field where hearing, speech, and language will play a significant part. Both Sam and Liam have been tremendous language models for Lewis. They have always been very verbal children, talking and reading early and having excellent vocabularies. Lewis is now learning language very naturally, and I'm often surprised — yes, even thrilled — to hear expressions such as, "What a piece of junk!" or, "Good-bye, you stupid!" Nothing makes me happier than to see Sam and Lewis sharing the Christmas catalog and talking about what they want for Christmas. I often wondered if this day would ever come. There are still plenty of frustrations, especially when Lewis can't express himself quickly enough, or the older boys are teasing him. The screaming begins, and they are all sent to their rooms. But this is a function of having three boys in the family, not necessarily of having a child who is deaf.

Lewis continues to make terrific progress, though I often feel that progress is slow and laborious, and wonder how we will overcome future obstacles. But I also wondered how he would ever make the transition from the *learning to listen* sounds to calling the animals by name! That was accomplished; I don't even remember when. The problems that once seemed insurmountable are insignificant or forgotten now.

In that same movie, *Before and After*, the closing narration went like this:

> I look at him now and I think about how different our lives might have been. And that's the saddest part of all. But lately, sometimes, I can feel myself starting to come alive again and it's scary, kind of. I don't know if that's even allowed. Maybe you can't expect to keep happiness out of your life forever, any more than trouble. Your whole life can change in a second and you never even know when it's coming.

Katie

Glynis Kilmartin

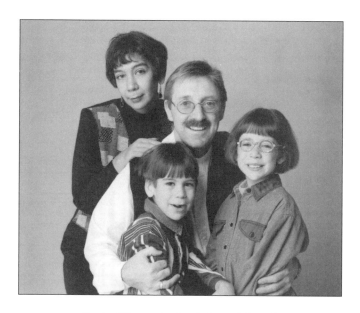

Katie Kilmartin (right) and family

One Special Kid

It is June 1995, exactly four years after our seven-and-a-half-year old daughter, Katie, received her cochlear implant. We're in the crowded gymnasium of our local school, and I'm fidgeting with a camera, getting ready to take her picture. Katie is about to receive the *Yes I Can* award for academic progress in math, from the Council for Exceptional Children. There's a huge lump in my throat, and I'm trying not to cry! She's sitting on the floor with my husband, John, at her side.

For a moment, I am lost in time, remembering another occasion: January 26, 1989, when our 14-month-old daughter and her father sat together, playing, in a waiting room. I sat to one side, fidgeting, waiting for the results of her first hearing test.

Now Katie stands and moves forward to receive her award, prompted by her father. The tears flow as I hurriedly start snapping.

"Profound Sensorineural Hearing Loss"

"...Severe-to-profound hearing loss." I'm staring blankly at the audiologist. She is instructing us to visit a hearing-aid dispenser and have molds made and hearing aids ordered. It's difficult to grasp what she is saying. John gets the details, and we set out for the earmold maker.

To say we were less than devastated by the results would be a gross understatement. We knew little about deafness and what it would mean for Katie. During the months that followed, she had other assessments and a brainstem response test, which confirmed a congenital, bilateral, profound sensorineural hearing loss.

Feelings

Those early months were an emotional roller coaster. We experienced feelings of sorrow, anger, fear, and depression. More than anything else, we were flooded with an overwhelming sense of *guilt* — we blamed ourselves. In retrospect, those were dark and confusing days. We eventually realized that in order to help Katie, we had to move forward and identify ways that would allow her to grow into a self-sufficient person.

Support

Joining the local chapter of a province-wide parent-support group proved to be our lifesaver. We got useful information on hearing impairment and its associated consequences. By attending a series of workshops organized by the group, we learned an enormous amount about aural, oral, and manual communication. One story in particular had a profound effect on us. A teenage boy spoke candidly, through an interpreter, about growing up hearing impaired. He told us he had been unable to "talk" to his father because his father had large hands and could not learn sign language! I went home that night and cried. It became clear to us then that, for our daughter to participate in the world as we knew it, she would need to use spoken language. Considering all available options, we chose an auditory-verbal program offered through a Toronto hospital.

Talk, Talk, Talk

Katie liked her weekly auditory-verbal lessons — she loved the attention and, of course, she played with great toys! We conducted our daily home lessons before we left for work and day care. At first, John and I felt self-conscious having to name every action or item that we touched, but gradually this became our way of life. Much of our time was spent walking around pointing and talking about everything in sight. We received our fair share of strange looks from passersby!

Change

Many changes occurred during that first year following Katie's diagnosis. We adjusted our work schedules to adapt to the weekly hospital visits. Katie's caregiver, a former Early Childhood Education teacher, was superb. She shared Katie's weekly lesson with all the children in her care. John and I began to feel that we had regained some control over our lives. He volunteered with the various parent-support committees. The parent-sharing meetings were invaluable — an opportunity to swap stories about whistling hearing aids and badly fitting earmolds, and to talk about the latest in hearing-aid technology. It felt comfortable to be in the company of others who shared the same experiences — to learn about coping strategies from parents with older children who were hearing impaired, and who were well on the road to integrating into their school settings and society.

Hardware Overload!

Katie continued to work enthusiastically through auditory-verbal therapy, but displayed a few signs of frustration in getting across her daily wants and needs. A breakthrough finally occurred in March 1990, when she managed to say a feeble "aaah" in response to a toy airplane. We were ecstatic; she'd "found" her voice, and she practiced that sound repeatedly.

Her monthly audiology tests produced inconsistent results. Although Katie understood the tasks, she just didn't hear! In August she received a tactile aid, and shortly after that an FM system was added. The hearing-aid dispenser, incredibly, managed to hook the systems together. The sight of our tiny, nearly three-year-old daughter wearing all this hardware was absurd, and we were not happy. She was, however, starting school in September — in an oral program for children who were hearing impaired — and needed all the help she could get.

By now, articles on cochlear implants had begun to surface. At the time of Katie's original diagnosis, an otolaryngologist told us that she would not be considered a candidate according to the criteria of the day. Some of the professionals we dealt with had conflicting feelings about this technology. We were interested! Although Katie had gained a few sounds in her repertoire, she mainly communicated through gestures, pointing, and lipreading.

We approached the cochlear implant center in London, Ontario. The team met with us and reviewed Katie's background. It was agreed that she appeared to be a likely implant candidate. However, funding for the Ontario program had temporarily been withdrawn. Katie was placed on the waiting list.

Right Place, Right Time

Until now we had been *reacting* to our circumstances. It was time to become proactive. We consulted the team we had come to rely on and trust with our daughter's communication development. They gave us the name of a surgeon in New York. After contacting our local health insurance office to find out about funding for out-of-province procedures, John met with the doctor who managed such cases. He said that funding for this procedure was "under consideration" and asked us to provide a letter about Katie with supporting medical information. That letter became the most important letter we have ever written. John delivered it on the day of the funding meeting. Unbelievably, two days later, we received a call from the doctor with permission to go ahead.

New York, New York

Although the cost of Katie's operation was funded, we still had to come up with the money to cover the cost of travel and accommodation. The airline confirmed our eligibility for a discount on travel for medical purposes, and for that, we are eternally grateful.

We flew to New York in March 1991 for a three-day assessment. The surgeon who would be performing the operation was extremely reassuring. He addressed our fears and provided a clear and honest picture of the surgery and its implications. We left his office with a thorough understanding of what our daughter would undergo, and supreme confidence in his abilities. Everyone we met who would be involved in this process inspired the same confidence. The criteria for candidacy were explained: a child with a profound hearing loss who was not able to benefit from the conventional use of hearing aids. Katie then received an extremely powerful FM system, which she had to wear for approximately two months. A surgery date was set for June 25, 1991, dependent on assessment results.

Meanwhile we talked to a family in Toronto whose daughter had received a cochlear implant the previous year. This family was a tremendous help in preparing us for what lay ahead.

Helicopters Flying

We returned to New York the afternoon before the operation and took care of the administrative details. We talked about everything *but* the operation. Our previous sense of confidence had seemingly evaporated! We now felt uncertain about this decision. John and I smiled and laughed a lot, but I think Katie sensed the underlying tension. She held on to her rabbit, "Hop-Hop," most of the time.

The following morning we walked with her down to the doors of the operating room. The smile on my face felt frozen, and my heart was beating wildly. John held onto her hand. We said our goodbyes and they wheeled her away.

We made our way into a garden on the hospital grounds that overlooked the Hudson River. It was a stunning, spectacular summer morning. We heard and watched the helicopters flying overhead, bringing business people into the city. We were both thinking, but were too scared to say, "Have we made the right choice? What if something goes wrong?" It was the longest four hours we've ever experienced.

Twenty-four hours later, Katie was looking at picture books and toddling around the hospital ward with her IV! Everything about that morning remains etched in my brain like a bizarre and vivid dream.

Adjusting

Five weeks later, we returned to New York to activate Katie's implant. Eleven electrodes one day, 11 the next: Katie responded well to the stimulation, which, we were told, would sound like a series of "whirrs, clicks, and buzzes." The next 12 months involved traveling back and forth, twice a month for the first two months, and then once every two months, or as needed. The follow-up team lived up to their promise and always made sure Katie left with the optimum in hearing ability.

Team members were readily available by phone if we had concerns or questions about the implant.

Katie, as usual, adjusted very well to wearing the processor. John and I watched her closely, looking for signs of change in her hearing ability. Five months later, she responded to her name! Her vocalizations started to increase, and she began to be aware of different sounds.

Blow to the Ear

In the summer of 1992, we had a terrible scare. Katie sustained a blow to her implanted ear. It immediately started to swell, and we rushed her to our local children's hospital. The otolaryngologist who saw her admitted her for surgery immediately. That evening Katie's ear was drained and she spent the night in hospital. The staff were amazed at her cooperation for an IV insertion. (She even displayed it proudly to friends who came to visit!) Meanwhile, we had contacted the hospital in New York, and they were ready to see Katie whenever we could get there.

Wishes Do Come True

Katie continued to do well in the self-contained program. Each week brought her recognition of new sounds. Her language started to develop. She didn't like the sound of water running; she was amazed that the kettle "clicked"; she became annoyed with the sound made by the lining of the cereal packet. She loved to make the cat say "meeoow." She told her brother, Nicholas, that he was too noisy! She relied less on gestures and started asking for things she wanted. It seemed that at long last our wish for our daughter to use language was finally being realized.

A move to a new house in 1993 meant a change in schools. Through the Toronto School Board's IPRC (Individual Placement and Review Committee, similar to the American IEP), Katie was placed in a self-contained class, with three other children who were hearing impaired, in the morning and then bused to our local school for integration into first grade. That year we noticed a huge change in her hearing and social development. She was fortunate to have two great teachers. Her self-contained class teacher liaised regularly with her first-grade teacher, and this gave Katie a sense of involvement in both classes. She had a lot of extracurricular work, though. As well, she continued with weekly auditory-verbal therapy and speech therapy.

Being a Kid

Katie's work and study habits were good. Each evening after supper, either John or I would sit with her to help with homework and have "fun" with the auditory-verbal lessons. These were now more informal and, quite often, included her three-year-old brother, Nicholas. Bedtime, though, was becoming later and later. In 1994, Nicholas was starting kindergarten and Katie moved into second grade. I wanted to be more available to *both* of them, so I started to work from home. This new arrangement helped: Katie was able to finish her work before supper and still have time to unwind and play.

By the time Katie reached third grade, her negotiating skills had sharpened. She declared Friday a "no homework" day, and I was happy to comply. She had also developed a steady friendship with a local school classmate that was extremely important to her, so weekly after-school play became part of her routine. Around this time I remember her auditory-verbal therapist asking her about her "hobbies." Katie didn't know what hobbies were. When the word was explained, she looked blank, but I think she did mention swimming!

Steady Development

Katie's speaking and listening skills are steadily increasing. It's difficult to remember when she stopped trying to *see* what we were saying and just started listening. Of course, her language skills are delayed compared to those of her hearing peers. However, the full-time use of the implant and her support programs work well towards bridging that gap. Her speech processor is now MAPped at the cochlear center of our local children's hospital, which also provides a forum for parents to come together once or twice a year for information and discussions on related hearing and social issues.

A Leap of Faith

This year, in fourth grade, Katie has made the transition to a fully mainstream setting. She was extremely happy to find out that she would be walking to school with Nicholas, who entered first grade. Further, her itinerant teacher, who works with her for one hour, three days a week, is the same teacher she has had for three years in the self-contained class. Katie absolutely adores her. This has made the transition to a fully mainstream setting much smoother than anticipated. The workload is still present, and the vocabulary is more complex, but she embraces the challenges and does the best she can.

Her auditory-verbal therapy has taken on a different slant: every two weeks she shares part of her session with another child, a friend from her former self-contained class, who also has a cochlear implant. This provides an opportunity for Katie to exchange ideas and information with a child of similar ability in a safe setting. Katie really looks forward to these twice-monthly sessions.

Lingo

John and I now take more of a back seat in Katie's daily life; Nicholas has assumed a larger role. He is her constant playmate and, more importantly, has become her mentor in matters of everyday "lingo" — "Don't bug me! Oh, that's cool! No way! Sooo! Yeah, sure." It's wonderful to hear Katie using language that hasn't been "taught," but that she hears and uses in a meaningful way.

Looking Back

Katie has now had her cochlear implant for five years. Quite often we find ourselves still focusing on what she doesn't know, hear, or say. So every now and then we deliberately stop and look back — she's come a long way. It goes without saying that all parents think their child is remarkable. I truly believe that Katie is blessed. Her keen intelligence and even temperament have served her well in coping with these turbulent years.

We can never be thankful enough to the professionals who have been, and continue to be, with Katie along the way, and who have helped shape the person she is today — a self-confident and sociable child who now speaks for herself.

Eric

Mike Sieloff

> "He is very intelligible — I have several children in the class who are harder to understand than Eric and they have normal hearing," the kindergarten teacher said. "And he's so attentive — during story time he just tunes right in. He's always among the first to answer questions. He's very assertive — doesn't seem to be self-conscious about his deafness or implant at all. The other children are very interested, very accepting."

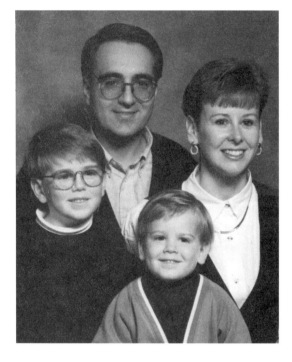

Eric Sieloff (left) and family

The Plan

Eric was born in February 1991. In October of the following year, we brought him home after three weeks of hospitalization due to pneumococcal meningitis. The meningitis had wreaked havoc on his little body. Clinically speaking, he was hypotonic. He had dysarthria, a right third nerve palsy, and a profound bilateral sensorineural hearing loss. He could not sit up or roll over. He could not eat solid food, move his tongue, or control the movement of his right eye. And he could not hear. We were just grateful his life had been spared!

During the drive home from the hospital we realized that Eric's deafness would be the greatest challenge for all of us. We equated hearing with communication, communication with education, and education with opportunities in adult life. Although the other conditions might not return to "normal" — indeed, they have not — we were optimistic that the healing powers of time and therapy would result in improvement. We knew, however, that his hearing loss would not spontaneously recover.

Shortly after returning from the hospital, we borrowed several books about deafness from the library. They were somewhat dated, and there certainly were no references to cochlear implants. Two, however, were helpful, and one in particular made a lasting impression on us. The first, *Choices in Deafness,* described three approaches to communication: a manual approach (Exact Signed English or, more typically, American Sign Language), an oral approach (maximizing aided residual hearing and supplementing it with lipreading), and cued speech, which we understood to be a unique combination of manual and oral methods. We were immediately drawn to the oral approach, as it seemed the most inclusive. Ours is a hearing world, and it seemed logical that maximizing Eric's capabilities would be the first and best choice. We were also realistic, however, and were prepared to switch to a manual approach if Eric was not succeeding.

The second book, the revised edition of *Learning to Listen,* contained stories by Toronto mothers of children who were deaf and who had followed the auditory-verbal approach. In these 200 pages, we found inspirational stories of courage and optimism, and felt we had found the path we would take with Eric. Although we did not appreciate this then, we now have a sense of how heroic these families were: these children grew up in the 1970s. The body-worn and behind-the-ear hearing aid, not the cochlear implant, were their technological breakthroughs; auditory-verbal therapy was not yet formally recognized, presumably considered to be an oxymoron by most of those who had heard of it at all!

By November 1992 we found, through a recommendation from a local parent of a child who was profoundly deaf, a wonderful audiologist at the nearby university who fitted Eric with a powerful set of hearing aids. We searched out an auditory-verbal therapy program at a clinic in a Toronto-area hospital for an initial visit and consultation, and we began. This was a big commitment. In addition to the daily auditory-verbal lessons, we — or rather my wife, Angela — would make the weekly drive from our home to Toronto and back (400 miles, round trip). So, starting in February 1993 the routine began: Angela would pack up Eric, who still wasn't walking, pack up the baby (Adam was five weeks old), the cellular phone, and winter emergency kit, and head off for therapy. Finally, after several months, we had a plan. In time, with hard work and commitment, Eric would learn to listen, and then, we were certain, he would learn to talk.

The Cochlear Implant

As it turned out, Eric did not learn to listen. For an hour a day, in a sit-down high-chair lesson and then throughout his waking hours, we worked on creating those all-important, meaningful auditory experiences. Our family and friends looked on in disbelief: it was not at all clear to them how "the cow says mmmmoooo" would result in Eric's speaking one day. We soldiered on, reminding ourselves over and over that receptive language always preceded expressive language.

Our audiologist encouraged us to work at play audiometry. The only sounds to which Eric would consistently respond were the banging of a large pot with a wooden spoon and the popping of a balloon behind his back. Sadly, Eric had virtually no awareness of sound. The few words he had known before his illness were becoming less intelligible, and by mid-March we thought that our goal of oral communication was becoming unrealistic. We began to investigate a cochlear implant.

At the time of Eric's hospital discharge, the otolaryngologist had dismissed a cochlear implant as an inappropriate option for Eric, since there was little evidence of any benefit from these devices, particularly in children. We, however, had seen the November 1992 episode of *60 Minutes* featuring cochlear implants for children, and we were intrigued by the possibilities. There were several children who had received implants in Eric's therapy program, and the therapist was aware of the great possibilities for access to spoken language through the implant. In April 1993, after several weeks of research and careful consideration, we applied directly to three pediatric cochlear implant centers for assessment: two in Ontario and a third in New York City. Funding for implants in Ontario by the provincial health insurance plan was imminent, we were told; however, political wrangling in the provincial legislature prevented local implant centers from even considering adding names to the waiting list. A formal assessment in Ontario was not possible at that time.

We therefore had Eric assessed in New York, where we were advised that he was, indeed, a suitable candidate. Because of the advanced ossification in both his cochleae, caused by the meningitis, we were advised to arrange Eric's surgery as soon as possible in order to ensure the likelihood of a full insertion (use of all 22 electrodes). We returned home and checked once again with our local implant centers: the funding situation had not changed. We rearranged our finances. The implant would be at our expense, with hopes of recovering costs from the provincial health insurance plan in the future, and we booked a surgery date.

Eric received his implant on May 18, 1993, at the age of 27 months. The surgery was stressful enough, since we were in a strange, big city; without the support of family and friends, it was an overwhelming experience. The five-hour operation went well, but the ossification had indeed progressed, and Eric received only a partial insertion with 11 or possibly 12 usable electrodes. We were devastated and wondered how his oral communication potential might be limited by a partial insertion and his oral motor weakness.

Eric bounced back quickly and was discharged two days later. We paid the bill, packed up our son, and drove 13 hours back home to Ontario.

Four weeks later we returned to New York for the initial stimulation. We were tense with anticipation! We were told that some children cried at initial stimulation, while others giggled; others were awe-struck as they absorbed sound for the first time in a long time, or perhaps for the first time ever. Eric cried. After eight and a half months he had forgotten all about sound, and he certainly didn't care for *this* sound. On the first day of stimulation, 10 of the 12 electrodes were activated at low levels.

We arrived back at our 30th floor hotel room and started experimenting. He consistently detected a squeaky alligator toy. He had sound awareness — our son could *hear!* A fire engine went past the building on the street far below. The wailing siren could be heard above the din of traffic. Eric heard that fire engine and looked around the room in panic. He could not identify or locate the sound, but he *heard* it!

The following day the remaining electrodes were activated and the MAP fine-tuned. All those play-audiometry sessions with the cooking spoon and the pot paid off. His detection responses were quite consistent, and his speech processor was relatively easy to MAP. Happily, the three of us left the implant center and returned home.

At home, we redoubled our efforts. Lessons were finally fun for all of us because Eric could hear. Three weeks after his implant was activated, Eric could detect the sounds of the Ling Six-Sound Test and could consistently identify the *learning to listen* sounds given a closed set of two choices. Our home had become a veritable barnyard: "The cow says mmmmoooo, the sheep goes baaaa, peep-peep-peep, says the hen." After months of little or no response, communication began again.

At five weeks post hook-up, Eric could identify the telephone ringing and was responding to his name. He had a receptive vocabulary of 50 words that he could identify through listening alone, and he was learning new words at a rate of about one per day. At eight weeks post stimulation, he reached 100 words of receptive vocabulary. We celebrated! In September, we proudly showed our therapist the product of our summer efforts: a receptive vocabulary of 250 words! September also marked the first year anniversary of the onset of Eric's deafness. His remarkable progress validated our choices and personal sacrifices.

No Looking Back Now

As Eric's receptive language grew, he began to communicate his wants and needs with words instead of the gestures he had used for the last year or so. Most of the words were intelligible only to Angela and myself. His single words were followed by two-word combinations and then simple sentences. As his word strings became longer his intelligibility deteriorated even further, but his single-word intelligibility slowly improved. By Christmas 1993, he knew all his colors and family members' names, and we were working on counting.

The next two years of our family life were highly disciplined, filled with auditory-verbal therapy. Angela continued her weekly sojourn to Toronto. By this time, she was working three days a week. Eric attended day care, where he also received a daily one-on-one lesson with the resource teacher, who followed our weekly auditory-verbal therapy objectives. Every day after supper Eric had another lesson with either myself or Angela. All waking hours were filled with creating meaningful auditory experiences. We seized any opportunity to talk with Eric. Consequently, his receptive language progressed rapidly.

Eric's articulation had always been hampered by dysarthria brought on by the meningitis. He was now processing information very well through listening, but his expressive language was still lagging. At this time, Eric began weekly speech therapy sessions in addition to his auditory-verbal session. Progress in articulation was not nearly as dramatic as the success we had enjoyed in language learning, but Eric's articulation slowly began to improve. One day, he explained to his therapist: *"Do you know what? My cat threw up in the family room! It had germs — blech. My cat lives in the basement. It's dirty."*

School Days

As Eric approached his fourth birthday, school options became paramount. Integrating Eric into a mainstream classroom was a logical step, but it was also a daunting proposition. We live in a small community; our local school boards had limited experience with children who are profoundly deaf, and no experience with cochlear implants. We were required, once again, to take the initiative. We were advocating on Eric's behalf. Eric could enter junior kindergarten at age four in September 1995, so we began discussions with the local school board late in 1994. We wanted to provide all parties with sufficient lead time to be able to prepare the necessary support services for Eric's success in a mainstream classroom:

- classroom acoustic assessment and modifications, as necessary.
- an FM system, appropriately modified for Eric's cochlear implant.
- services of an itinerant teacher consistent with those provided for all children who are profoundly deaf.
- an educational assistant for the classroom teacher.
- speech therapy services.
- a school placement meeting scheduled at the earliest opportunity.

As it turned out, the school board was unable to commit to several of these items, so we kept Eric in day care that year and planned to renew discussions with the school board the following year. Eric had made good progress at his day care in the areas of communication and socialization. Although he was the only child with a hearing loss, the staff was adaptive, flexible, and accommodating. One more year really prepared him for starting school.

In the fall of the following year, we initiated discussions with another school board. The special-education supervisor was straightforward and very professional. To our relief, the board was able to commit to substantially all our requests, but speech therapy would be available only in first grade. After visits to our local school and meetings with the kindergarten teacher, principal, and itinerant teacher, we decided that Eric would begin senior kindergarten in September 1996. Now we just had nine months to wait!

Although we had had our share of stressful experiences, the first day of school was very challenging! There Eric went, up the steps of the school bus, by himself, off to school. He arrived to find several people awaiting him: his classroom teacher, his educational assistant, even his principal. They had all met Eric and knew him by name! We certainly could not have been more prepared.

Eric could not have been more prepared, either. He had been using his implant for over three years and had several years of auditory-verbal therapy. He had age-appropriate vocabulary and language comprehension. His intelligibility had improved, but his dysarthria continued to be a challenge.

His teacher tells us Eric has excellent basic skills in counting, phonics, spelling, and emerging reading skills, and he has an excellent attention span. He also has good lipreading skills for coping in situations with high background noise, and he readily asks for clarification when he has not heard or understood.

He is confident and well adjusted, and appears to have healthy self-esteem. He is not self-conscious about his hearing loss or his cochlear implant. He goes to swimming lessons and has recently joined Beaver Scouts. While these challenges may prove to be more significant than the academic ones in the future, he appears to be off to a good start!

Our Lessons

Our experiences with hearing loss and the cochlear implant have helped us to make a few observations:

- There are some excellent practitioners in the professions of medicine and education who are knowledgeable and compassionate. We need to seek them out to help our children and our families.

- Success of children with cochlear implants is not predictable, and several factors contribute to the probability of success:
  - Children who are candidates should receive implants at a young age to minimize the duration of deafness.
  - Even though cochlear ossification can occur very soon after meningitis, children with partial insertions of cochlear implant electrodes can be very successful users. It seems reasonable, however, that hearing sensation is enhanced with full insertion.

- Helping a child who is deaf to become an effective oral communicator is a lot of hard work. Ironically, the more successful a child becomes, the more average the child appears. Such a paradox! It is difficult to describe the effort and personal sacrifice parents are required to make in order to help their children who have cochlear implants. The therapist said, "The implant is just a thing — a wonderful, marvelous device that opens up all sorts of opportunities — but it's just a thing."

- Videotaping weekly therapy sessions is highly recommended.
  - Our therapy was parent-centered; fathers (typically, mothers take children to therapy), grandparents, aunts, uncles, siblings and other caregivers, such as day care staff, could learn therapy techniques and strategies.
  - Videos are a wonderful way of sharing a child's progress with out-of-town family members and of looking back after several months (or even years) to monitor progress. Videos were especially helpful when we were having a bad week or waiting for the next language breakthrough.
- Joining parent and professional organizations can maximize learning opportunities through conferences, workshops, periodicals, and newsletters. We have benefited tremendously from organizations such as Voice for Hearing Impaired Children, the Robarts School Home Visiting Program, A.G. Bell Association for the Deaf, Auditory-Verbal International, and Cochlear Implant Club International. Through these organizations, families can forge valuable friendships with others in similar circumstances.
- When making arrangements for mainstreaming, contact the school board or school principal very early. It will take several discussions to communicate the nature of your child's hearing loss and the implications of a cochlear implant.

Not Fair!

"Mommy?" Eric asked one day, "Will I have to wear my implant when I grow up? I don't want to be deaf. I want my ears to work. I want to be like Adam. It's not fair!" By now, tears were streaming down his face.

Of course it's not fair. Despite the technology available today relative to even five years ago, and despite the great lengths to which we parents go to help our kids, it *is* patently unfair. We are thankful for the cochlear implant, thankful for the many excellent professionals we have had in our lives, and thankful that Eric has made a good start — a second start, really. In the end, however, it is still unfair. While our five-year-old doesn't dwell on it, I suspect that before long we will need to come up with some good answers to the "fairness" question. When that time comes we will do as we have done in the past: talk with other parents and professionals, do some research, and then do what we can — our best.

Alana

Joanna Nichols

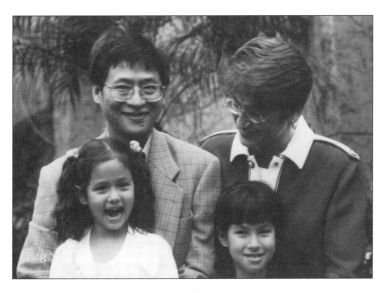

Alana Nichols (left) and family

Wait Until…

When Alana was born, three years after our first child, deafness never entered our minds. What a "good" baby she was, sleeping peacefully for long periods during the day. At night, however, she had a distressing habit of waking up and crying — not the usual fretful, demanding-to-be-picked-up cry, but more like terrified screaming. Later — after her profound deafness was diagnosed — we wondered if she cried because she felt so alone in the dark, deprived of the reassuring sounds that would comfort a child with hearing.

By eight months of age, Alana was not babbling the way our older daughter had, and uneasy questions began to form in our minds. We did take her to see doctors; one of the most prominent said, "Wait till she's three, then worry about it." Looking back, I realize we wished ourselves into believing that Alana did hear us call her name, at least once in a while. She might turn around when we played a game; but she never seemed to hear the phone ring, the dogs bark, or the birds sing. She had a strangely detached expression on her face, as if she were swathed in cotton wool, not in full touch with her surroundings.

When Alana was 11 months old, the thought finally surfaced: "I think Alana is deaf!"

Alana Is Deaf

An auditory brainstem response (ABR) test at a large hospital in Taipei showed that Alana had little or no hearing, at least in the high frequencies. Absolute disbelief! There must be some mistake. Neither my husband, Kenny, nor myself had any history of deafness in our families. I had had a model pregnancy: exercising, watching my diet scrupulously, visiting my doctor regularly; everything always checked out normal. Without preparation or warning, our family was suddenly plunged into the frightening unknown, with a very uncertain future for our baby.

Educating Ourselves

Kenny and I were determined to find a solution. Despite our sorrow, we began the search for answers and to educate ourselves. We made telephone calls, wrote letters, and visited many clinics and professionals on three continents. The professionals in Taiwan, North America, and Australia sincerely cared and desired to help. We focused on oral approaches rather than sign language because we believed these would give Alana many professional, educational, and social opportunities, and be easier on our whole family.

The professional advice was contradictory and ultimately distressing: "Cued speech, total communication, signing, lipreading; send her to a boarding school, send her to a day school; be firm, don't be too hard on her." Each experienced professional was confident that his or her particular approach was the best. We began to realize that there was no definitive answer. It became clear that it was up to us, Alana's parents, to make these decisions, and we were determined to do this by evaluating the results. We listened to how the children in the various programs spoke and communicated.

Audiograms and Hearing Aids

Alana's audiological results were inconclusive and inconsistent, and this contributed to our confusion. Sometimes she seemed to have some low-frequency hearing, and other times almost nothing. Her hearing aids were also distressing and frustrating to us because of the constant feedback; we had many sets of earmolds made during that first year.

There were indications, nevertheless, that Alana had begun to hear something. Before getting her hearing aids, she would gently bang her head on the table, an action that, according to one psychologist, was a "substitute stimulus for hearing." After she received hearing aids, this behavior disappeared. The hearing aids also made a difference in her vocalizations. Previously, she had never made more than a "throaty" sound, yet only a few days after getting her hearing aids, she thrilled us by saying, "Amamam." Because of Alana's very profound hearing loss, however, amplification did not help beyond this stage.

We experienced many moments of grief and confusion. How could we help Alana to live successfully in a hearing world and to realize her complete potential? To make life more complex, we live in a Chinese-speaking society where English-speaking teachers of the deaf are nonexistent. We decided to teach Alana in English because it is the language used in our home, and we felt it would be of more practical use worldwide. We needed to find a teacher who would live with us to help with the day-to-day, hour-to-hour therapy and provide guidance.

Through friends, we found a highly experienced teacher in Australia who devoted herself to us for six months, when Alana was 16 months through 22 months of age. Alana's cognitive development was good, but in she had not progressed at all in hearing, speech, or language. While Alana didn't demonstrate any consistent signs of hearing, we had heard it takes time for children who are profoundly deaf to learn to use their residual hearing. So, we kept waiting and hoping.

Colorado, USA '93

The Alexander Graham Bell Association held a seminar in Denver, Colorado in October 1993, focusing on children from birth to six years of age. Our entire family attended. In a session about the auditory-verbal approach, a lecturer showed videos of children who were profoundly deaf, like Alana. Most had hearing aids, and a few had cochlear implants. These children spoke, sang, laughed, and above all, communicated intelligibly and confidently. After two hours of private consultation that evening, we grew more hopeful because of the high standards of speech, language, natural communication, and educational performance expected with this approach. We said to ourselves, emphatically, *"This is what we want for Alana."*

At the same time, we wondered if Alana's progress, or lack thereof, was normal. The lecturer agreed to visit Taiwan over the Christmas holidays to assess her.

That visit was a turning point in our lives. Other than the occasional "amamam," the only sound Alana made was a guttural, grunting noise; she could not understand or speak a single word. She communicated entirely through gestures. After a few days of observation and sound field testing, the consultant said, "I see no responses to sound."

A Cochlear Implant

Two or three professionals had previously mentioned the cochlear implant, but I had rejected that option, saying to myself, "Our daughter can't be *that* deaf." This therapist, however, enthusiastically explained the excellent results being obtained with the cochlear implant. Encouraged by the consultant's positive attitude, we began looking for an implant center.

It was not simple! There were many criteria, regulations, restrictions, and demands to be met, the most important of which was being *absolutely certain* that Alana had little or no residual hearing. Most clinics required a hearing-aid trial of many months before agreeing to give a child an implant, and we did not want to waste any more of the critical language-learning months. We were able to put together a convincing case, including audiograms over the 15-month period that Alana had worn hearing aids, and a 10-minute video showing her lack of response to any sound and her limited range of utterances. Both the Australian teacher and the auditory-verbal consultant wrote letters stating their opinions that Alana was probably a good cochlear implant candidate. We had made arrangements for "long-distance therapy," either in Taiwan or Canada, every two to three months, with phone calls and faxes in between.

After exploring several excellent implant centers, we decided to go to Melbourne, Australia, where the clinic agreed to accept Alana if their evaluation confirmed her lack of hearing potential. We made the trip to Melbourne, prepared for a stay of about two months.

The CT Scan Shock!

Alana's tests in Melbourne showed hearing only at vibration levels, and the team therefore agreed that she could receive an implant. Then came another shock: the CT scan revealed that Alana had a condition called "common cavities," a severe malformation of the cochleae. A normal cochlea has two and a half turns, and the electrode array of the implant is threaded through the outer turns. Alana's cochlea, however, was nothing but a small hole. The very kind surgeon explained that it had stopped developing at about four weeks into gestation: he said, "I am not saying I won't operate on Alana, but there is no telling what, if any, benefit she will receive."

That day is vivid in my mind! It seemed as though our last hope for Alana to hear went up in smoke. As my father and I left the doctor's office, I broke down and cried for the first time since her diagnosis. Neither of us spoke. Thankfully, my inner determination took over again, and the only thought I allowed myself was how to maximize our chances of success.

I obtained the names of six surgeons in North America and Europe who had performed operations on children with Alana's condition. I phoned each of them and, without exception, they shared their time and expert advice freely. I became familiar with the medical terms and possible complications involved in implanting a common cavity. Kenny and I typed up detailed notes of each useful consultation and presented them to our surgeon, who read them all. He, in turn, telephoned several of the doctors. His dedication and kindness, coupled with the competent support of the entire Melbourne team, gave us confidence. Finally, the surgery was performed on March 16, 1994. Fourteen of the 22 electrodes were successfully inserted into Alana's tiny cochlea, and 12 of the 14 electrodes have been activated.

Alana's recovery was uneventful. In Melbourne, "switch-on" takes place two weeks after surgery, as long as the incision has healed well. The suspense was intense. We had been counseled that Alana may have no response at all, or that a response could merely mean a physical rather than a hearing sensation. Early in the MAPping, however, an alarmed look came over Alana's face, and she ran over to me for comfort and protection. We were ecstatic!

After two weeks, when 10 of the 14 electrodes had been switched on, we were convinced Alana was hearing sounds, and she appeared to turn to her name. There was a marked difference as soon as 10 electrodes were activated and the SPEAK strategy was employed.

Some family members expected that Alana would hear normally as soon as she received the implant. Nonetheless, the professionals had advised us that progress would be gradual, like the development of a newborn's language.

Learning to Listen

Our auditory-verbal therapist prepared a six-month plan for Alana, with goals, instructions, and expectations. We saw the therapist every two months for a week or so. During this time Alana would have therapy once or twice a day. She loved it! The entire family was coached so that every member of the household could contribute to Alana's communication development. It was clear that we, the parents, were Alana's primary teachers, and the therapist's job was to teach us, set new goals, and ensure that Alana's progress was on target. During the intervals between therapy visits, I gave Alana therapy each day to reinforce specific goals. Every household activity was turned into a learning opportunity.

We learned many new techniques: to speak to Alana from beside or behind her, and to cover our mouths if she was looking directly at us when we were speaking. Listening became more important than lipreading. Soon, we ceased to marvel at what had seemed impossible a month or two earlier. We turned eagerly to the next "impossible" sound or target on the lesson plan.

Gradually, Alana began to imitate certain sounds and to turn frequently to the sound of her name. I clearly remember the thrill of hearing her first word: "ow" for "sit down," as she motioned for me to join her at the dining table. Little milestones boosted our morale, and we felt, "Everything's going to be all right."

A few months later, we returned to Melbourne for a check-up. We took Alana to visit the surgeon, to share our excitement at her progress. I told him she could hear, but he was still skeptical. I held Alana so she could not see me, and asked her to repeat several sounds. He looked at her in joyful surprise and said, "We may have to rethink our criteria in these cases!"

Perhaps Alana's case would eventually prove to be a blessing for many other children! Perhaps that was when the seed was planted to begin a foundation in Taiwan to help other children have the chance to hear, listen, and speak.

More Therapy

I did not feel at all like a natural teacher. This was a new experience, but like most parents, the determination to help my child made me nearly oblivious to the feeling of burden. My main fear was that perhaps I wasn't doing enough to help Alana; perhaps I didn't know enough, perhaps it wouldn't work. Little by little, however, a feeling of personal competence developed. I was comforted by the knowledge that many parents had accomplished great things for their children.

Every six months, we received a new long-term plan: new goals, new sounds, and additional techniques. We learned that there is a definite order in which sounds are introduced. Insisting that the child make these sounds before he or she is ready can lead to frustration and discouragement. A primary goal was to help Alana to feel happy and to enjoy the sessions. Learning could then occur. Much to our surprise, one of the most valuable lessons we learned was that behavior management was key to Alana's development. We learned not to feel sorry for her because of her deafness, and not to give in to her because "she didn't understand what was required." We also learned to have the same expectations of obedience and behavior that we had for our elder daughter. This encouraged Alana to develop a sense of responsibility for her actions, and an inner control that will serve her well for the rest of her life.

About 10 months post implant, Alana's spontaneous use of vocabulary and speech sounds began to develop. It was exciting to see her making quick progress. Two years post implant, she was speaking in short, complete sentences, rather than just phrases. In a surprisingly short period of perhaps three or four months, her speech became very natural, and her language was often near to grammatical perfection. This gives us great joy, and we never take it for granted.

Alana was very passive as an infant, and some well-meaning friends had thought she might be mentally handicapped! But first with the hearing aids, and then more obviously with the implant, Alana's personality blossomed. Today she is an outgoing, intelligent, effervescent child. The mother of a six-year-old child with a cochlear implant once said, "You are wondering if Alana will ever learn to talk. Believe me, the time will come when you will say, 'Alana, will you please be quiet!'" How very true!

Looking Back

Two and a half years after Alana received her cochlear implant, our family looks back and remarks, "Remember when she couldn't say 't' or 'k' or 'the'?" Alana can now talk on the phone and hold a conversation with the driver from the back seat of a car. She even corrected a Chinese friend whose English is somewhat hesitant: "When you say 'mother,' you must stick your tongue out, like this!" Alana now puts her thoughts into words. She asks questions about the world, about ethics, and the reasons for behavior and about human relationships.

At an auditory-verbal conference in Taiwan, I introduced Alana to two Chinese friends. "Say hello, Alana," I urged. Without hesitation she responded, "Nee how," which is "hello" in Chinese. She understands that Chinese people require a different greeting than her Western friends. Our older daughter is bilingual, speaking both English and Chinese, and attends a Chinese school.

Like a house of bricks, Alana's hearing, speech, language, and cognition have been constructed, painstakingly, one brick at a time. Alana began attending a regular preschool about four months post implant, and is now enrolled in a mainstream kindergarten at an international, English-speaking school. The teachers and principals have been understanding, cooperative, and very helpful.

Alana, my parents, and I recently had lunch in Hong Kong with an old friend, whom we hadn't seen for many years. We all had been chatting for about 10 minutes, when the friend said, "I understand your *other* daughter has a hearing problem?" She couldn't believe, even after several minutes of conversation with Alana, that *she* was that child!

Helping Others

As a result of our good fortune, we have established a foundation to help children who are hearing impaired in Taiwan and Asia. A friend remarked recently, "There are so few things people can do to make their own lives worth living, things that will have a positive effect in other peoples' lives. Helping these children is certainly one of them." We are fortunate to be able to help others receive the support, information, encouragement, and guidance we have found.

In spite of the trials, stress, and hard work, having a child who is hearing impaired has added immeasurably to our lives. We have been blessed with dedicated professionals and caring friends who have entered our experience through Alana's deafness, and I no longer look upon "handicapped" people as being "different" from myself. We are all just human beings.

Patrick

Eva Quateman

There are certain things you never forget when it comes to your children. I remember every detail about the day Patrick was born, especially how perfect and healthy he was; I also remember the day he almost died, and how it changed our lives forever. There was very

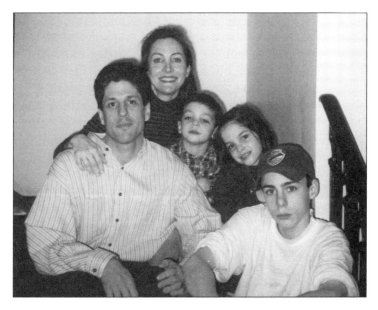

Patrick Quateman (far right) and family

little time between those two events, only four and a half months. And it's difficult to recall the few carefree, happy days, because what followed was a nightmare.

June 1983

On Saturday, June 2, 1983, I put Patrick down for his nap and went to a neighborhood antique fair. After I came home, he awoke, burning with a high fever. He was inconsolable. I immediately called our pediatrician, who said that he was on his way to dinner, but that I should meet him in the hospital emergency room. After examining Patrick, he sent us home with instructions to take Tylenol and Pedialite, as needed.

There was nothing I could do to make Patrick happy — he wouldn't eat, sleep, or drink. In the middle of the night he began projectile vomiting. I was scared to death, and at 2:00 a.m. I got in a cab and went back to the hospital. An intern examined Patrick, couldn't find anything wrong beyond the fever, and we were again sent home. I felt safer in the hospital, but I had no choice.

On Sunday, Patrick became increasingly lethargic. He still wouldn't eat, drink, or sleep; he was badly distressed and very uncomfortable. I remember being sleep starved myself, walking him from room to room, sitting when he wasn't too fussy, but mostly standing and swaying back and forth, trying to give him some small comfort. I was frightened all that day, but come nightfall, I was panic-stricken. There was something about the darkness that made everything seem much worse.

Around midnight, I was in a cab again, off to the hospital. By this time Patrick, dehydrated from lack of fluids and vomiting, hadn't had a wet diaper for a day and a half. He took a little Pedialite, and his fever went down slightly. The intern again told me to go home, in spite of my begging her please to let us stay. Later, when I reflected on that weekend, Sunday in particular, I realized that I had learned three important lessons:

- Never get sick on the weekend.
- Doctors are not always right.
- Nobody loves you, or knows you, like your mother.

Monday morning I was back in our pediatrician's office. He said to me quite off-handedly, "Maybe Patrick has meningitis. There's a bit of it going around." Naturally I was alarmed, but the doctor seemed so calm that I just assured myself that Patrick didn't have it! Finally, after a whole weekend of my wanting the safe haven of the hospital, Patrick was admitted. As there wasn't a bed available on the infectious disease floor, up we went to the orthopedic floor.

One intern after another was sent to question me. Nobody asked appropriate questions, and I was completely frustrated. I did feel somewhat better, however, being in the hospital, because Patrick was looking worse and worse.

Tuesday at about 6:30 a.m., my husband (also named Patrick) came by on his way to work. He never dealt well with things like this, and I could tell that he was scared but he, too, expected things to get better now that the baby had been admitted. No sooner had my husband left the hospital then I looked at the baby and noticed his skin color had turned gray. He'd gone from a rosy-cheeked, chubby, happy baby to a gray, thin, lethargic wet noodle. I snapped.

I went to the nurse's station and demanded action of some kind. Everyone acted as though I was just a nuisance and ignored me until I had an honest-to-goodness temper tantrum, kicking and screaming on the floor. This is not a personal habit but, at this point, I hadn't slept in three nights!

One of the nurses said, "Really, Mrs. Grafft, children get fevers and the flu all the time. Get hold of yourself." Feeling embarrassed, I retreated to the bathroom to splash water on my face and get a grip on myself. I came out of the bathroom to see so many white coats surrounding Patrick's crib that I couldn't see or get to him. Someone unlocked the gurney and they took off, running past me, crib and all. I ran after them, asking questions that nobody would answer. Finally, I grabbed one of those white coats and a woman whirled round and told me Patrick might not make it through the day! I found out later that by the time they did a spinal tap, with one look at the milky fluid, there was no longer any question: the diagnosis was bad.

I called my husband and our family priest, and we went to the Intensive Care Unit. Patrick was put in isolation and started on an IV of general antibiotics while medical staff tried to discover what type of meningitis he had. Within an hour, my family arrived, and we began the long wait. Would Patrick live or die?

About three series of antibiotics later, it became clear that Patrick was responding. He was so much improved that we all thought he would certainly survive. My cousins stayed behind to sit with Patrick while he had his first quiet sleep in days. My husband, my brother-in-law, and my second husband (more on that later) went to the local pub to toast Patrick's life to come. Little did we know what that life would be!

Every day in the hospital, Patrick got better, but things were not the same. I could see differences in his eating and sleeping habits and especially in his personality. No longer was he bubbly and cuddly. He didn't like to be picked up at all, arching his back and fussing until I put him down. Towards the middle of his 12-day hospital stay, tests were begun to determine what damage might have occurred.

Diagnosis

On day 10, standing by the nurse's station, I was told that my pediatrician needed to talk to me. I picked up the telephone, and he proceeded to tell me that Patrick was now deaf and that he would not be able to attend a regular school. Why he felt he should add that tidbit about school, I'll never know! In my mind this incompetent, lackadaisical approach to pediatric medicine nearly cost my baby his life, and it was difficult to understand how this man felt expert enough to determine Patrick's future. Later, upon reflection, I thought perhaps the doctor's attitude was what drove me so hard to help Patrick succeed in a mainstream school.

Deaf? I didn't know anyone that was deaf. I didn't know about "deaf" at all. I just wanted my son to have an abundant life; together, we would deal with deafness.

We came home from the hospital on Saturday, June 16. As we were about to turn off the telephones, my brother-in-law called and told us to turn on the television. There, on the *Wide World of Sports,* speaking very clearly, was a young gold-medal hopeful, who had lost his hearing as a baby due to meningitis. At that moment, we were too full of denial and self-pity to be inspired, but later, we realized it was a sign from God.

Choices

Education for the deaf in Chicago at that time strongly favored total communication. It sounded like a good idea, but I wanted something different. One program director told me of a clinic in Pennsylvania where auditory-verbal therapy was practiced. She told me she didn't believe the program worked and that it took a lot of time and probably a lot of money.

Fitted with a body aid and much hope for the future, Patrick and I got on a plane in August and headed for Pennsylvania. One week there was all I needed to be sure that I had to give this auditory-verbal approach a shot, even if there was nobody in Chicago to help me. The therapist I had consulted in Chicago was unable to embrace the idea, and so we parted ways.

I came home with all sorts of ideas and inspiration from a mother I had met there. Her son was attending Harvard University, and I had seen a videotape of him talking about his college experiences. His speech seemed good, and I was determined that Patrick could do as well.

I kept talking and playing games, talking and taking photos, talking and taking field trips, talking and building models of our home and surroundings, talking and making experience books, talking and playing listening games with my whole family — and talking, talking, talking. At first a lot was going in, but nothing was coming out. Somewhat discouraged, we questioned the effects of meningitis on Patrick's cognitive abilities. More evaluations indicated that Patrick had some sensory-integration and balance problems.

It's difficult to keep something going, doing it more or less alone. My husband encouraged my efforts and participated when I asked, but took no initiative to do his own listening activities. My family thought I couldn't face reality. The only one I could find to help was an audiologist who believed in auditory-verbal therapy, but she lived far away and her time was stretched as it was. By February, I needed a boost, and I headed back to Pennsylvania.

There was an occupational therapist working at the clinic who told me about her 11-year-old son, adopted at age four. Nobody wanted him because he "seemed somewhat retarded and couldn't talk." After testing showed that he was severely hearing impaired, she obtained hearing aids and got on with the process. At age 11, he was listening, talking, and functioning well, even with a learning disability. This was an against-all-odds story that I needed to hear!

Inspired again, I got back to work. Patrick, fortunately, would sit in a high chair for hours, which made it easy to do structured listening games with him. Sure enough, he began to listen! He was able to do very difficult puzzles, and I began to realize that he was a really smart kid! Finally, when he did begin to walk, he became a whirling dervish and a behavioral problem. Gone were the days of sitting and listening!

I went to my first A.G. Bell Convention in Portland, Oregon, where I met many professionals who have helped us over the years. There were two therapists in particular who would come and stay in our home, evaluate Patrick, and give me new ideas for his therapy. Eventually, one of these people moved to Chicago and became our therapist, our liaison to mainstream education, our good friend, and a member of our extended family. Thank God I had these people, because when Patrick was 34 months old, his father died at the age of 30.

Our lives fell apart for a while. Patrick was talking a little now, but only his therapist and I could make out what he was saying. He was in a mainstream preschool where the staff was becoming increasingly annoyed by his behavior. At the A.G. Bell Convention in Chicago I took him around to everyone I could, hoping to get some encouraging words, but his behavior was so stinky, it was hard to get past it. I needed a new focus!

About a year after my husband died, I started dating Gary. He had been my husband's best friend, the best man at my wedding, and Patrick's godfather. He wanted both of us, problems and all. Not surprisingly, not everyone could deal with a "handicapped" child, especially one with behavioral problems. Knowing I wasn't braving it alone anymore made it easier to get back in gear.

School

Patrick was expelled from preschool, which made the decision to go to a behavior-modification preschool easy. We no longer had a choice. In January 1987 I took Patrick to Canada to see a therapist who had raised a son who was hearing impaired. She was tough with Patrick and showed me that much of his slow progress in listening and speech was due to his behavioral problems. I needed to spend more time on this issue and get some communication going. So that's what we did!

Gary and I were married in March 1987, and the countdown for kindergarten began. We had 18 months to get Patrick ready for a mainstream school program. Patrick, Gary, and I played hundreds of listening games. In a short time, Patrick started calling Uncle Gary "Daddy Gary" and then "Daddy." Patrick was well liked at the preschool. His behavior was less of an issue because that's why he was there.

Then the best thing happened: Sacred Heart School was willing to give Patrick a desk when not many other schools were. They knew he had behavioral problems, knew his language was delayed, and yet took a giant leap of faith by giving him a chance.

One day while we were playing, I noticed that Pat couldn't answer a question that normally wouldn't have given him difficulty. I took him to the audiologist who found that he'd had a drop in hearing! He'd lost some middle and high frequencies, enough to make complicated listening games impossible. Even some of the simpler games had become difficult.

We went to a specialist in meningitic hearing losses in Alabama; we also went to an audiologist in Louisiana who specialized in hearing aids. I wanted someone to fix the problem, but it wasn't possible. While in Louisiana, Patrick developed an ear infection, and we had to take the train home.

That night, while Patrick slept in the upper berth, I let go of my dream that he would be like that boy who went to Harvard. I decided that I would be happy if he could get a cab and tell the driver, "Airport, please" and the driver would go to the airport, or go to the cleaners and say, "No starch, please!" and have his shirts come back with no starch.

After that, we started stressing natural language and social skills and eased up on intensive auditory development. Soon, I was pregnant and too "morning sick" to keep up the pace. September came and we weren't so nervous. We felt we had done our homework.

During Patrick's first school years, everything had to be "spoon fed" before, during, and after classes. Behavior was still an issue, but Patrick clearly was a very smart boy.

Third grade was a turning point in Patrick's behavior. We thought that perhaps he should repeat second grade because he had done well with that teacher and her class had fewer boys. Patrick thought otherwise; the idea mortified him. He knew he had to toe the line and improve his behavior fast. We hired a reading specialist, and things began to improve. Somehow, we squeaked through third grade.

Cochlear Implant

We had heard about cochlear implants, mostly from professionals, but we didn't want to be the "first ones on the block." Finally, we made plans to attend every seminar about cochlear implants at the A.G. Bell Convention in San Diego. There, we would find out about the current implant procedures and results, and then we would decide.

If the device had been FDA approved for children when Patrick had lost his hearing in infancy, we would have requested an implant without agonizing over it. But Patrick had already been using hearing aids somewhat successfully in the mainstream for over nine years.

We decided that we wanted Patrick to have the implant, but that he had to want it, too. He didn't want any part of it. Perhaps his resistance stemmed from his needle phobia and his illness as a baby. However, a friend from Canada visited us and spent half an hour talking with Patrick about the device. Patrick decided then that he wanted to have a cochlear implant.

We went to Indiana for evaluation. Patrick was considered a "silver" hearing-aid user — someone who is functioning well with the use of hearing aids. Nonetheless, the professionals agreed to give him an implant, and we agreed to be part of their government study. The doctor set a surgery date over the Christmas recess so that Patrick wouldn't miss even one day of school.

Just before we were to leave, Patrick's school had a Christmas pageant. Events like this were usually painful for us, as Patrick would stand staring out at the audience every year while all the other kids sang. But this year was different. He was master of ceremonies, and he introduced the play. Many mothers turned to look at Gary and me with tears in their eyes, and later told us how great it was that they understood every word he said. Normally this would have made us rejoice, but now it only served to add to our already-high anxiety. Were we making a mistake? Wasn't Patrick doing well enough?

Patrick, my aunt, and I got on a plane bound for Indiana, and Gary drove there to meet us the following day.

Patrick was given a sedative, and the nurses wheeled my baby away. My Aunt Sally calmed me down with good old-fashioned prayer, and we all settled down for what we thought would be at least a three-hour operation. I was much more relaxed during the surgery than I had been the previous two months. It's amazing how powerful my aunt's prayer can be!

A little less than two hours later, someone came to tell us that the operation was completed. All the electrodes were inserted, and Patrick was fine. When he woke up, he was such a pain in the butt that I knew he was OK! Christmas Eve we all drove home to await January 13, his "turn-on" date.

January 13 is also Patrick's birthday, and we foolishly looked at the coincidence as a sign of the beginning of a new era. Patrick looked at it as birthday sabotage. Everyone told us not to expect too much at first, but I didn't believe them. I was wrong. Patrick had some head noise for about two days, and he didn't recognize the sound of his own name or most other words. Needless to say, we went home disappointed.

That night at dinner, Patrick kept tapping his fork on his plate — *tap, tap, tap, tap* — driving us crazy. I demanded he stop. He said, "But Mom, listen to the sound my fork makes!" Needless to say, our disappointment evaporated!

Progress after that was very fast. After his six-month evaluation, one professional on the evaluation team in Indiana wrote us a letter saying that Patrick's progress was amazing, and explained that she would like to refer to his case in the future.

We had felt all along that all Patrick needed was to *hear* more. He already had the therapy, and he was prepared to benefit. In fact, Patrick complained the instant his battery ran out! He was attending a mainstream school, needing less help from us. His reading took off, along with his confidence and his grades. Suddenly, he had a few friends!

As time passed and Patrick became accustomed to processing all the extra input provided through the implant and therapy, his listening skills improved. Now, he frequently holds conversations without even looking at us. He and his friends phone one another constantly. We never thought he would be able to use the telephone unassisted. What a gift!

Today

We're always bragging about our son: Every time something great happens, I call everybody in my family to let them know. When Patrick graduated from sixth grade, I sat in the audience shedding tears of joy to watch him and nine other boys earn academic first honors.

In seventh grade he made first honors every semester, and did so well on the Stanford Achievement Test that he qualified to participate in Northwestern University's talent search for academic excellence for the Midwest states. Gary and I now spend little time preparing Pat for school. He is flying on his own.

As eighth grade progresses and we look ahead to high school, have we come to take all this for granted? Not really! I was not looking forward to going to Indiana for Patrick's three-year evaluation, but I had agreed to help, so off we went. While there, I was approached by a woman from the National Institutes of Health, who asked if I would answer some questions. She sought us out because Patrick placed in the upper 10 percent, nationally, of performance of children who had cochlear implants! Needless to say, that news made me happy to answer any questions, and happy about coming for that final evaluation.

This year Patrick's goal was to make it to the State Science Fair. His project was titled, "Comparing the performance of the cochlear implant to hearing aids in prelingual deafened children." Guess what; he made it! He has been invited to represent the Academy of the Sacred Heart at the Museum of Science and Industry next March. Whoever thought that he would?!

Leah

Reba Demeter

My husband Milan and I first met in my father's medical office. I adored my dad, an ear, nose, and throat doctor, and often dropped in to visit him at work. One day a few of the nurses sent a Dr. Milan J. Demeter to Dad's office to meet me. He was a good-looking young bachelor in the department, and the nurses saw it as their duty to look out for him, mother him, and perhaps discover a good match for him. We met, married, and the rest is history.

I had everything planned for the next decade. Milan didn't want the responsibility of children right away, so that he could complete his ENT residency at the Los Angeles County Hospital. I chose to complete my BFA in photography from the prestigious Art Center College of Design in Pasadena. I particularly enjoyed documentary and journalistic photography, especially when children were part of the story.

Milan eventually joined the practice of another ENT doctor in Glendale, California, and I began working for a Hollywood photographer. Everything fell into place. We even got pregnant on schedule,

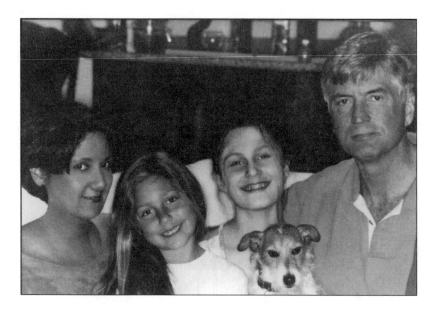

Leah Demeter (holding dog) and family

about a year into my job, and I worked until the delivery. We were very happy.

A Perfect Pregnancy
It was a perfect, healthy pregnancy, and I did all those right things that women are supposed to do: I ate healthy foods, never took medication, never had caffeine, diet cokes, nor chocolate, and I regularly exercised. I even drove 20 miles out to Beverly Hills once a week to the Jane Fonda Pregnancy Workout. Milan and I diligently went to our Lamaze classes together and were committed to having this baby drug-free and *au naturel* — and we did.

The look of total bliss on Milan's face when he first held our new daughter, Leah Suzanne Demeter, is emblazoned in my mind. Following Jewish tradition, we chose the name Leah in memory of my beloved grandmother, and Suzanne in memory of Milan's. With a smile of deep happiness, Milan whispered, "This is the best thing that has ever happened to me... Everyone should have one." He instantly bonded with Leah, his perfect daughter. Later, on the very afternoon of Leah's birth, Milan returned to the hospital to see his new family. Holding Leah in his arms, he looked up at me and said, "I don't think she can hear." I thought he was just being an overly sensitive ENT dad. I wondered if, had he been an eye doctor, he would have said, "I don't think she can see."

The baby came home to family and friends and, except for my having to be up every few hours throughout the night to feed Leah, everything seemed great. Surely she must hear! She was an easy-going baby, happy to socialize, and she made the usual baby sounds. We did remark that we could play music quite loudly and yet Leah would peacefully nap on. During the fourth week following her birth, I stood by the side of the crib and made some noises. She didn't wake up. In a panic, I telephoned my sister, Esther, in desperate need of her experienced years of motherhood.

"Esther, I even screamed and still Leah didn't move! She just keeps sleeping." Esther pointed out that many newborns can sleep through a lot of noise.

This was the beginning of months of agony for Milan and me. We would stand beside Leah's crib with noisemakers. Even the ringing of a huge bell didn't work. Once in a while she would open an eye and acknowledge our presence with gurgling baby sounds.

Hearing Tests

Milan suggested that Leah have an auditory brainstem response (ABR) test. It would relieve our ridiculous and impossible thoughts that our daughter couldn't hear. The results of the ABR were interpreted by the audiologist while we observed the monitor. After much time and effort trying to get the magical wave V (5) on the screen, the audiologist told us how sorry he was: our gorgeous, perfect baby was probably deaf.

Devastated, but determined to prove the test wrong, we flew to Stanford University to see its highly recommended and experienced brainstem doctor. He ordered us not to give Leah any medication to make her sleepy; instead, we had to keep her awake before the test. That night was one of torture. Each time Leah began to sleep, Milan picked her up, tossed her in the air above his head, and then caught her. This game worked at first, but by the early hours of the morning, Leah slept soundly even while traveling through the air.

In the morning the ABR was administered. Leah was immediately whisked away to a booth for another test, where loud and ugly sounds were made, sounds that did not wake our exhausted baby.

When the doctor told us Leah was deaf, Milan and I protested. She was just exhausted from a night of little sleep. This doctor said that Leah could have a bright future because today's hearing aids were very powerful. She might even learn to communicate through the use of speech. He advised us to "slip in" some sign language because it would be easier and less frustrating for Leah.

Devastated and in shock, Milan, Leah, and I headed back home. We agreed that the professionals must have been mistaken. Milan felt that our final and best option was the House Ear Institute, where he had spent part of his residency. This group of doctors were known throughout the world for their achievements in otology, and the medical community recognized the many years of work by Dr. William House on the cochlear implant.

Upon arrival, Leah was sedated before the brainstem test. My mother and father were there to give us much-needed support. Leah's grandfather and Milan agreed that we would accept the results of this test, no matter what the outcome.

All I can remember is Milan and me standing in the middle of a busy room, with doctors and nurses bustling about. We held on to each other tightly, crying as if we were one connected soul. It was as if the entire world had separated from us. Never before, nor since, have I felt so close to another human being.

Our drive home was like a strange dream. It was as if the three of us had remained the same, while the whole world had become an unfamiliar place. As Leah rested in my arms, with not a care in the world, I silently wondered at the sadness of her not hearing all the sounds that meant so much to me: the chirping of crickets at night, leaves rustling in the wind, the sweet song of the mourning dove as the sun comes up. Later, I learned that all those sounds were "icing on the cake" — nice to hear but not necessary for survival. The impact of a profound hearing loss, in a child that had not yet learned to talk, was incomprehensible.

Hearing Aids

The audiologist in Milan's office informed us that it was vital to get hearing aids for Leah, and begin a habilitation program, as soon as possible. "The earlier the diagnosis, the better," she told us. So Leah got appropriate amplification and started on her journey of learning to listen.

In the first year of Leah's life, things happened very fast. We seemed to be on "automatic pilot," traveling on the freeway from one appointment to the next, doing all the required things. Yet, we were unable to comprehend the total picture of where we were and where we were going. In shock, we went through all the phases of having experienced a great loss, and we grieved. Even in all the commotion, Leah was our pride and our joy. She was a happy baby, always smiling and attracting people. God had given her a gift, something special in her spirit that would carry us through this challenging journey.

Life did not have a perfect fit anymore, and we were no longer making plans a decade in advance. I accepted that there were no guarantees for the future. We would always be reevaluating our successes and failures. Our love for Leah was the guiding light through dark moments and difficult decisions. We researched every possible option and obtained information as quickly as possible, so that we could make critical decisions. I found unknown strength within Milan and myself that enabled us to do our best, no matter how difficult the task.

Two years earlier, while finishing my graduate year at Art Center, I had spent weeks completing a photographic documentary project at the John Tracy Clinic. I had enjoyed photographing the children and the dedicated teachers of the program, which was designed to help youngsters who are hearing impaired learn to speak, with an emphasis on lipreading. Now I was back again, not as a photographer but as a mom with a child who was hearing impaired.

My mother met us at the clinic each and every week. Without her support, her kind and joyful heart, and her love for Leah, our days would have been bleak, indeed! I will carry her love with me forever.

Education and Decisions

Milan and I quickly informed ourselves in order to make the important decisions that would affect our daughter's entire life. Leah's future opportunities hinged on our early decisions. The critical questions were: How will she learn to communicate? Will she learn to listen, and then to talk, with the help of powerful hearing aids and a therapist? Will she be integrated into the hearing world? Will she learn sign language, go to a school for children who are deaf, and become a part of the Deaf world and its culture?

We fell victim to many well-meaning professionals who felt that their way was the only right way. We were told that not to teach Leah sign language was cruel and even abusive, an indication that we were unwilling to accept our child's deafness. We learned about total communication, visual-oral, cued speech, manual-oral, auditory-verbal, and on and on. We sifted through each of these approaches by reading, making telephone calls, and visiting schools, therapists, and clinics. Most importantly, we observed *the children* in all these places. We spoke to many parents and professionals, and concluded that the "right way" to teach our child was by using whatever would work for Leah and our family. We finally chose the auditory-verbal approach, which we felt would provide a life as normal as possible and would allow her many opportunities to fulfill her potential. We wanted Leah to grow up with high expectations.

Learning to Listen

I became Leah's primary teacher, which was natural since any child's first teacher is usually the parent. We went to auditory-verbal therapy twice a week and were given specific goals to incorporate into her play. Listening was emphasized. Milan and I didn't have any preconceived ideas about normal speech and language development. Leah was our only child at that time. Thus, her progress was always exciting, and we never had to compare her to an older sibling.

After intense hearing-aid evaluations, Leah was aided with proper amplification. I learned how the hearing aids worked and how to keep them functioning at peak performance. At first, our primary goal was to help Leah become aware of the noisy world around her, and "I hear that!" became a common phrase in our home. Leah was soon pointing to her ear whenever she heard a sound.

At eight months of age, she said her first word. I was sitting on the bedroom floor with Leah playing behind me when I suddenly heard a little voice say, "Eye." She pointed to the eye on her stuffed animal and said it again: "Eye." That was the small miracle we had been praying for, and it was the key that unlocked the door to spoken language. Soon after, Leah was connecting words and objects. The sounds she had heard repeated, hundreds of times, every day, for hundreds of days, now had some meaning.

In many respects, Leah's development progressed similarly to that of a child with typical hearing. However, she did not learn language in the same easy and natural ways that others did — by hearing conversations, the TV or radio, or her parents chatting in the next room. Instead, all words, all phrases, sentences, and verbal thoughts were consciously presented to her, close up, within her earshot. But Leah did learn. Life seemed bittersweet. Learning to listen and talk, she moved at a constant pace, sometimes reaching plateaus, then moving forward again — but we knew she would get to her destination.

School

After looking at many preschools, we enrolled Leah at one in the neighborhood that emphasized social skills through play. I casually mentioned to the director of the school that Leah had a hearing loss. She had no idea what that meant, or how her deafness would affect our child's relationships in this new environment. Welcomed with open arms, Leah had entered the mainstream of life.

We quickly came face to face with the painful truth that our daughter was significantly delayed in language. She was three years old, and most of the kids her own age and even younger were talking in complete sentences, while Leah spoke in one-word utterances or simple phrases. Sometimes, she did not talk in school at all. The first time Milan went to observe Leah at school, he left in tears. Fortunately, our therapist got us back on track by reminding us to keep everything in perspective. Actually, Leah was making daily progress. But sometimes I was so angry that I wanted to shout at the world that my daughter was smarter than anyone else's kid, even though her speech was delayed!

Nevertheless, Leah enjoyed her days at preschool and soon made friends. We visited their homes, and they visited ours. However, playing with just one friend at a time has always been more comfortable for Leah than playing in a group.

Changes in Hearing

Shortly after she entered preschool, I noticed a change in Leah's hearing, one so subtle that no one noticed but me. She was not hearing from the same distances as she had, nor was she hearing soft sounds. We went for an audiological assessment and hearing-aid check. The audiologist said that everything was the same and that no changes were apparent on the audiogram. I am sure everyone thought I was obsessed with Leah's hearing and that I was a bit nutty. Unfortunately, I proved them wrong. Her hearing progressively deteriorated in the high frequencies, and later also in the low frequencies, leaving her with a "cookie-bite" audiogram and aided thresholds that soon fell outside the "speech banana." Her voice was no longer the *pretty voice* upon which most professionals commented. She could no longer hear herself talking, and the sounds she did hear were even further distorted. The floor fell from beneath our feet, and I panicked! Leah was prescribed large doses of steroids to bring down any swelling that might be causing pressure on her auditory nerves, and she was given more powerful hearing aids.

At the onset of her fluctuating and diminishing hearing, her dad inserted PE tubes to keep her ears clear of fluid. She had such precious little hearing that the slightest amount of fluid could temporarily wipe it out.

Milan saw no relief with the tubes. I expected him to be a miracle worker and demanded that he get her hearing back. He was even harder on himself. The frustrations of not being able to make a difference hurt him terribly. We agreed that treating his own child was too much of an emotional strain and that he would not do it again.

Soon Leah had two exploratory surgeries on her left ear, the only ear with hearing. The surgeon felt that he had successfully patched a tiny fistula that allowed leakage to the inner-ear hair cells. To complicate the medical problems even further, Leah's "better" ear began to drain. She was immediately prescribed antibiotics, and a culture was taken. Within days she was hospitalized for a nasty, unusual bacterial infection called pseudomonas. Various intravenous antibiotics were tried. Each time the prescribed drug appeared to be doing its job, the bacteria would mysteriously change form, and the drug would no longer work. We tried all the antibiotics that were not ototoxic. When those ran out, she was prescribed experimental drugs.

During all this, Leah's voice quality and speech deteriorated. She heard nothing without her hearing aid in the left ear.

Two doctors, my father and my husband, each felt very differently about the course of action. My father wanted mastoid surgery performed immediately to clear the infection and stop further hearing loss, while my husband felt that the possibility for further hearing loss would be increased with this surgery. We were torn apart, terrified of making the wrong decision. After another week of aggressive intravenous drugs, her grandfather and dad agreed to go ahead with the mastoidectomy.

We were holding on by a thread when Leah was released from the hospital a couple of days following her surgery. When the swelling subsided and her ear healed, the hearing aids were finally back on. Leah's hearing did not return. We were told it could take a while! The idea of Leah's losing her hearing entirely was unthinkable.

We continued therapy but no longer restricted lipreading. Temporarily, I lost our vision of Leah's future. Amazingly, her language skills kept progressing, but her speech had become unintelligible to anyone other than her immediate family and her therapist, who kept our dream alive during those days of despair. Somehow, Leah continued to absorb information from her world. Her sweet, positive nature helped her still to find therapy and language learning pleasurable.

Another Precious Child

I learned to be flexible in a world that seemed uncertain and full of unpleasant surprises. Milan and I had delayed having another child, waiting for a day when our lives would be more stable and manageable. A dear friend, the mother of two children who are hearing impaired, pointed out, "If you're waiting for things to be perfect, you may end up waiting forever."

On April 7, 1988 Rachel Lill Demeter was born, filling our home with happiness and laughter. She has brought much love to each of us. But the unexpected happened once again: Rachel was born with transposition of the great arteries and faced major open-heart surgery at the age of six months. Happily, today she is a thriving eight-year-old with boundless energy and amazing creative and intellectual abilities. Leah and Rachel play hard, fight a lot, talk all the time, and love each other. Leah has clearly benefited from having a younger sister.

Two Years Later

Two years had passed, and Leah's hearing was never again the same. When Milan was invited to speak at an Alexander Graham Bell Association conference in Ottawa, Canada, Leah and I accompanied him, while Rachel stayed with her grandparents. After the conference we saw an auditory-verbal therapist herself who had a son who was profoundly hearing impaired. She gave us the wake-up call we desperately needed. Leah would not regain her hearing. At the time, I felt anger and resentment. The pain was barely tolerable, but we left Canada accepting the truth.

Leah continued to work on her listening skills during therapy sessions. In her daily life, she used whatever little hearing remained and became more and more dependent upon her eyes. She was attending a wonderful kindergarten class in a private elementary school where the class size was much smaller than in the public schools. The older she became, the more difficult and tiring classes were for her. Leah did not have the luxury of resting her eyes and mind and daydream, not even for an instant. If she did, she had trouble finding her place again in the lesson. Attention and focus were paramount. But school was tough, and Leah was exhausted.

The Cochlear Implant

Milan and I knew the current information about the cochlear implant. The Nucleus 22-channel implant had been approved for about two years for children who were prelingually deafened. We spoke to auditory-verbal therapists from all over the world and got the names and telephone numbers of families who had children close to Leah's age with similar hearing losses and auditory-verbal backgrounds. We were confident that Leah would be a good candidate because she had the memory of sounds that she had processed through her hearing aids, and she had worked hard to become a good listener. By now, Leah was no longer able to hear low-frequency sounds or discriminate between vowels; earlier, she had lost the ability to hear many of the consonants. We knew that if the implant could help to furnish more spoken information, she would use this new hearing sensation for great benefit.

Leah would be nine years old that year, old enough to grasp the amount of time and effort that it would take to learn to listen again. She needed to know that the implant wasn't something that she would just put on and suddenly hear everything, and that the electrical stimulation she would receive would not recreate sounds as she had known them before. There would be no progress without her commitment. She was shown the processor and all the equipment worn outside the body. Leah desperately wanted to hear, and therefore agreed to continue auditory-verbal therapy. Although she didn't like the equipment that she'd have to wear, she would do so. We all hoped that she would hear better, but once again, no promises were made.

On May 6, 1992, one day after her ninth birthday, Leah had successful cochlear implant surgery. Three weeks later the processor was connected and turned on. The unbelievable happened! Everything was too loud for her. Even the sound of a piece of cellophane being unwrapped from a candy was too uncomfortable to tolerate. That day we all had to whisper. But when Leah woke up the next morning and put on her implant, the sounds that had been too loud were no longer so. We were later told that her brain had learned to process the sounds and had adapted to them. In three days Leah's implant was MAPped to comfortable levels of sounds. In less than a year, her processor was improved and replaced by the SPEAK system.

Today

Leah is now 13 years old and has worn her cochlear implant for four years. Her perseverance, intelligence, and love for people, along with the implant, have contributed to her success. Her speech has improved enormously. She is intelligible, her "pretty voice" has returned, and she can even understand me on the telephone.

Thirteen is a difficult age for any teenager: no one wants to stand out because of a difference, so it's natural that Leah wants to be just like her friends and classmates. Most 13-year-olds do not realize how much they have in common with their friends! Today Leah is a much sought-after left-handed fastball pitcher in the girls' softball league; she has won many blue ribbons for riding and jumping in horse shows, and she maintains a high grade-point average at school.

Leah, our beloved daughter, please take a close look, a very close look. It is your spirit that makes you the very special person that you are. For this, your friends and family love you! Many professionals and your family have provided you with skills to live your life to the fullest. But it is you who has used these skills to become such a vital part of this wonderful world. We thank God every day for the blessing of your presence.

Guilherme

Marta Salvucci

Não pode!

"Não pode!"

When I hear my six-year-old son, Guilherme, shouting these words out loud at me, I think to myself, "Yes, you're right, dear, não pode." In Brazilian Portuguese, "não pode" may have two meanings: "You can't do that," which certainly is what my son means, or "This is incredible, unbelievable," which, of course, is what I mean!

Guilherme is the second child of a family of three children. Our eldest daughter is nine years old, and our youngest girl is three. Guilherme is the only boy, a middle child, and also the only one who is hearing impaired. We are unsure of the cause for his profound hearing loss. There were several possibilities, one being that he was born prematurely. During the early months after his birth, we did not suspect anything. We found all his reactions quite normal, but we did notice that he seemed a little "slower" in his development than his sister had been. We attributed that to premature birth.

By the time Guilherme was eight months old, however, it was impossible not to notice that he did not respond to his own name, he

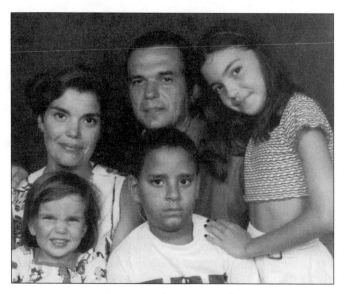

Guilherme Salvucci and family

would not wake up at the sound of the doorbell, he was not bothered by the ringing of the telephone, he would not dance or sing to sounds on television, he would not look at the TV screen, and was not frightened by loud noises, such as the explosion of fireworks.

Hearing Loss!

After having spent too much time blaming all this on his lack of attention or immaturity, we finally took Guilherme for an audiological assessment. He was just 11 months old when I heard the words that would haunt me for a long time: "Your son has a hearing loss." I did not have the slightest idea how that diagnosis would change the life of my entire family.

I thought wearing hearing aids was similar to wearing glasses: I would simply put them on and all our problems would be solved. I understand now all the hard work, all the time, and all the dedication required to help my Guilherme.

I got other opinions! I took him to seven specialists, until the final verdict was rendered: Guilherme had a congenital, bilateral, profound hearing loss, etiology unknown. From the moment of diagnosis, I became obsessed with one thought: Would my son be able to speak? I have a strong background in language teaching, and was aware of the importance of hearing in the development of speech and language.

A week after the initial diagnosis, Guilherme started speech therapy. My husband and I had no doubt in choosing an oral approach. We are not against sign language, but we thought that, although we knew it would be difficult for Guilherme to learn to talk and for the family to help him learn, we all wanted to try. In Brazil, there are very few therapists who specialize in the rehabilitation of children or adults who are hearing impaired. Schools are not equipped with adequate sound systems or FM systems, and there are not many qualified professionals in the schools to work with any special-needs children. In Brazil, prejudice against "handicapped" people is, unfortunately, still a reality.

Hearing Aids

It took a long time but, on November 14, 1991, at 16 months, Guilherme was fitted with his first pair of hearing aids, the most powerful ones existing in the market. His adaptation to wearing the aids was not difficult, even though he did experiment with floating them in the toilet bowl and throwing them the farthest distance he could manage. He was showing some progress in therapy and could approximate some simple words, such as "papa" ("daddy"), "dá" ("give"), "pão" ("bread"), but he depended on lipreading. He even learned more complex words like "sorvete" ("ice cream"), which he would pronounce "tovete," but it took him, the speech therapist, and us an enormous effort to achieve such results. It was such a slow pace! Even with the very powerful hearing aids and speech therapy, he still did not react to most sounds, and he could never detect human speech.

Right after I learned Guilherme was hearing impaired, I read a newspaper article about the cochlear implant, which was proving to bring good results to people with profound hearing losses. I remember that I asked the therapist if the cochlear implant would be applicable for my son. She told me that, unfortunately, in Brazil, at that time, surgery was being recommended only for adults or children with postlingual hearing losses. Nonetheless, I never stopped considering the eventual possibility of a cochlear implant for Guilherme.

In November 1993, we got the marvelous news that a cochlear implant center in Brazil had successfully performed the first cochlear implant in a three-year-old child with a congenital, bilateral, profound hearing loss. "Well," I thought, "if they did that first surgery, they might be willing to try another; why not Guilherme?"

My younger daughter was only 15 days old at that time, and I was nursing her. My husband had to start the evaluation procedures. As we live in Rio de Janeiro and the surgeon's office is in São Paulo, Gui and his dad took trips there during November and December 1993 for the primary evaluation tests. The audiological assessments revealed what we had already suspected; Gui's hearing aids would enable him to hear only at low frequencies (250 Hz and 500 Hz) at levels of 85 dB HL and 90 dB HL, respectively. At all other frequencies, his responses were nonexistent! Those results indicated that he was a candidate for cochlear implantation. Other evaluations, nonetheless, were still to come, including several audiological evaluations, psychological assessments, and computerized tomography. We discovered a problem with Gui's central nervous system, and perhaps a cochlear implant would have no effect. Picture this: 400 km away from my boy, caring for a 15-day-old baby, receiving news only by phone, and learning that what I had expected and longed for so much as the "light at the end of the tunnel" was probably going to be ruled out!

A Cochlear Implant!

I believe that Guilherme is surrounded by a legion of guardian angels, not just one! Luckily, the surgeon decided to continue Gui's evaluation process for the implant. He ordered a neurological assessment and a magnetic field scan to decide whether my boy would be an acceptable candidate for surgery. The results of the magnetic field scan, though more positive, were still inconclusive. The surgeon decided to take my boy's exams and evaluations to discuss with other surgeons in the United States. Meanwhile, Gui and my husband went to Bauru, a city in the inland of the state of São Paulo, where the implant center is located, for more tests.

In February 1994, we had the final answer: Yes, Guilherme would have his cochlear implant. Can you guess how I felt? I had great hopes for the effectiveness of this surgery, even though I knew it was not supposed to be a miracle! The electrode array would not replace my son's hearing, but it was something! My husband and I never had doubts concerning the surgery; we just waited for the surgeon to tell us when to take Gui to hospital. Some other parents called us crazy, because we were going to expose our almost four-year-old son to another general anesthetic (he had already had five for previous exams and surgeries) and a procedure that could not promise any improvement. To those who thought us mad we said, "We believe in the professionals who are assisting our child and, above all, we believe in God."

On April 29, 1994, Guilherme received a cochlear implant in the hospital in Bauru, Brazil. The whole family went together with Gui to Bauru for the surgery, including the six-month-old baby. We are convinced that the presence of both mother and father and his two sisters was fundamental for his fast recovery. The procedure was successful. The surgeon was able to implant the entire array (22 electrodes) in Guilherme's cochlea. A week later, we took the long trip back home to Rio to wait for the activation, which occurred a month later.

At first, Gui did not want to wear the device. It was very different from his hearing aids, since it has wires and a small speech processor, worn on the body. It was not difficult, however, to convince him to keep the system on. In exchange for two plastic toy swords he had been asking us to buy, he wore the system. He did not immediately become aware of sounds the moment the audiologist activated the system. It took a lot of training, effort, and patience to help him learn to listen through his cochlear implant.

Discipline?

Gui is not a highly disciplined child. He is very stubborn, and he will accomplish only the tasks he is interested in doing. In the past, he has thrown away the exercises from speech therapy and his homework assignments. He has pulled out the microphone and coil of the implant system to demonstrate that he did not care to hear or listen to what we were saying. He once ran away from the audiologist's office in Bauru, trying to escape a MAPping, which is a procedure he does not like, and he has shouted at his therapist. We have had several moments in which Guilherme did not cooperate with either the professionals or us! But I thank God for the angels around my son: his speech therapist, his audiologist, his psychologist, his surgeon, his pediatrician, and many more throughout these years. Maybe he listens because of their patience and dedication!

Today

There have also been wonderfully rewarding and happy times. Once Guilherme was three rooms away from the room of Bia, his sister, when she cried. He looked up at me, and said, "Mama, Bia chora," which means, "Mom, Bia is crying." For the first time in his life, at the age of four and a half years, he heard a distant sound and he recognized it! Another unforgettable moment happened in July 1996, when Guilherme went to the telephone to receive congratulations for his sixth birthday. He listened, heard, and recognized the words that were being said — simple things, such as "Guilherme, congratulations, a kiss." He repeated the words out loud and was clearly delighted to realize that the telephone he now heard ringing really did have a purpose!

Guilherme has now had his cochlear implant for 30 months, and his progress has been steady, if not fast. Among other things, he is able to recognize his name being called in any environment, even the noisiest ones, like Disney World; he does not depend on lipreading for daily questions or instructions, such as "Let's have lunch, now," or, "Gui, it is time for your shower" (to which he immediately answers, "Mom, I'm going soon, OK? Wait"). We think that's pretty good! Guilherme has also learned some colloquial expressions without having been taught them during therapy sessions.

It is obvious for people who meet my son for the first time that he is hearing impaired. People look curiously at his implant and, though they rarely ask, I explain what that "strange" device is. In Brazil, I would guess that fewer than 100 people have received cochlear implants, so it is not difficult to understand such curiosity. Thankfully, my husband and I, Guilherme himself, and God do not care about such things!

It is really incredible that, after so many hopeless moments, doubts, wonderings, and suffering, we can finally see Guilherme's progress, not only in learning to listen, but in the acquisition of language. The quality of his language and the intelligibility of his speech are certainly not perfect, but they are much better than before the implant. We feel his hearing ability improves with intensive therapy sessions and with additional MAPping. We know we still have a long, long way to go, especially in a country like ours, where, unfortunately, children such as Guilherme do not have all the support they need and deserve. But technology is improving and Guilherme is still a boy. There will be many new and wider paths opened for him.

To Guilherme: "Pode, Sim!"

Well, Guilherme, when I hear you shout "Não pode!" because I did something you did not like, I have mixed feelings. On the one hand, I agree with you, because it is almost unbelievable that you are arguing with me. On the other hand I disagree, my son. "Pode, sim" — it is possible, with the help and dedication of all the wonderful people that surround you in your life. And with God's blessing, you can be a happy and fulfilled person!

Julie

Karen Sworik

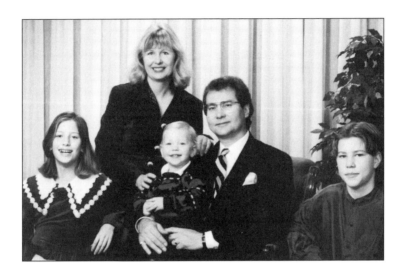

Julie Sworik (left) and family

Recently, our 13-year-old daughter, Juliane, sat on a panel of students who were hearing impaired, fielding questions about her deafness and implications for her studies and goals. One of the questions was, "Have you decided on a career?" Without hesitation Julie responded, "Either a model or a doctor." I am surprised by neither.

This past summer, while peers participated in camps and team sports, Julie completed two modeling courses. The highlight was being selected a finalist in a major department-store model search contest! A career in medicine would present rigorous academic challenges, yet we admire Julie's recent award for "academic achievement and effort" and recognize that this choice too, is not an impossibility. School success has not come easily for Julie; determination has taken her farther than "school smarts" alone ever could.

Diagnosis

Not so many years ago, we were thrilled to hear our doctor announce, "You have a beautiful, perfect daughter." A year later, we learned our beautiful, perfect daughter was deaf. Over the years, we have come to realize that our early experiences — where both the family doctor and pediatrician dismissed our concerns about Julie's hearing — are repeated in families all over the world.

When Julie's diagnosis of profound bilateral sensorineural deafness was finally confirmed, it was done without compassion or satisfactory explanation. We were advised to contact the local school for the deaf, which provided a home-visiting program for newly diagnosed children. There were assurances that educational worries would be eliminated as Julie blended into the school's total communication program. Would Julie talk? The possibility of this was about the same as the one-in-a-thousand odds that we would have a child who was deaf. Through our sadness, my husband Bruce jokingly assured me that we had already been blessed with that first lottery; maybe we could win again!

Julie is our second child, three years younger than her older brother, Dylan. I had not returned to work after her birth, deciding to remain a stay-at-home mom. Little did I know the implications of this decision! As Bruce returned to the business of working and providing for our family, I became absorbed in the topic of deafness. The public library and the Canadian Hearing Society were my first sources. Through books and publications, I was able to obtain many other contacts and organizations. Soon our mailbox was filled with information from the Alexander Graham Bell Association for the Deaf, the John Tracy Clinic, and a Canadian organization — Voice for Hearing Impaired Children.

The Early Years

Dr. Daniel Ling, renowned international expert in the field of speech and language development of the hearing impaired, was the keynote speaker at a meeting we attended one month after Julie's diagnosis. We heard children who were deaf speaking! Not much later, the Voice organization put us in touch with our therapist, who works at a hospital in Toronto, many miles away. We began *learning to listen* when Julie was 17 months old.

We embraced the motto, "A little bit of hearing can go a long way," and auditory-verbal therapy became our way of life. The six-to-seven-hour round trip to Toronto, in fair and foul weather, became routine. The car seemed to head there on auto pilot week after week, year after year! We worked faithfully and diligently. Often, I begrudged my husband his "paid" job. My hours were long, the preparations for lesson materials extensive, and the frustrations many. The compensation often seemed elusive. But then a little miracle would happen, and another, and another. With each one, I felt rekindled and renewed that this was the right approach for us!

Lottery Win Eludes Us!

Still, we had to face our doubts, and ultimately the reality. By the time Julie was five years old, she had great receptive language, acquired primarily through vision and reading. Our therapist recognized that, even amplified, Julie's hearing was insufficient to perceive sound in the speech range. For all intents and purposes, her speech was unintelligible except to her therapist, family, close friends, and Snowball the cat.

Waves of stress and anxiety filled our household. Julie did understand the English language; she could read and was a good lipreader. But speak, no: at least not in a language the world understood! In 1988 we faced a choice between the total communication approach or a cochlear implant. We have never opposed sign language, but we felt it would limit the number of people with whom Julie would be able to communicate. Clearly, it would be unfair to continue without offering her the tool of expressive language. Would it be through signing or the possibility of acquiring hearing sensation and speech through a cochlear implant? We had struggled too long, fought too hard, cried too many tears to abandon our dream of having Julie function in the hearing world to give up without exploring this last chance.

A Cochlear Implant

Today, cochlear implants have become a successful surgical procedure for individuals who are profoundly deaf. But when we began investigating this option, these devices were largely experimental. Clinical trials for children were just being completed in the United States, and only adults had received implants in our home province of Ontario, Canada.

We began the candidate selection process at a hospital in New York City. The screening included extensive hearing, psychological, and neurological testing which was thorough and exhausting, taking two separate visits of a couple of days' duration each. We visited other families whose children had received cochlear implants; their encouraging stories and delightful children inspired us. We were relieved to learn, shortly thereafter, that Julie had been approved!

Amazingly, at the same time, the surgeon who was currently providing implants for postlingually deafened adults in our community learned of our out-of-province arrangements, and requested a meeting with us. He was willing to accept Julie as his first pediatric patient. What good fortune! Not only would we be relieved of the expense and time involved in traveling out of the country, but the numerous postoperative visits for the programming and fine-tuning of the speech processor could be done right at home.

Implantation

Julie received her implant on July 4, 1989, four days after her sixth birthday. The surgery was not entirely routine. The surgeon emerged from the operating room three hours into surgery and informed us that he was having difficulty inserting the electrode array. He was prepared to drill a little further, but did not want to get anywhere close to the facial nerve. My husband and I were in tears! When our child was on the operating table, we were tempted to say, "Stop right now," but we didn't. Instead, we assured the doctor that we had confidence in his judgment, either to go ahead if the drilling was safe or to conclude the surgery without implantation. A few hours later, we all met again. The doctor was satisfied that the majority of the electrodes had been inserted into the cochlea. The remainder had been laid in the drilled cavity.

You can imagine that the month-long wait before the device could be activated was a worrisome time for us all — for everyone except Julie. She bounced back from surgery as though it were a cut finger. In her usual fearless manner, she would jump on her two-wheeler or climb to the highest rung of the climber. (Child, don't you realize what could happen if you injure your head? No, and who cares, anyway! Life is too much fun!) The hardest thing to do was forbidding her to swim in what was probably the hottest summer on record. In the water, Julie was a mermaid. Swimming has always soothed and exhilarated her, and having to wait for those staples to come out was brutal.

At last, the activation day arrived. It was tense as we waited for Julie to show some sign of hearing. Finally, there it was: a broad smile with the words, "I heard that!" As the audiologist proceeded through the channels, the words were repeated 19 times. Of the 22 electrodes, 19 were activated.

Julie Listens!

In the first days and weeks at home, Julie heard our voices but was not discriminating speech. Her first responses were to environmental sounds, and we were kept busy identifying all of them: lawnmowers and motorcycles, as well as the household noises of doorbells, dishwashers, telephones, and Dad's pager, among many others.

Over the months that followed, Julie's speech discrimination improved significantly. She was finally a listening child! We could call her from the top or bottom of the stairs of our two-storey home, and she would respond. If she was outdoors, we could call her in for dinner from the doorway. We were becoming more relaxed as she bicycled around the block, because the sounds of approaching vehicles were now audible to her. Julie loved extracurricular sports and activities with neighborhood children, and her confidence grew as she became more proficient at communicating. She learned to ski, and continues to do so avidly. She also excels at swimming.

Julie's growing independence was increasingly evident. She could order her own fries and Coke at a concession booth, and the attendants understood her. She could talk to her ski instructor or a sales clerk. Her improved communication skills opened pathways to new adventures. Mom, Dad, or her close friends no longer had to act as her oral interpreters.

A Deaf Sibling?

When Julie was eight, our family received a second miracle: her little brother and our son, Alexander. Since neither medical examination nor genetic testing had explained Julie's congenital deafness, we awaited Alexander's birth with some anxiety. As his birth grew closer, I was amazed that the possibility of raising another child who was hearing impaired no longer terrified me. As a family, we felt that we were experts, and knowledge certainly dispels fear. We knew that if this child was deaf, he would not have to wait six years in silence. He would have cochlear implantation as early as possible.

Fortunately, our now four-year-old boy hears perfectly and has exceptional expressive abilities. We joke that years of auditory-verbal therapy had become such a part of our parenting that we unconsciously gave Alexander "mini lessons." Moreover, big sister Julie, having been subjected to her share of lessons, promptly took over the teaching role, and Alexander became convinced that all preschool children did lessons and homework! A standard poodle joined our family this spring, and now Julie is determined to train Niko! Even dogs need lessons, right?

Teenhood: Triumphs and Trials

Julie is currently in eighth grade at a school where there is a cluster of children who are hearing impaired. All are integrated into mainstream classes. Julie takes all subjects, except French, with her peers. She receives tutorial support services from a teacher of the deaf and a teaching assistant, as well as the mainstream classroom teacher. Unfortunately, speech therapy has been available only on a limited and often sporadic schedule, over the years.

Currently, we are focusing on speech production. Even though Julie can be quite intelligible, her speech is not always at its best.

While the improvement of Julie's hearing sensation with her cochlear implant has been amazing, those first six years of silence have yet to be fully overcome. Julie is presently working privately with a speech pathologist who shares her interest in fashion, nails, and make-up, so they are hitting it off splendidly and making progress! The challenge is to fine-tune Julie's speech production.

While the cochlear implant has helped to improve her listening and speaking abilities, Julie does remain a "visual" child. The first six years of watching became an integral part of her being. Julie is a phenomenal lipreader, and she continues to rely on combined auditory and visual information. She is also a compulsive writer, whether it be notes or letters to friends and family, messages on the whiteboard, or hours spent at the computer. Even in junior kindergarten, her teacher was amazed that she rarely painted pictures, but painted words instead. We have read stories about teenagers who are deaf and use the oral approach; some have learned sign language later on. If Julie chooses sign language, not French, as her second language, that will be her choice.

It Takes a Village

In the coming year Julie will be required to leave the familiar and venture into new life experiences. The comfort and security of her elementary school will be replaced by the challenges of new teachers and new expectations in high school. Also, we are leaving our home of 15 years to settle in an area closer to Julie's secondary school and that of our older son. She will be leaving the familiarity of a neighborhood that knows and loves her. It has been said that it takes a village to raise a child, and we often felt that our very dedicated friends and neighbors played a significant role in shaping our daughter. Hopefully, Julie's new-found independence with the local transit system will enable her to maintain these special friendships. Happily, her school friends will be nearer, so she is excited about the prospect of spending more time with the girls, and yes, boys!

Julie wholeheartedly reassures us that she is happy to have received a cochlear implant. Like us, she is hopeful that future technology will bring improvements, making the external device smaller and even more effective. But had we waited for the "perfect" device, Julie's formative years would have gone by very differently. We are proud to be the parents of a young teen who inspires everyone with her enviable love of life and learning! For Julie, the cochlear implant has been a sixth sense. It certainly isn't hearing like anything we know or can imagine. But we do know it has been a blessing, like the blessing of our beautiful and perfect daughter!

Justin

Cheryl Exner

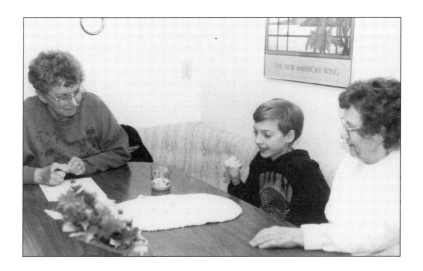

Justin Exner and grandmas

Diagnosis and Despair

In Justin's first months, our concerns for him centered, contentedly, around sleeping schedules and diaper rash. By his eighth month, we wondered. The suspicion of deafness began to dominate our lives. At the time, public health services in Regina, Saskatchewan were slow to respond. Twice, in a government clinic filled with parents and children, I waited. Twice, they had no time for us.

I approached our new general practitioner and asked for help. Her preliminary checkup confirmed our fears. A whirlwind of activity followed, yet all action seemed incredibly slow. Screening, a specialist's visit, travel to a city two hours away for brainstem testing, discovery of a profound hearing loss, further testing and fitting for an FM system — the professional's device of choice — took months. Justin received his FM just before his first birthday.

I have no words to describe the ache of loss. Nothing prepares parents for this. We felt desperation as we attempted to maintain control, to comprehend the implications of the word "deaf."

Despair followed as I floundered in my understanding of God. The crisis in diagnosis matched my crisis in faith. Why had this happened? Coming to peace with this question took time.

When Justin was almost two, I read something that suggested God searched to find suitable parents for a "disabled" child, parents of strong character and full of love.

The story troubled me, so I prayed. After some time, I understood my feelings. If God *chose* us for this, then God was either exceedingly cruel or horribly controlling! In my belief, God is neither. Justin is deaf because Justin is deaf. The deafness just "is." In fact, God has very much sustained us in our care for our child.

Hearing Aids

Justin's fitting with hearing aids brought us some assistance. Many services, however, did not match our needs.

What was missing? An acknowledgment of grief, private talks about how to move through the grieving process, a description of *all* types of therapy and communication methods, and an offer to *teach us* how we could help Justin. In a province with funding that extended more to sign-language services than oral services, I faltered. My research skills and quest for "something more" led me to a route we have followed for years — auditory-verbal therapy.

The book *Learning to Listen,* edited by Pat Vaughan, was my introduction. A professional willingly lent me this book, assuring me that Regina's services were quite similar to those described but that the children in the book were exceptional; I should not hope that Justin would accomplish what they had.

I contacted an auditory-verbal therapist who reported that, in Ottawa, there was a program for out-of-province children. I discovered I could take advantage of it, with Saskatchewan Health covering the therapy, though not the travel and accommodation costs — an excellent opportunity. Soon Justin, my mother, and I were in Ottawa!

Hearing and seeing children who were profoundly deaf talking with enough clarity that I could understand them was intoxicating. Our first therapist, who had a son who was hearing impaired, tempered my enthusiasm with a strong dash of common sense — nothing would come easily. I would have to be creative, think of games, use all my teaching talents, and make learning to listen *fun!*

But learning is not always fun. Recently, I asked Justin how much fun he thought he had in lessons. He was kind. Although I was sometimes "boring," the lessons were "mostly fun" but "too long." Knowing when to quit has never been my forte.

After three weeks, we arrived home and continued to try the therapy with the support of local professionals. We faced two problems. Some professionals here did not believe auditory-verbal therapy was significantly different from their own, and, more importantly, Justin simply did not make progress.

The Choice

We visited Ottawa again when Justin was two and a half, having brought audiological testing to show Justin's responses at 60 dB HL. He was retested. Result: Justin had no residual hearing. He was smart; he had fooled everyone, but he could not hear. We were given two choices: learn sign language or cued speech. A cochlear implant was suggested, with reservations by the therapist because she knew of only one prelingually deafened child who was experiencing success with it, a boy in Toronto.

We ruled surgery out, for it seemed too drastic. For two weeks I learned about cued speech with a therapist from Australia who was in Ottawa on a practicum. I practiced and returned to Regina only to find that no school would support cued speech. We turned to sign language as a final option.

Statistics on the average reading levels of children who sign were part of our concern, but we were distressed also that family members might not learn sign language, even when they said they would. For us, this meant many limitations.

The choice of a cochlear implant remained, yet I was emotionally exhausted. Empty, I began half-hearted research. So much effort; so much pain.

To our dismay, no center in Canada would take us. Justin was prelingually deafened and the consensus from Canadian centers was that his chances for learning language through the implant were slim. Such children rarely received implants.

I telephoned our therapist, who directed us to the United States. Ultimately, the choice narrowed between a center in New York and one in Denver. New York seemed too exotic, and Denver was closer. We chose Denver.

The Cochlear Implant

The professionals who assessed Justin in Denver did not want our expectations to exceed the implant's potential. To expect more of Justin than he could deliver would have hurt, not helped, him. I insisted that I would be happy if he were limited to hearing sounds that would alert him to danger and distinguishing some environmental sounds. In my heart, however, I knew I wanted more. If the implant could be activated, more use of audition alone *could be* the goal. I didn't care if the implant provided sound quality equivalent to that of an out-of-tune radio. If he could obtain enough hearing sensation, listening and speaking would be our goals. I would not push Justin beyond where he could go, yet I could not ask him to accept less than our best efforts.

Some people believed that speech for a child with a cochlear implant who was prelingually deafened was possible, but that there would have to be some memory of sound. Justin had none. In fact, the physicians wondered if he even had an auditory nerve.

Surgery

Not knowing if Justin had a functioning auditory nerve was one of the worst parts of the surgery. There was no way to test for this, except through surgery. In the summer of 1989, Justin had many tests and evaluations. Psychological evaluation, speech and language testing, audiological and medical visits all combined to confirm that Justin was a good candidate for the implant. Throughout the assessments, we were calm. We knew we were doing the right thing.

Professionals involved with the cochlear implant cautioned us; they were honest about all possible complications — temporary paralysis of the facial nerve, use of an anesthetic, head incision, and pain. It was a comfort that few children experienced such complications. We were alerted to potential problems: MAPs change, processors fail, cords break, and microphones become silent. Children can reject their processors. Knowing all this, we chose surgery.

Justin's surgery was scheduled for October 3, 1989, at 6:30 p.m. During the day, people at home said prayers for Justin. That afternoon, I panicked. We met with the surgeon one last time. Everything became terrifyingly real and at one point, I suggested we just go home. But Howard — up to this point, the skeptical parent — was now certain we should press ahead.

Preparation for the surgery was filled with fun for Justin. A nurse with a fantastic knack for entertaining children played with him while we composed ourselves. The needle to relax Justin was a temporary nightmare, since he tried to escape it! Mercifully, it was the worst part of the entire procedure.

During the surgery, we were in a state of high anxiety. I went to the chapel to pray. When the surgeon came out and announced that Justin had a functioning auditory nerve and all electrodes were in correctly, my prayers were answered.

Recovery was swift and easy. Howard stayed with Justin overnight while I snoozed at the hostel. On October 4, Justin was discharged. He experienced little pain and didn't want the medication after the third day. We flew home October 6.

Therapy

We could not know the cochlear implant would provide Justin with so much. Through faith and work he has learned spoken language. What luck that we were not only provided with an exceptional implant center, but also with therapists who helped us realize our dream.

Justin's implant was first MAPped when he was three and a half years old, one month after surgery. I was unable to be there since our funds were low, but Howard took him. On our video of the event, one can see the miracle begin. At one point, the audiologist comments that Justin is beginning to babble. It was true: the silent child who boarded a plane to Denver, deplaned in Regina, already verbalizing.

Intense daily therapy began. As in most auditory-verbal families, one parent became dominant in encouraging listening, speech, and language development. I worked mornings only to allow time to be with Justin in the afternoons. Because of my Ottawa experiences, I could focus clearly on the goals.

The early stages were demanding, for I wasn't sure what to expect. Unfortunately, the Ontario program was now closed to out-of-province children. Because I knew how to begin auditory-verbal therapy, the Ontario therapist guided my work at long distance. She was also helping two young girls who had received implants. One had a history similar to Justin's; the other had contracted meningitis. With their parents' permission, I received videos of their therapy. We followed their progress and used many ideas on the tapes to help Justin. In turn, I sent some of our videos to the therapist. Her return letters and comments assured me that we were moving forward.

When Justin began therapy at three and a half, he had little vocabulary and spoke in one-word utterances; his language was signed. Soon after we began therapy, we dropped sign. In his preschool for children who were hearing impaired, the teachers agreed to work on our language program, but they felt sign was necessary in the school.

In the first three months, Justin was given nine goals by the audiologist in Denver. He achieved 23. By February, he had an auditory-only vocabulary of 42 words. His first words were *bow-wow, meow, up, round-and-round,* and other such language. As the school switched him to an oral program, our therapist in Ontario told us of an auditory-verbal program, which parents had struggled successfully to begin, in Winnipeg, six hours from us. We arranged to go there during Easter break. I was floundering. The therapist in Winnipeg — experienced, supportive, and directive — put us on track. At four years old, with a hearing age of six months, Justin spoke in two-word phrases.

Our kitchen and multiuse spare room/computer room/therapy room/junk room were always a mess of games, toys, and files. I haunted church and garage sales for more treasures, such as dolls and small furniture. My sisters became my secondary bargain hunters. The furnace room became an extension of our spare room.

Daily, we worked. When Justin slept, I made lesson plans, gathered pictures, made games, analyzed his progress, and watched videos. While he was awake, we talked in appropriate language to help him understand and expand what he already knew. We visited, played, shopped, and cleaned — always with language in mind.

Parent Contacts

We knew no other families in Saskatchewan who used auditory-verbal therapy. I felt isolated. When Justin turned four, I contacted the mothers of the two girls whose tapes I had received. I thought the kids could be "picture pals." Tentative correspondence began, but was minimal. As other children in Alberta and Manitoba, neighboring provinces, received implants, we developed more parent contact. To combat our isolation, I relied on the telephone. Talking to other parents helped.

School

In April 1991, while preparing for Justin's fifth birthday party, we had more to decide than what decorations to put on the cake: Justin was to move from the half-day preschool to a full day (half preschool and half kindergarten) in the fall.

A new task fell to us: what to do about schooling? Our neighborhood Catholic school posed major problems. Justin would have to cross a busy street each day, the school had never worked with children who are hearing impaired, and his friends went to the public school. If he stayed in the public school system, he would be placed in a school outside the neighborhood. We had to move — but where?

Following a spring concert, the parents of a boy who went to the preschool told us their son would attend kindergarten at his neighborhood school, where there already was a student who was profoundly deaf. This school, 10 minutes outside Regina, seemed to have a good environment.

We contacted the director of student services, sold our house, and bought another, all within 15 days. The move meant I had to return to work full time.

There are no absolutes when considering a school. We have been fortunate that our new neighborhood school and the school division supported our wishes for Justin. From the beginning, the resource room teacher has supported Justin's language development.

Justin's teachers have focused on his abilities rather than his "disability." They expect of him what they expect from the other children. Placing him front and center, they wear the FM system and insist he listen and pay attention.

The use of the FM was a given for us. When we discovered Justin would not be able to hear his own voice because the processor microphone silences external sound when something is plugged into it, I balked. I telephoned the FM company, got FM specifications, contacted a parent of a boy in Toronto who had a cochlear implant to get ideas, and lobbied for an FM option that would allow the child to use an external microphone to hear his own voice. The company made the modification.

Justin's first classroom had no carpet. We purchased a remnant and the teacher installed it! Justin knew no children in the community; we arranged visits and held parties at every conceivable time to enhance his social circle. Once, when Howard went to Edmonton, he brought Justin and me each a present. Justin received a sweatshirt with his picture on it. I got a book with children's game ideas!

Through kindergarten and first grade, Justin moved ahead in both language and academics. He read above grade level and was developing better speech. In March 1993, in a classroom with a superb teacher, his talk was full of "comets" and "vipers." I could not have anticipated the setback that was shortly to bring all our progress to a crashing halt.

A Second Implant

I was truly pleased for Justin when, as we paid for our groceries one evening, he carried on a conversation with the clerk: "Could we get the number? You know, when you give us a number and put a number on the cart and then the man takes it back there and we drive in the car and we get our groceries back there?"

Smiling, the clerk said, "You mean parcel pick-up?"

"Yes," replied Justin, "parcel pick-up. Can we have that?"

The feeling of pride I had was overwhelming. She understood him! He had used both his speech and his listening to request something of a complete stranger. It epitomized our goal — independence to communicate with anyone, without written messages. We celebrated by going for a doughnut!

It was then, at this moment of deep joy, that Justin yelled, "Ow!" and whipped his coil off his head. Though he replaced it, he said it didn't "work right." Our son could not understand the six sounds! I felt ill, for I suspected the problem was not the processor. A complete change of headset, cords, and processor proved my theory correct.

A frantic call preceded the drive to Winnipeg, where Justin's therapist worked through the weekend and into the next week trying to reMAP the processor. Our belief was that Justin's MAP had simply changed. Nothing helped. In fact, Justin began to experience noises so loud they caused pain. As our therapist shut down electrodes in search of the sensitive ones, we saw his hearing evaporate.

The therapist, constantly in contact with our implant center, finally told us we would have to travel to Denver. It seemed the implant had failed.

When I telephoned the implant center, the already-informed director was reassuring. Testing and possible surgery could be completed within a week. Time was vital, for Justin was missing school! More importantly, we could not live with the uncertainty; we needed to know.

Difficulties faced us. Application for medical funding in the United States had to be approved since, by this time, implants were being performed in Canada. The telephone, again, became our ally as we contacted Saskatchewan Health from Winnipeg. The person in charge understood the situation and approved.

To reimplant: a serious decision. We asked Justin what he wanted. He was not thrilled with the thought of another surgery, but he was not content to remain in a silent world. The sharing of secrets and bedtime stories won. We chose to make the trip to Denver together.

The original implant proved faulty; it powered up at odd times, then didn't work at other times. Justin's pain was the result of setting a new MAP with loudness comfort levels too high, since they were set when the implant was low in power.

Surgery was again uneventful. Both Howard and I were more relaxed. All 22 electrodes were inserted. Computer testing showed the new implant to be fully functional. We received a perk when we were told Justin could return after three and a half weeks. If he healed well, his implant could be MAPped in time for his seventh birthday on April 26!

Justin's party was sensational and, yes, he heard the kids chattering. He happily went back to school, caught up easily on his work (after missing nearly a month), and was promoted to second grade. It took him only two-and-a-half weeks to get back to his previous level of comprehension. Though we have had trouble with external parts, we have never experienced another internal problem.

Today

We feel the implant has provided Justin with choices. He may speak; he may sign. It's his choice, not ours. Do we think all profoundly hearing-impaired children or adults should have implants? Of course not. Each family must examine its resources and desires. No choice is more right than another.

In Canada, we are fortunate to be covered by publicly funded health care. When Howard and I had limited resources and needed funds for travel and accommodation, we applied to community groups, but the bulk of our expenses were paid by the health care system. We are grateful!

Justin continues to work hard. He remains in a mainstream school and, at age 11, is in sixth grade. He has a minor balance problem, poor muscle tone, and mild allergies and, up until fourth grade, he was restless in school.

Interventions such as vestibular stimulation and regular swimming classes help. Justin is a happy boy whose concerns center around what clothes he will wear, winning at SEGA™, playing with friends, and collecting Spiderman comics. School is going well, and the restlessness is resolved. Justin is able to use the phone, shop on his own, order his own food in restaurants, and argue.

Things have not always been smooth. Cords, coils, and microphones have failed. When the improved Spectra 22 processor came out, it took Justin weeks to get used to the sound. Today, he considers it "the best processor in the entire universe." Last summer, we put Justin on a bipolar MAP. He didn't like it, so we switched back to common ground. We are considering the purchase of a processor that would allow him to use the FM with no external microphone, but it is very expensive.

Much of what we fear has not come to pass. Justin has fallen many times, once striking his head right above the implant. No problem. He swims well and experiences no difficulties. Cords last a long time. With his processor hidden under his clothes, on a belt around his waist, he finds it easy to adjust to the FM (on the same belt), and has complete control over sound. When the Spectra 22 came out, our school division paid for the upgrade. We have been fortunate.

Would we replace Justin's implant when the next generation of devices comes along? When I discussed it with Justin, he stopped me, patted my arm, and said, "Let's think about it when it happens, OK?"

Bria

Gael Cole

"I will find a way for her to hear again." Those were the first words I remember speaking after being told that my daughter had been deafened from meningitis when she was two years old. We have never looked back. At that time, cochlear implants were something very new. Yet if anybody had asked me eight years ago if I thought that Bria would be where she is today, I would have answered, "Without a doubt." Even then, I firmly believed that the cochlear implant would work when most people did not.

When Bria lost her hearing, she went from being a happy-go-lucky little girl to a frustrated, angry child who was, at most times, uncontrollable. Our life together that following year was full of constant tantrums and confrontations. Our only method of communication was through lipreading and cued speech. Meanwhile, I was researching the

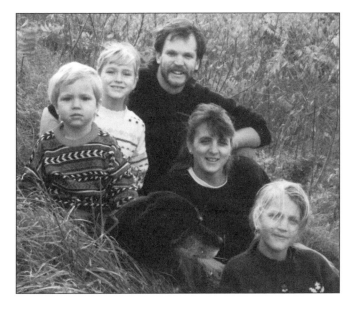

Bria Cole (far right) and family

implant, and doing everything in my power to get it. After a year of testing Bria with high-powered hearing aids, working with an auditory-verbal therapist, lobbying the government for funding, and meeting with doctors, the day of Bria's surgery arrived. Following the successful four-hour operation, my husband and I went to the cafeteria, laughing and crying in the same moment.

Commitment

For the three years following the surgery, I lived, ate, and breathed "cochlear implant." Commitment to success was critical! My life was put on hold. Today, I feel no resentment, because the rewards for my efforts have been bountiful.

Life was definitely not a picnic during those first few years. Programming the implant was nerve-wracking, and we had to travel seven hours every two weeks for six months. There were days when I didn't like anything involved with the implant or dealing with a child who was deaf. Numerous times, I wanted to throw in the towel and just get on with my life. Few people understood. Family and friends expected Bria to hear and speak normally right away.

Learning to listen with a cochlear implant is not an easy process, nor are there results overnight. There may be innumerable complications: financial, programming, technical breakdowns, broken cords, and interpreting what the child is actually hearing. We encountered many technical frustrations, including the need for reimplantation three years after Bria's first surgery, due to the failure of her internal device. Even though we would have chosen reimplantation right away, that time it was Bria's choice. We were relieved when she informed us that, without a doubt, she wanted the operation!

Not only did I have to deal with the challenge of helping the implant "work," but Bria had a very challenging personality. Her stubborn streak, however, has benefited her, even if it has just about done in her parents! She is full of character and drive, which has helped her to excel in using the implant. A similar stubborn streak in her mother has allowed us, as a family, to dedicate the hours and commitment that have resulted in her success.

The Process

It took about a year of listening to sounds before Bria started to produce any sort of sophisticated speech. At that time, I saw the "lights start to go on." A major milestone! Her language improved steadily after that.

I am a firm believer in "tough love," and made no concessions for Bria. She was given practically no lipreading, and rarely a day passed when we did not do a one-on-one lesson. We saw an auditory-verbal therapist every week for three years. I set high expectations and weekly goals, without doubting that Bria would meet them. When she achieved those goals I would push her a little bit more. I always kept notes to review, and also to record how far we had come.

The biggest challenge for me was learning to integrate lessons into everyday life. I had to train myself to be mindful to reinforce all language opportunities, especially vocabulary! Over time, this process became more and more natural, and my skills in learning to listen to speech and to analyze it became more acute. I acquired a thorough knowledge of all the different characteristics of speech production, and I researched all the material I could get my hands on, including newsletters, teaching materials, and information about other people's experiences. Knowing the material inside and out increased my confidence. I also had to learn to troubleshoot complications with the implant.

I sat through every MAPping, and still do. No one knows my child as well as I do. I know when she is giving a true response just by watching her eyes. I learned to understand and to monitor the MAPs and to tell if we had a good program. We worked until I felt the MAP was perfect and until I was confident that Bria's responses were accurate. Relentless as I was, Bria says she is happy with the work we have done and how she can hear and speak today.

Professionals have played a crucial role in this process; the surgeon, the programmers, the audiologists, the auditory-verbal therapist, the teachers of the hearing impaired, the mainstream teachers, and teachers' aides are all part of the team. Also, we joined a very enriching parent-support group. The dedication of our family to reinforce consistently everything we taught was critical. We made many sacrifices, but we have no regrets. The commitment was 100 percent.

Lessons

For home lessons I used lots of paper and pencils, and we had pages of stuff covering the walls. Including brothers and sisters was a great tactic. Everything I bought — puzzles, props, tapes, and games galore — was educational or vocabulary enriching. Garage sales were goldmines! We found things that we would never have thought to use for lessons. We got a TV compatible with closed-captioning before Bria could even read, and we used many books. Reading is an essential tool, not only to expand language, but to introduce ideas and social skills that otherwise could be missed. Even today, although she hears very well, Bria does miss a lot of information in day-to-day conversations. We read labels, cereal boxes, newspapers, magazines, and picture books. We visited the library and countless bookstores, and I encouraged more complex reading as Bria got older.

We encouraged any venture. We visited museums, art galleries, maple syrup farms, the cottage, and "Hallowe'en" farms. Today Bria participates in sports, art classes, French classes, school choir, swimming, and many other activities; these functions allow her to learn with joy and develop independence. Fortunately, we have found that most people are very willing to help a kid with special needs. We don't discount anything she can do with the implant. She has a passion for music, and the thought that she might not sing in key never enters her mind. Actually, the best learning activities are real-life situations and whatever engages us as a family. It is to everyone's benefit to look at the world as one huge learning experience. In search of opportunities to develop language, we have talked about and discovered in depth many wonders that might otherwise have passed us by.

School

I first recognized Bria's developing independence when she was in first grade. I was expecting my third child, and our family business was having its busiest season ever. I was exhausted! Fortunately, Bria had an excellent teacher and an indispensable teacher's aide. I developed a great rapport with them and was able to teach them many things that helped them to reinforce Bria's speech and language. We kept a home and school book in which the teacher's aide and I wrote faithfully every day. A teacher of the hearing impaired came to the mainstream classroom twice a week, and I was in the school at least once a week. When the other kids went to French class, Bria spent one-on-one time with her aide. This help came as great relief to me.

Bria's personality began to blossom. Her temperament became more bearable and more mature and, by gaining independence, she was taking control of her own life. She started to accept responsibilities, such as changing her own batteries, taking care of her home and school books, obtaining proper information from school, and doing chores around the house.

Mainstreaming in the public school system is challenging for any child with a cochlear implant. I remain very polite and appreciative of the school and, at the same time, I am determined to ensure that Bria's needs are met. Each spring, I meet with the new teacher for the following school year and present a set of reading materials about cochlear implants and about teaching children who are hearing impaired. Over the summer, the teacher can become acquainted with the whole concept. I encourage the teacher to talk to me at any time about Bria. The school knows that I am willing to help in any capacity, without stepping on teachers' toes. These factors have created an atmosphere free from the intimidation of working with a "special-needs child." We work very closely with a teacher of the hearing impaired who is not only Bria's teacher, but also a friend. She monitors Bria's progress, continues to set goals, and acts as a liaison between the family and the school. I still continue to go to the school and work with the itinerant teacher. This keeps me on top of Bria's progress and gives me a boost when I need it.

Developing Bria's social skills and her relationship with peers was also challenging. Bria was teased and rebuffed by some children, and she was not aware of some of the subtler niceties when interacting with so many kids. We needed to pinpoint the skills she was lacking and to try to teach her the expected behaviors, especially appropriate ways to resolve conflict. We had to foster her self-esteem and to reinforce her confidence, especially in regard to the teasing. We still keep a "current events book" and try to keep abreast of what is "hip" in order to help Bria mix more easily with her peers. Each year becomes easier, as Bria becomes more independent and socially astute. She seems to have many friends and is learning to socialize quite effectively.

Reflections

In hindsight, one of my most significant thoughts is that I wish we had had more of a sense of humor about several incidents. As a family, we were perhaps too wrapped up in the intensity of our experience that we missed many humorous situations, but our extended family and the professionals helped us to laugh. Today, some of those frustrations seem quite funny. We did not let anything become an obstacle. *We truly believed that we could do anything and we accepted nothing else.* We wanted Bria to have this characteristic so she would benefit from everything she strives to do in life.

As time goes on, hard work and determination continue, but it has become easier! Independently, Bria has begun to use many strategies to communicate effectively and we, as parents, have started to "let go" — a difficult process after having played such a pivotal role in her progress. Fostering independence is nonetheless a very gratifying experience. We are developing a more relaxed friendship with our daughter, and the physical and emotional stresses have eased.

My biggest jobs are staying in touch with the school and the itinerant teacher; the integration of speech, language, and social skills in daily life; and being aware of Bria's frame of mind. I still remind Bria about her speech, and I expect her to correct herself. I continue to have high expectations for her. These expectations have encouraged her to excel in anything she chooses, including using her cochlear implant. Even though Bria and I have had many good battles, there is now a lot of time to be friends with her. I believe that our demands and commitments have fostered Bria's solid learning skills, self-assertion, appropriate attention span, and attention to tasks, as well as her tremendous success in her use of the implant. I am able to see my child for who she really is and to accept her eccentricities. I have achieved that with the help of my friends, family, and professionals. I put myself in Bria's shoes every once in awhile, and try to imagine what a day in her life is really like.

Greater acceptance of the cochlear implant has resulted in the creation of more centers. Consequently, I now have access to one in our own city. I feel the cochlear implant is truly miraculous technology, and I have never regretted making the choice. Bria says she loves it and would never want to be without it.

The doors to the future are wide open, and Bria may choose what she wants to do and what she wants to be in her own life.

Alex

Theresa Spraggon

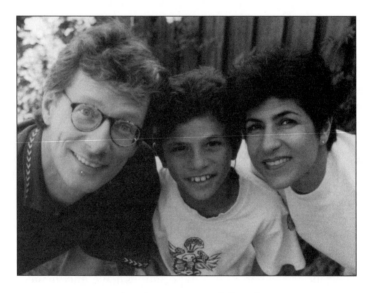

Alex Spraggon and family

I hear Alex say to Chris, "Come on Dad, you know that's against the rules... no crossing of fingers or toes or any other part of your body. You know that's not allowed." This string of words, a natural part of a 10-year-old Australian boy's banter, brought home to me how natural our family life is, and I reflect on the early years of Alex's life and how far we have come.

Despair

It was exactly 10 years ago that our lives were crumbling around us. Our eight-week-old son Alex had just had an auditory brainstem response (ABR) test, which confirmed he had a profound hearing loss. That same afternoon he was being fitted with his first set of earmolds. Hearing aids for our baby!

With the audiologist's words, "he's pretty close to stone deaf," ringing in our ears, I sat in the back seat of the car, breast-feeding Alex, with my heart breaking and my husband Chris covering his pain to give me the support I so desperately needed.

My usual control and common sense went absolutely haywire as I tried to imagine what Alex's life would be like. What difficulties would he face at school and work? What would his relationships be like with family and strangers? Would he ever have a family of his own? We knew nothing about deafness! We could think only in negatives: our tiny, otherwise perfect baby had such an uncertain future, and so did we.

Initial Action

At first we were overwhelmed with all the information about hearing loss, hearing aids, and educational options, but we hungrily sought more. We often couldn't see past the next day, let alone make decisions on issues that would have a profound effect on Alex's future.

We were lucky. We had a wonderful marriage; Alex had been diagnosed and given hearing aids at a very early age; he was our only child and didn't appear to have any additional "handicaps," and I didn't have to go back to work. We would be completely dedicated to helping Alex. Our quest for information revealed that there were other kids and young adults who communicated and functioned well in the hearing world even though they were deaf. Although the future promised hard work, our personal commitment meant that if others had succeeded, we could as well.

Options

Our lives became a whirlwind of appointments, with reams of information to read and understand, hearing aids that drove us crazy with nonstop whistling, and the agony of educational options.

Alex has a classic "left-hand corner audiogram," with an average loss of 113 dB HL in his better ear and hearing to 1000 Hz. With few exceptions, the majority of professionals urged us to enter a total communication program. We could see the attractions of this, but we set out to inform ourselves about all the alternatives, and we visited several different programs.

At this time we had the good fortune to meet a family with a five-year-old who had a very profound hearing loss and could talk. We were inspired to seek the same option and decided to join a well-established oral program which had a strong parent-support group and provided sound technical information. We also had the opportunity to meet other children who were hearing impaired and their families. We were starting to find some direction.

I threw myself into the task of educating Alex. We were rewarded with slow but steady progress. At times progress was so slow that we wondered whether we had made the right decision. On more than one occasion I said to Chris, "I don't want this job anymore — I don't want to be a teacher!" — a sentiment often expressed by other mothers of children who are deaf or hard of hearing.

I had to be very disciplined, because there were a hundred things that I would rather have been doing than Alex's lessons. I tried to get his daily lessons out of the way first thing in the morning so that the rest of the day I wouldn't feel guilty. I drew attention to every sound, created experience books, went on excursions, filled my bag with little toy animals and a variety of tiny models, and my Polaroid camera was always at hand. When Alex wouldn't attend, his lifelike friend Mick (a doll) would be ready and anxious to join lessons. Mick developed bat-like hearing. Mick has been Alex's lifelong friend, and his image has changed several times to suit Alex's maturity. In recent times, Mick has become a face-painted, tattooed wrestler.

We knew the importance of reading. As soon as Alex could sit, Chris followed my instructions, "Read to him each evening and just have fun." By the amount of noise coming from Alex's bedroom, I have no doubt he did a fantastic job. This daily reading routine fitted well with Chris's evenings after work, and I really valued the contribution, not only for Alex but for me. It was their special time together. But there were times when it felt as though everything we were doing was not enough.

We had some wonderful teachers, audiologists, doctors, other parents, and friends, but I still felt that I was Alex's main educator and that his development lay squarely on my shoulders.

A Valuable Lesson

One of the most valuable experiences I had was when Alex was about two. After a harrowing day with one thing or another, I wanted Alex to do a particular task and he stubbornly refused. I felt myself begin to boil to the point of exploding but then I looked at Alex and thought, "What the hell am I doing?" I sat down on the carpet, completely deflated, and Alex came over and started playing. We sat for ages just enjoying being together — it was *my* lesson. Yes, we had to teach Alex to speak. But there had to be those times when we could all "chill out." Even now, I call on this experience to keep things in perspective.

After two and a half years we changed programs to one offering the auditory-verbal approach. Making the most of a child's audition to obtain language made sense to us.

During this period Alex attended his local preschool, fitting in nicely, proving himself to be a bright, communicative, strong-willed child with a lively sense of humor, who made friends easily.

Cochlear Implants

We had always followed the progress of the cochlear implant, especially since the first congenitally deaf child received one in 1987. Parents of children who are profoundly deaf are quite a small community, and we became friends with many people involved with cochlear implants. The device seemed to hold some promise, but we decided that it wasn't for us at that time, as Alex was making good progress and there was no firm evidence that an implant would improve his situation.

We decided that we would look at the implant again before Alex started formal schooling at five and a half years of age.

Alex's language at five years of age was better than age appropriate. Much of his speech, however, was difficult to understand. He made good use of his limited hearing using hearing aids, and we knew that he enjoyed listening, talking, shouting, and laughing. He was oral! We wanted to improve Alex's hearing sensitivity to take the edge off the heavy effort that he always had to make. We knew that school work would become very demanding. If a cochlear implant would make it easier, we needed to consider it.

We knew a lot about implants by this stage, and we knew a number of children who had received them.

We all had come so far with Alex's limited residual hearing. Could we gamble with this? What if something went wrong and he lost that hearing? There would be no way he would be able to progress as well with any less. What about the crucial months of auditory input he would lose following the implant while he was adapting to the new signal? He was about to start school — a critical time. There were no guarantees.

Chris and I understood everything about hearing aids; we could listen to them and identify a problem quickly. This would not be the case with the implant, and this bothered us. If we proceeded, our vigilance to changes or problems with Alex's hearing would need to be heightened.

Plagued with these doubts, we enrolled in the 10-week hearing-aid trial at the cochlear implant center in Sydney. The center evaluated and monitored Alex's audition and assessed whether an implant would be a better listening device for him. He underwent a battery of tests to determine his listening abilities and the auditory functioning of each ear. Some children who had received implants had more hearing than Alex, but none had achieved such high test scores requiring the use of audition alone, prior to implantation. The implant team was having difficulty recommending him because he was doing so well with his hearing aids.

Towards the end of the trial, we decided to give ourselves a break and clear our heads. We had been running on overload for a long time. We visited friends and family in Europe and America and spoke to members of various implant teams and programs. We were urged to proceed carefully, but many saw great promise with the implant, and were impressed by this little chap from "down under." "If he is a good hearing-aid user, chances are he will be a good implant user," was a phrase that stuck in our minds.

To Implant or Not to Implant

Chris and I returned to Australia and had our final assessment meeting with the implant team. The clinical staff was divided. The decision was left to us. As informed as we were, it was the hardest decision we had ever made. We went ahead.

As part of the center's protocol, Alex had to have electrocochleography testing, an objective measurement of mid-to-high audiometric frequencies performed under light anesthetic. Alex contracted pseudomonas, a virulent infection, arising from this procedure and was without hearing aids for over a month. Lipreading became our way of communicating.

Throughout the entire implant evaluation and decision process, Alex was informed of what was going on; he was always given the opportunity to ask questions and tell us what he thought. We have always felt Alex should be included in any decisions about his future. Although he was anxious about going into hospital, he knew that the implant could help him hear a little more and could make things a little easier. We were never troubled that perhaps Alex might resent this decision later in life.

The original operation date was postponed for two months because of an ear infection. We were also anticipating an extended postoperative stay in hospital to administer antibiotics intravenously as a precautionary measure, given Alex's previous infection.

The new school term was looming closer, and on December 7, 1991, Alexander Edmund Giles Spraggon was admitted to hospital for a cochlear implant. We were plagued with second thoughts right up to the moment the hospital staff came to collect him for the surgery. We had confidence in the ability of the surgeon but nonetheless, we sought last-minute reassurances even outside the operating room doors. We carried Alex crying into the operating room and lay him on the table. He received the anesthetic mask and we quickly left. Our hearts were pounding and our nerves were on edge as we took to pacing and drinking coffee.

When the surgeon emerged from the operating room three hours later with a smile on his face and a spring in his step, we knew the operation had been a success. Our spirits soared!

Alex entered the recovery ward with his head bandaged. The following day he took life easily, became pals with the kid in the next bed, and found some action with the other kids on the ward. Alex's spirit and adaptability amazed us throughout his four days in hospital.

Our Christmas photo of 1991 shows Alex on Santa's knee with a big bandage on his head covering his 17 stitches. He went back to wearing his hearing aid in his unimplanted ear and took everything in stride. Yes, it was difficult, but he seemed to cope.

I Heard That

Four weeks after surgery Alex's implant was switched on. His discipline and all our early preparation paid off. He knew exactly what to do. We both felt relieved and excited when his first sound was followed with "I heard that." He started to imitate the sounds he was hearing right away.

All the electrodes were activated over two weeks. We were in no hurry, happy to take things slowly to ensure Alex had plenty of time to grow accustomed to the new sounds. We had confidence in his ability to assess acceptable loudness levels, and we encouraged him to extend those levels daily. We couldn't know exactly what he was hearing, so we had to rely on what he told us.

Alex started school two weeks later and, like all parents, it was important to us that his first experience at school be encouraging. With the help of his itinerant teacher of the deaf and a brilliant classroom teacher, Alex progressed well.

However, after we had worked so hard to help Alex use his hearing, now with the implant he couldn't distinguish among the basic six or seven sounds nor could he tell the difference between Chris's voice and mine. He told me, with great amusement, that I sounded like our dog, Jassie! Every sound had to be heard and identified again. We listened to everything; "What was that?" became our most-asked question. Alex could at last hear "sh" and "s" easily, but "ee" sounded like a growl.

Alex was well positioned academically in his class, and this meant he could now concentrate on listening and making friends. There was good communication among Alex's itinerant teacher, his classroom teacher, and us. No problem seemed insurmountable! Chris and I have maintained regular, open communication with professionals and have not shied away from criticizing them constructively, if necessary.

About seven months after Alex's implant was switched on, he was listening and understanding at his previous levels, and it was quite clear that he could hear much more than previously. Speech targets that were difficult prior to implantation were easier to attain. "McDogall's," a pronunciation we found highly comical, finally became "McDonald's." Alex started to use the telephone, having conversations with his nanna in England about the next load of comics she was going to send, and television became easier to understand.

Alex's implant was MAPped at least 15 times in the first 18 months. We were vigilant for any problems or changes in his speech or hearing. He detested MAPping; the sessions were long and boring. He also disliked the sound of new MAPs, so we again had to take things slowly. Treats were freely given to encourage patience!

About 18 months after Alex received his implant, Chris completely lost the hearing in his right ear. This happened virtually overnight and although the cause was uncertain, either a virus or an aneurism was suspected. Chris now had single-ear hearing, and it was interesting listening to Alex offer him advice that he should move his head around to know where sound was coming from. We have a very old dog who has now become almost totally deaf, and sometimes I feel the odd one out, as I'm sure all three of them become selectively deafer when it suits them!

Choosing Schools

It was time to choose a primary school for Alex. Once again, we had a big decision. Everything seemed to be a compromise. We wanted him to have an up-to-date education, but one with a traditional approach and a quiet, structured classroom. State schools seemed to have variable standards but private schools, although they maintained consistent standards, were very expensive. As Alex is an only child, we would have preferred him to go to a co-ed school, but the local ones seemed large and impersonal. Alex finally started third grade at a smaller, private all-boys school that followed a traditional, structured teaching style. It was at this time that he decided to exchange his chest-worn, bra-like harness for a belt.

Even now Alex dislikes wearing an FM with his implant, reporting he hears an odd "shooshing" sound. What a shame, since he used an FM system with his hearing aids so effectively. Alex recognizes his limitations within the classroom, and with the help of his itinerant teacher is learning to assert himself. This is not so easy when all he wants is to be like the rest of the guys!

Sports play a big part in Alex's life. This is his opportunity to participate on equal footing with his peers. He has developed some good friendships on the sports fields, and he is popular at school. Things can still be tough though, like the time Alex's teacher forgot to tap him at the start of a swimming race and Alex didn't dive until he saw the other kids hit the water.

Reflections

Alex had now had his cochlear implant for five years and yes, we made the right decision. The implant has helped him hear better, which has led to better speech and a more integrated life. He is an avid reader and does well academically. Would we ever have dreamed this 10 years ago?

Alex is still a child who is hearing impaired, and it still requires a great deal of effort from lots of people to make sure he is given the same opportunities as other children.

He has matured a great deal in the last year. Although he still doesn't like MAPing, he willingly accepts it as something that needs to be done. When he says, "I think I need to pay attention to the way I speak," Chris and I swell with pride at the way he approaches the challenge. When we talk about the future of the implant he knows that engineers and scientists are working on a smaller, smarter processor. His dream is "something just to stick on the back of my ear like a hearing aid", but for now, Alex, dressed in surf shirt, boogie shorts, and "No Fear" sports cap, is growing up to be a real cool kid.

Tim

Gaby Thierbach

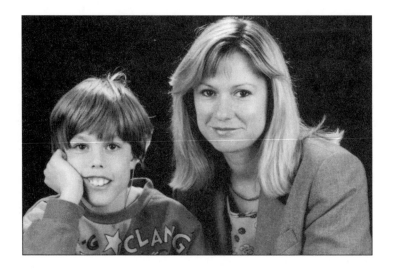

Tim Thierbach and mom

"**M**ama, today is Wednesday," said Tim. He was looking into his monthly diary, which we created for his daily activities some years ago. His diary lets him know exactly what we have planned and what will happen every day. Today we want to go to the cinema.

"We will see the film with the goose. What is the name of this film, Tim? Do you remember?" I asked. "With the goose," he replied.

"Amy and the Wild Geese," I added.

"I'm looking forward to the film!" exclaimed Tim. We looked again in the program, and I explained what the film was all about. He gave me his version of the story in short and simple sentences, so I knew he could understand what I had told him. Today, Tim is nine years old.

When Tim was born, the doctors told me that everything was okay. My husband and I were very happy with our little boy. On the same day, five other children were born in the same hospital. As soon as one baby started to cry, every other baby followed suit. But not Tim; he just slept through it all.

"Why doesn't he wake up?" I asked the doctor.

"He is very tired from the birth," replied the doctor.

"Can't my baby hear?" was my instinctive question. But the doctor laughed at my fears. I suppose he thought I was being an overanxious mother. Once I was at home, I forgot all about the idea that my child might have a hearing problem. No one in either of our families had ever had hearing problems.

When Tim was eight months old, my husband died in an accident. I was only 22 years old and a single mother. I wanted to learn about the development of children, so I bought some books to read all about it. I didn't want to make any mistakes. I could already see that Tim was a late developer. He hadn't started to play with his voice, babble, or crawl around. In fact, he was totally limp. When he tried to sit, he would fall over, as he couldn't support himself. I went to seek the advice of a pediatrician, who diagnosed Tim with muscular hypotonia. He recommended special therapy with a physiotherapist. Tim didn't like this at all. He had to sit on top of a big ball, but he had no balance and fell off all the time. Consequently, Tim became very anxious about falling down, and would start to cry frantically. The therapist didn't seem to know what to do. After awhile, I felt angry and frustrated that we weren't going anywhere with the treatment.

Sensory Integration Therapy

I was lucky to discover a book by a pediatric psychologist about the milestones of a child's development. The author described a special kind of therapy that she had developed for multihandicapped children. The goal of this therapy is to stimulate all available senses so that the child can become aware of all parts of his or her body. I began trying this therapy with Tim. Every day, Tim would sit naked on a rug on the bathroom floor with a jar of cream. I took the cream and massaged his whole body, at times softly, and at times quite strongly. Tim liked this very much and began to do the same, stroking and searching his body. By this time, he was 14 months old.

Later, when he was wearing hearing aids at the age of 18 months, I tried to teach him about every part of his body: "This is your foot, your arm, your leg." By doing this I was trying to combine the information he could get through his hearing aids with the tactile sensations through the sensory-integration therapy. On one occasion I took a piece of fine sandpaper and rubbed it gently on his body. Tim immediately didn't like that. Afterwards I took a feather, and did the same, stroking his body with it gently. He was able to distinguish the difference between textures and demonstrated the different sensations through the emotions he expressed. Clearly, the sensory-integration therapy greatly stimulated his senses, and at the same time, fatigued him very quickly. He often needed a small break between sessions.

Diagnosis of Hearing Loss

An additional problem caused by the lack of muscle tone was Tim's lack of movement. He wouldn't crawl. To encourage him, I bought him a small toy car, which, unfortunately, he liked to drive very fast. This was a tough time for me, as I would cry out to Tim, "Stop, wait!" — to no avail, as he would not react. I started to think again that maybe he didn't hear me. I also thought that maybe he just didn't want to! I had to be sure, so I took Tim to the hospital for a hearing evaluation. The diagnosis: Tim had a bilateral hearing loss of 90 dB HL and was prescribed two hearing aids. He was profoundly deaf! I couldn't understand how the pediatrician whom we had consulted regularly had never picked up on his hearing loss!

Following the diagnosis, Tim had a routine checkup with his regular pediatrician. I decided not to mention anything about the diagnosis of Tim's hearing impairment. After the examination, the doctor happily informed me that Tim was a healthy little boy with the exception of the *already diagnosed* muscular hypotonia. I told him that my son had just been diagnosed with a profound hearing loss! I wanted to know why he wasn't able to diagnose Tim's hearing problem before. His answer was quite short and simple, *"It's very difficult to diagnose a hearing loss in very small children."* He called two other doctors in to the room to confirm his explanation. I was angry because Tim had lost some precious months without hearing aids and consequently the benefits of sound.

Hearing Aids and Speech Therapy

After the hearing-aid fitting, Tim and I were scheduled for weekly speech therapy at the hospital. The speech therapist played with him and began to teach Tim about colors. "Look, this is blue; this is green." Tim didn't react.

At home I tried to capture Tim's interest in sounds by playing musical instruments. This was interesting for Tim for a very short time. He didn't seem to want to interact. Half a year went by! We had speech therapy regularly, but I didn't notice Tim reacting to any sounds. The doctor said, "Yes, yes, he has made progress." I just couldn't see it, so I couldn't agree with him or feel satisfied.

Tim became very aggressive. Everybody expected him to hear and thought he could, but I felt he wasn't hearing anything at all and that his hearing aids weren't helping him. The speech therapist recommended that we try sign language to help Tim's communication and to prevent him from becoming frustrated. I still wasn't satisfied, and asked my doctor again if there was another kind of therapy.

"No," was his answer. "There is nothing." But I would not and could not accept the thought that my child would grow up in silence.

Besides Tim's hearing problem, he still wasn't able to walk and continued to have difficulties with his balance. In the meantime, we developed our own sign language. Tim was able to communicate to me that he could not hear, and often took out his hearing aids. I knew he wasn't hearing anything through them.

In Search of an Alternative

After my husband died, Tim and I went to live with my parents. Everyone in the family was naturally drawn into our situation and very saddened by it all. I bought special medical journals to obtain more information about hearing impairment. To my surprise, I found an article about a doctor who surgically placed a cochlear implant in a small boy who was deaf. The headline read, "My Deaf Child Can Hear Now." This gave me new hope. I called that very doctor to arrange an appointment for him to see Tim.

We spent three days in the hospital, where Tim underwent many different examinations. The team told me that there was no response from the hearing nerve to the stimulations. Tim was close to being totally deaf.

It was then that the doctor explained the cochlear implant. He was the pioneer surgeon in Germany who had successfully placed the new implants in children as well as adults. He explained that there was opposition to the operation, but at the time, about 25 children had already received implants in Germany, many of whom attended the rehabilitation center linked to the hospital. I had the opportunity to talk with the parents of some of these children, and also had the opportunity to see the children themselves.

The speech processor and headset looked so big and uncomfortable for such small children. I couldn't imagine my little boy wearing something like that. But these children were reacting to sound. It wasn't necessary to speak very loudly, and they were *listening*. They understood when their names were called; they were talking, and they understood one another. The parents told me that they expected that their children would go to a mainstream school in the future. To me, this meant that the children could have close to a normal life.

The Decision Is Made

"I would like to try this for Tim," I told the doctor. After the final examination, the doctor told me that Tim was indeed a candidate for the cochlear implant. I met with the parents at the center twice more before finally deciding that a cochlear implant was the only possibility to help Tim learn to listen and talk. I was very anxious about the operation, but the doctor anticipated no complications. The surgery was scheduled for a few weeks later.

Full of hope, we drove to the hospital for the surgery, which was completed without any complications. After the operation, the doctor told me that the device was in place and working, and that Tim would have every opportunity to learn to hear. All the stress from the previous weeks dissolved, and I cried.

Switch-on to Sound

Tim was two and a half years old at the time of the operation. Four weeks later we went to the rehabilitation center for the first stimulation of Tim's speech processor. That was a great day for me. I was very nervous. Would Tim react? Would I be able to see that he can hear?

The team included a teacher of the deaf, an audiologist, and a speech therapist. Tim seemed very proud to be such an important person. The audiologist gave him some stones and told him that the sound that he would hear would come from the stone. With a very serious face, Tim placed the stone near his ear and waited. Suddenly he looked very anxious and had tears in his eyes. At that time I also picked up a stone and told him we would hear it together. Tim concentrated very hard. I could see that he could hear. In the first session they were able to program 12 electrodes.

I had assumed that Tim's progress would be very fast, and that he would react to his name almost immediately. But this was not the case. We had to spend 12 weeks during the first two years undergoing special rehabilitation at the hospital center.

Speech Therapy

I needed to find a very determined and engaging speech therapist who could show me how I could teach my son to listen and to talk. Many therapists had said, "Your child has a cochlear implant; we have no experience with this device. Sorry, we can't teach your child."

I decided to move with Tim to Hannover, Germany where I could be close to the rehabilitation center for children with cochlear implants. We stayed at the center one week every three months. This was a tough time for us, as we lived together with so many other children day and night, and they had their own problems. Despite this, one big advantage was that in the evenings the parents had the opportunity to discuss their concerns and problems together.

At this time, in 1990, no one knew much about cochlear implants and the therapy involved. I still needed more information, so I decided to visit a few scientific meetings and conferences specifically on cochlear implants in children.

The Founding of a Self-Help Group

Parents needed to share information. What could I do? I decided to take action by founding a self-help group for parents of children with cochlear implants. My aim was to open the eyes and ears of all parents to the potential benefits offered by an implant for a child who is hearing impaired. Self-help group members could then act as a resource and enable their child to grow up in a regular learning and living environment and become independent citizens in the community.

Auditory-Verbal Therapy

During a conference in Regensburg, Germany, I listened to a presentation about auditory-verbal therapy. It was my first opportunity to hear anything about this approach. I was impressed with the success and progress of the children receiving this type of therapy, and asked the speaker to recommend a speech therapist in Germany who could help me, which he did. Initially, the therapist developed a six-month program for us to follow. A new program was developed every subsequent 6 months, based on Tim's progress. This was very motivating for me.

Half a year after Tim's implant was first stimulated, he suddenly reacted to voices and noises. He was standing at the window. He indicated that he had heard something and asked what it was. He gestured towards what he had heard and at the same time said, *"Peep-peep."* This was the first time that he heard birds singing. I was very happy. I took a toy plane and flew it in the air whilst saying "a-a-a-a," followed by Tim imitating that sound.

Trying to teach Tim by sitting at the table proved unproductive. He was very active and wasn't able to concentrate for very long. Instead, we played on the floor together. I would teach him about sounds using whatever toys and materials he was interested in at the time. We created a farm, and I would say noises for each of the animals. Tim found this to be lots of fun. He built fences and tried to mimic the animal noises. Steadily his interest in sounds began to grow. I used small sheets of paper with pictures of furniture. *Everything* had a label. Each time Tim was close to or sat on a piece of furniture I would say "chair" or "table" and draw his attention to it. It was much easier for him to identify and remember the word if he could visualize the object *and* hear the name. At this time his difficulties with balance also improved, and by the age of three years, he was able to walk much better. We continued to make regular weekly visits to the speech therapist and the physiotherapist.

Kindergarten

At the age of three-and-a-half years, Tim went to kindergarten. I wanted him to attend a mainstream kindergarten, so I requested a list of all the kindergartens in Hannover and was successful in obtaining a place for Tim in a neighboring suburb. The group was quite large with 25 children, so the teacher wasn't able to devote much individual time to Tim. I felt as though I had to be at his side the whole time. Tim was happy to play with other children and tried to communicate with them, but the children didn't readily accept Tim in return. I tried to explain to them that Tim was hearing impaired and what that meant, but the children were too young to understand. Tim could speak in short three-word sentences, and most of his sentences were not grammatically correct. It was also difficult for him to understand the other children and to participate in the sing-along or storytelling. This made him very frustrated and aggressive, and on occasion he would strike out at the other children. I finally removed Tim from the kindergarten. My attempt to integrate him into a mainstream classroom was unfortunately not successful. Following this experience, Tim was enrolled in a kindergarten for children who are hearing impaired. There were two teachers and six children in the group. This was a better choice for Tim.

At home I continued using the auditory-verbal approach. I learned to be very patient with Tim, to respect that he needed time and a lot of practice to learn and understand sounds.

We began a diary in which we wrote about every important event. We took photos or made pictures related to our activities, and I would write some short, simple sentences under each picture to describe what we had done. Tim used the diary to explain his experiences to others. Although he couldn't read, he could recognize the words we used in the diary to help him talk. He was very proud to tell his grandparents about his weekend activities. It was important for him to have such a sense of achievement. Through listening and talking, he learned that he was able to interact with other people, and he was greatly satisfied.

Once a week, Tim attended a local sports club, where he enjoyed playing with other children and was able to wear his speech processor and headset even while playing ball games. Tim was six years old and still had difficulty integrating socially, as he wasn't always the most cooperative of little boys. I felt Tim needed more time to mature before going to school, so I decided that he stay in kindergarten for one more year.

Full-Time School!

In the spring of 1995, I visited schools all over Germany, and Tim came along. I discovered that Montessori schools integrated handicapped children, so for a trial period of one week, Tim attended a Montessori school. Each morning the children were allowed free work time of three hours, in which they elected what they wanted to do. During this time they were not permitted to talk to one another; the classroom was in total silence. Tim was surprised and couldn't understand or accept that he wasn't allowed to talk during this time. The teacher suggested that Tim might not be the right type of child for this kind of school. I went in search of a more appropriate educational setting.

The schools for the hearing impaired that I visited didn't appeal to me. They were in large cities with large classes, and the main mode of communication was sign language. I was in contact with the director of a private school for hearing-impaired children in Switzerland, and I sought her advice. I drove from Germany to Switzerland to discuss the possibilities. By this time I was in great despair as there were only a few months until summer, and I had to make my decision before school started. I immediately warmed to the small town where the school was located. Each class consisted of only three to four children and the teacher used an auditory approach. Tim's level of communication and use of hearing were evaluated, and he was judged to be a good candidate for the style of education offered at the school. The atmosphere was one of harmony and peace, and I was convinced that this was the place for Tim.

Two months later, after quite some reorganization and changes in our lifestyle, we moved to Switzerland, where Tim would go to school.

Looking Back

Today, we have been living in Switzerland for three years. Tim is now able to write and read very well. When he speaks, his sentences are grammatically correct and everyone is able to understand him.

The road from "Tim then" to "Tim now," from Germany to Switzerland, from hearing aids to cochlear implant, has been long and hard, but success confirms that I made good decisions. Choosing cochlear implantation for Tim was a great thing.

My message to parents of children who are hearing impaired is, "Don't give up. The process of learning to listen and talk does not happen overnight. Be excited about every little step your child makes. Learning through listening develops over time — and natural, spoken communication with parents, family, and friends is cause for celebration."

Joshua

Susan Silver Schonfeld

The night Josh was born, I was upstairs in the room that was to be his, when I caught a glimpse of my huge stomach in the full-length bathroom mirror. I remember being awed that at any moment, my life would be swiftly and irrevocably changed as I was thrust into parenthood.

Josh was a sweet-natured baby with huge brown eyes, and he had a keen sense of his environment. His first few months were idyllic, but by the time Josh was seven and a half months old my husband, Alvin, had a disturbing suspicion that Josh did not hear well. When Josh was nine months old, despite everyone's skepticism, he had Josh tested. Much to our delight, the first results were fine! After awhile, nonethe-

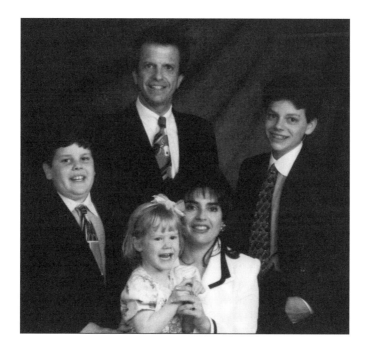

Joshua Schonfeld (right) and family

less, we found ourselves banging pots behind Josh's head, slamming doors when his back was turned, and letting the phone ring 16 times, just to watch him continue his play and display no reaction.

Diagnosis
At 11 months, Joshua was definitively diagnosed with a severe-to-profound bilateral sensorineural hearing loss. "He can't hear a thing and will probably never speak. He could probably go to some residential state school for the deaf where he could learn sign language," said the pediatric neurologist.

I have never forgotten nor forgiven that clinical coldness. I felt totally lost, having no idea of what to do except to get hearing aids.

My only brush with deafness was in high school. My school played volleyball against the Lexington School for the Deaf and in the locker room, many of my teammates and I imitated the sign language we observed. At Josh's diagnosis I said to myself, "Is God punishing me for this childhood unkindness of long ago?"

We decided to try the only two approaches we had heard about, acknowledging that we did not know enough to make an informed decision. Josh started with sign language in a program for children who were hearing impaired and also went to Northwestern University in Chicago for oral rehabilitation.

When Josh was 13 months old, we attended an educational fair for the deaf. We were on our way out the door when a woman, who had noticed Josh's hearing aids, asked how old he was. This led to a discussion about educational options. When it became obvious that we were floundering, she suggested we contact the Alexander Graham Bell Association for the Deaf. Later, we met this woman's daughter, who was 15 and deaf since age two from spinal meningitis. We were astonished that Betsy could speak and that we could understand her!

Shortly after this fateful meeting, we received a letter from a wonderful woman at the Bell Association, suggesting we consider attending the 1984 A. G. Bell convention in Portland, Oregon to learn about oral and auditory education.

Portland, Oregon

In Portland fate again intervened, when I haphazardly walked into a short course about children who had learned to talk through listening. How was it possible that these children could have such profound hearing losses and speak the way they did? On one screen there was a "profound" audiogram, and on the other the corresponding child was talking. I even heard about one child being bar mitzvahed, a dream for Josh that we thought was shattered. I drove everyone crazy with incessant questions. I called my husband and tried to explain my experiences. The road had now become clear.

At the same conference, fate led me into the opening session where, feeling rather lost, I found an empty seat next to a regal-looking woman and a vivacious curly-haired woman, who both became future lifelines. The former was a pioneer in teaching children who are hearing impaired to listen and speak; the other became Josh's auditory-verbal therapist from the age of two and a half to the present day. This approach was what we wanted for Josh, but my biggest hesitation was the leap of faith required. Though I had seen "the proof of the pudding," I worried that maybe I had seen "miracle" kids. I read everything available about the auditory-verbal approach but still did not understand how the process developed over the long term. Nevertheless, we took the leap!

Therapy

We quickly learned that the children we had seen in Portland were not *miracle kids* and that the auditory-verbal process involved long, hard work. Back in Chicago we did not have an auditory-verbal therapist, so we imported one. We began working with Josh and luckily, he responded immediately to therapy. He was about 17 months old when he began to model "m" and "ah," but he had a very high-pitched voice. It was difficult for us to understand the importance of pitch, duration, and intonation. I wanted to correct his speech to make him more understandable rather than work on these other vital components. We encouraged and rewarded any vocalization. I was getting parent training and found it harder than any job I had ever had. I constantly did therapy; in retrospect, I wish I had relaxed more and had more pure fun with my firstborn. But we were treading unknown waters and worried about the outcome.

At 23 months Josh was babbling and imitating, but his high-frequency sounds were like fingernails on the chalkboard. We learned that children with typical hearing may hear a word only two or three times before they begin to repeat and use it, whereas a child who is deaf or hard of hearing needs to hear the word 20, 50, 100 times or more. For example, while playing ball we would use the word "ball" hundreds of times: "Josh, throw me the ball. OK. You catch the ball now. Oh, no! What a dirty ball. Let's go clean the ball."

I got frustrated with my husband for not sticking to this teaching mode. Alvin was a good a teacher, however, as he engaged Josh in meaningful activities and capitalized on the accompanying language. This was a good division of responsibilities!

At about 27 months, Josh appeared bored, and his behavior was deteriorating. We gave him higher-level tasks as our expectations rose. He knew it and became devilish and manipulative. At the same time, he was displaying big shifts from receptive to expressive language, and at 32 months he was repeating a great deal and asking many questions. We focused on complete sentences. As soon as he was saying three-word utterances with some regularity, we pushed him to four and then to five.

After a couple of years, I declared myself a graduate of therapy. I did try sitting at the table for about a year and a half before I opted to be Josh's mother and not his formal therapist. But Josh was now doing better without my presence, and his behavior was much improved. Informal therapy, of course, had never stopped, but the change made us all a lot happier. Today, Josh and I are very close but, by mutual agreement, I have distanced myself from those parts of his life where he wants to be independent.

Even though many variables affect speech and language development, all kids go through the same stages, although not at the same times. Josh passed through these various stages too, and I was thrilled that he was making such great strides, but it was difficult for him and for us that he was not understood more often. To compensate, he used a combination of skills to get his point across.

On a camping trip, when he was almost four years old, Josh wanted a particular bag of candy from the general store. We gave him money and told him he could have it if he went in and asked for it himself. He came out, in fairly short order, with the candy he wanted. Similarly, we always looked for situations in which we could develop his independence, confidence, and self-esteem. He always ordered for himself in restaurants, even if we had to *fill in* for the waitress. Also, he had to explain the rules of games so we all could play.

At four years old, while at a Montessori School, Josh started to use an FM system. This was helpful even though it involved a lot of paraphernalia. We endeavored to enrich his vocabulary by expanding on words and ideas. For example, we followed *Ling's Thesaurus* and expanded words such as "coat" to include: *lapel, sleeve, collar, button, snap, hook, cuff, hem, seam* and *waterproof,* as he was well beyond a basic vocabulary .

At age five, Josh could express whole thoughts understandably and at six, he was doing high-level work through listening, even using the telephone. Josh was studying Hebrew, and he had become a competent reader. We now knew he would be bar mitzvahed!

At age seven Josh began speech therapy in earnest, as we wanted to enhance the fluidity of his conversations while maintaining natural rhythm and pitch, and, by age nine, he was completely understandable, although we continued to strive for more natural-sounding speech.

Children who are deaf miss a great deal by not overhearing TV, radio, and other people's conversations. Closed captioning on our TV has been a lifeline to the world. When Josh was young I would turn the TV on so he could get accustomed to it. TV provided excellent pre-reading skills and helped fill many gaps.

When Josh had a cold, he would lose 10-15 dB HL of hearing, and we always panicked. This transformed him from a "gold" hearing-aid user to someone whose favorite word was, "What?" He was not sure what he was hearing, and this played havoc with his confidence. After a cold, his hearing appeared to bounce back. There is such a close threshold between oblivion and being in touch. That not-so-little bit of hearing made an enormous difference.

At about age nine Josh's hearing seemed to change. He was not turning as readily when called, he questioned what he heard more often, and his limited use of the telephone became increasingly difficult. The audiograms confirmed that Josh appeared to have permanently lost more hearing.

The Cochlear Implant

We had always been told that a cochlear implant was not for someone like Josh, who managed so well with hearing aids. Initially we accepted that, but as time went on we started to question. We heard about children with cochlear implants who could now hear the toilet flushing and birds chirping, neither of which Josh could hear. We sought other opinions and could not understand why, if such children could hear at that level, could Josh not also benefit from this technology.

Josh and his dad consulted several physicians. Alvin felt that one physician would have operated on anyone, and Josh fell outside of another center's definitive criteria. We obtained another opinion in Iowa where the surgeon, after examining Josh and obtaining a detailed history, felt that our son would most likely benefit from the implant. There were, however, no guarantees. We had confidence in the doctor, but we wanted a crystal ball! Surgery was scheduled for September 1993.

As the date grew closer, Alvin and I panicked. What if we were making the wrong decision for Josh? What if it didn't work? What if the ear was damaged for future technological advancements? Would Josh ever forgive us? Overwhelmed by these unanswerable questions, we decided to postpone the surgery.

All along we discussed the implant with Josh and listened to his perspective, trying not to be too obsessive. He was, after all, only 10 years old. His final answer was, "I don't know how to decide something like this. You and Daddy have to do it for me." Had it been a couple of years later, he undoubtedly would have expressed a more definite opinion. Even as a preteen, Josh was concerned about wires and external paraphernalia. He didn't like his auditory trainer, and he lumped the cochlear implant in the same category.

By December of the same year, we had spoken with many parents from different parts of the country whose children's hearing losses most closely approximated Josh's and who had received cochlear implants. The kids could hear a multitude of new things, and their responses to environmental happenings were much keener. They appeared to be thriving. We could no longer postpone cochlear implant surgery. We made another appointment and kept it!

We drove to Iowa a day before the surgery for psychological testing and blood work. The following day, just outside the operating room, Josh met with the anesthesiologist, who put some medicine in a container of apple juice to make Josh sleep. Alvin went with Josh into the operating room, where he stayed until Josh was sleeping. This was a tremendous comfort for Josh. We were surrounded by kind and caring professionals who all seemed to have great empathy for how difficult this was for my husband and me.

The operation was performed quickly and without complications. All 22 electrodes were successfully inserted. I burst into tears, confounding the doctor, who reiterated he had just delivered great news! We were to share the good news with close family and friends who had kept a vigilant watch on Josh's adventure.

Josh wore an inordinately large bandage on his head to put pressure on the incision. Although not in pain, he spent the rest of Thursday dozing. On Friday, he was greatly recovered. We even ventured into an art class for children who were mostly cancer patients — a sobering experience. On Saturday, Josh was eating well and doing fine. The dressing was changed, we obtained our medicines, and began the four-hour drive home. Amazingly, all this was just 48 hours later!

Over the weekend, Josh held court, receiving one visitor after another, and he received more gifts than on his birthday. On Monday, he returned to school with a ski band covering his bandages and with answers to a myriad of questions. Three weeks later, we were on our way back to Iowa to have the implant turned on.

After two or three months, Josh was understanding spoken language well. Initially, when asked what speech sounded like through the cochlear implant, he replied, "strange." When asked the same question a few months later, he replied "It sounds just like speech has always sounded!" This was undoubtedly due to his extensive auditory-verbal therapy and his brain's ability to remember language.

Independently, Josh made the decision to wear the hearing aid in his right ear. When he is tested today, there is not much difference with just the cochlear implant than with the cochlear implant and hearing-aid combination. But Josh finds some security in wearing both. He seems to obtain more environmental information and is able to localize sound more easily than without the hearing aid.

Sixth grade, Josh's first full school year with the implant, was very successful. He had a tough teacher who was a strong advocate for him and who stressed high-level academic and organizational skills. There was an excellent liaison between this teacher and the auditory-verbal therapist, who continues to play a critical role in Josh's life today. He did, however, stop speech therapy and did not resume until the beginning of eighth grade.

One of Josh's greatest strengths is his social skills. He's very kind and happy and has many friends, including a couple of very special ones. His schoolmates have always been kind and helpful too, and Josh has integrated extremely well. The attitude of our school is largely responsible for this, in that its missions include academic excellence, kindness, empathy, and tolerance.

In sixth grade, Josh was the class representative for student council. At the end of the year, he announced that he wanted to run for president of the student council for seventh grade. He wrote a speech, made campaign posters with his grandfather, and won the election! He ran the student council with dedication and strong leadership, and publicly addressed the entire school community every week. His picture, taking ballroom dancing, was on the front page of the *Chicago Tribune,* and he went to Portland, Oregon to receive his 75 Stars Award from Miss America. At age 12, Josh emceed a special assembly in front of 800 people and, with far less nervousness and more aplomb than I would have had, introduced newscaster Bill Curtis and recounted Bill's biography. Later, Josh shot the breeze with him in the men's room. What a year!

Today

With each passing month, life becomes easier. While far from perfect, it is not such a struggle. It is easier for Josh to follow the dialog of teachers and conversations with other children. In fact, he now often overhears, so I have to be careful what I say! Josh has stopped continually asking "what?" and has much more confidence in his ability to hear and listen. The most wonderful change is in his use of the telephone. Before receiving the cochlear implant, Josh was able to answer some yes/no questions and obtain minimal information. Today I have to pry him off the phone. He still has to listen very carefully and occasionally may not understand, but otherwise he is independent on the phone, no longer needing me as his oral interpreter. When the time comes for Josh to exchange sweet nothings with his girlfriends, I am happy he'll be able to do so privately!

Recently, Josh's school soccer team had a match against another team that also had a player with a cochlear implant. It was a miserable day — cold, windy, rainy. Unbeknownst to the others, the two boys had taken off their implants to avoid moisture damage. All of a sudden, the spectators and the rest of their teams were scratching their heads. In the corner of the field the two boys were fighting over the ball, but the referee had blown the whistle, ending the play, some time ago! These two were oblivious! In such situations, sense of humor goes a long way.

Josh's recent bar mitzvah seemed unattainable many years ago. The cochlear implant certainly helped him to learn Hebrew and to prepare for that special event. Many people who had been with us from the beginning, when we were told our child was deaf and would never talk, were with us on that day, to see our handsome, confident, capable son delivering his bar mitzvah speech and reading beautifully from the Torah. Those who shared our pain were now sharing our joy!

Today Josh's life is in full swing. The cochlear implant has deepened his appreciation and understanding of life. To our son we say, "Congratulations as you listen, talk, and live life to its fullest."

Dana & Tamar

Elaine Matlow Tal-El

Twins!

The biggest surprise of my life — or so I thought then — was finding out that I was having twins.

Our eldest daughter, Michal, was four and a half years old, and Noa, our second daughter, was almost three when I gave birth to two beautiful baby girls — Dana and Tamar. I remember walking down the streets of my neighborhood in Jerusalem with the twins in the double stroller, flanked by Michal and Noa, thinking what a perfect family I had — four beautiful, healthy girls.

Only when Dana and Tamar were a year and a half old did I suspect that something was not right. Although they made all kinds of noises, they did not say any recognizable words. No "Ima," no "Aba" (Mom and Dad in Hebrew). I raised my fears with our pediatrician who,

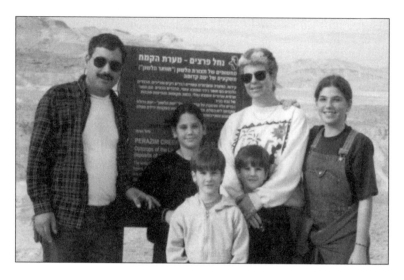

Dana and Tamar Tal-El (center front) and family

like others with whom I discussed my suspicions, only remarked — "It takes longer for twins to speak. They have their own language." We are a bilingual household, speaking both Hebrew and English, and for this reason also, everyone said that the twins' speech would be delayed.

I was happy to live with this delusion for a few more months. After all, I had my hands full with four children under five years old. Further, Dana and Tamar's hearing impairment was not readily evident, at first. They were extremely sociable, always connecting with people. They picked up every cue, from bringing their sandals, to going outside, to getting their coats. They just figured everything out on their own. Later, after the diagnosis of their severe-to-profound hearing loss, when asked if I hadn't noticed if the girls jumped when the door slammed, or other tell-tale signs, I responded that with four small children, I was happy just to get through the day.

But when the girls had reached the age of two, I couldn't avoid "the subject" any longer. I remember taking Tamar by herself (or was it Dana?) to the supermarket. It was rare for me to be out with only one girl at a time, and it was in the supermarket that I realized there was a real problem. After we packed our bag of groceries, Tamar took it and began to leave the supermarket. I called out, "Tamar! Wait! Don't go without me!" When she kept going, I called out in Hebrew, hoping that she hadn't understood the English. When she ignored me again, I called out, "Dana and Tamar!," a desperate last attempt to catch her attention, thinking then that perhaps she didn't know what *her* name was, spending so much time with her sister.

Needless to say, I knew as I walked home that it was time for some serious action!

I told my husband, Eli, the supermarket story, and he just wouldn't or couldn't accept it. He would not even come with me to the audiologist, thinking or hoping that I was just wasting my time. I remember sharing my impressions with the audiologist, including the girls' "normal" behavior and their speech and language delays.

Reality Bites!

The diagnosis confirmed my suspicions: severe-to-profound hearing loss. We were asked to come to the hospital for a more conclusive battery of tests. My husband joined me this time. The reality hit him as he sat with one of the girls in the sound chamber and witnessed for himself the lack of responses to what were unbearably loud noises to his ears. This was it — the *real* surprise of my life, which made the first surprise seem pale.

What to Do? Where to Go?

Once the test established that both girls had a severe-to-profound sensorineural bilateral hearing loss, we got into gear. We immediately ordered hearing aids, and informed our network of family and friends to see what they could find for us. Within three weeks, the girls received powerful ear-level hearing aids. We were advised to choose one language for the home, as the girls had missed some critical time for acquiring language. We chose Hebrew, a confirmation of my commitment to the life I had chosen to live in Israel. We were told to make sure that the girls looked at us at all times, so that they would begin to read our lips. We were also told to beware of our older girls' choice of husbands (the girls were by this time seven and five, respectively), as their sisters' hearing impairment might indicate a genetic defect!

The Jerusalem center for rehabilitation of children who are deaf contacted us and set up an appointment together with the girls. My husband and I observed a kindergarten with seven three-year-olds playing in total silence. Clearly, this was not what we wanted. What were the alternatives? The Jerusalem professionals focused on lipreading and a half-week self-contained program. As far as they were concerned, there were no other options.

Then, two miracles happened. First, my sister explored a Toronto hospital where auditory-verbal therapy is provided. She bought us our first books, as well as rubber ducks, airplanes, cats, and a dog. The *learning to listen* sounds began! The second miracle was acquiring membership in Auditory-Verbal International (AVI), a simple act that changed our lives.

Later, I received a phone call from a family from Mexico visiting Jerusalem who had obtained our number through the AVI membership list. They wanted to see what was happening for auditory-verbal children in Jerusalem. We didn't have much to tell them; we were fledglings ourselves. The mother of this then seven-year-old Mexican girl responded, "I thought that you could help us, but I see now that I can help you. Come over and meet our daughter." This meeting turned out to be the most formative experience of our new lives — the stuff that hopes and dreams are made of — a child who is deaf, yet speaking two languages, answering her mother while playing. Watching her, my husband and I cried. We decided then and there that somehow, auditory-verbal therapy would happen for Dana and Tamar.

Right after the diagnosis, we made contact with a private speech therapist who has continued lovingly to teach Dana and Tamar, as well as support and instruct us throughout our journey. She, too, was anxious to meet this Mexican family. She had never seen anything like this girl's achievements, despite her 10 years of teaching children who are deaf in Jerusalem. We decided to help her train in Canada to become an auditory-verbal therapist, and thereby help Dana and Tamar to reach their fullest listening and language potential.

Meanwhile, we chose to send our girls to a mainstream school in Jerusalem with the support of professional therapy. This was unheard of in Jerusalem, but we did it anyway. The twins were registered in the same kindergarten that the older girls had attended, and they have been following in their sisters' footsteps ever since.

Learning to Listen!

We spent that first year bathing the twins in sounds. We listened for every bark of a dog and every meow of a cat. We live beside train tracks, and would stop regularly to ask the girls, "Do you hear that?" as the train blew its horn. We were the only people in the neighborhood who sought out dog droppings to add another word to their tiny vocabulary! I attended our therapist's lessons three times a week, and did my own follow-up lessons at home the other days. We learned the *learning to listen* sounds, the names of family members, and environmental sounds. Despite a bit of progress, after a few months we came to a standstill. The biggest down side of being a pioneer was charting the unknown territory. Had we just plateaued before a great breakthrough? Was there another learning problem we didn't know about?

On my birthday the following July, a consultant in auditory-verbal practice arrived in Jerusalem. He loved Dana and Tamar. What was not to love? Two happy, sparkling, angelic blond girls. In the therapy session, he was impressed by what our clinician had learned and he joined in the session. I had hoped that he would say, "Keep it up; you're on the right track." No such luck! Based on their behavior in lessons — their difficulty in anticipating activities and their lack of response to many sounds — he felt that the girls were simply not hearing and listening. He said, "You might investigate a cochlear implant for your girls." In fact, later assessments by Real-Ear Measurement (REM), performed in Canada, verified that the girls did not hear enough.

Wearing hearing aids, Dana and Tamar responded to their names, understood some of the *learning to listen* sounds, and answered the doorbell. They made noises. They had about fifty "words" in their vocabulary. And yet, in light of the rigorous auditory program, they should have been farther ahead. They needed to develop more language, and we believed that auditory-verbal therapy after cochlear implantation would allow them access to the world of hearing, to speech, language, music, and to telephones (we do have four girls!) — in short, to that world in which we, as a family, live.

Happy New Ear!

Where to do the implant became a major decision. Dana and Tamar were in the "silver" category of profound hearing loss. That means that they were not unresponsive to sound with their hearing aids — they were not in the "gold" category, in which little or no benefit is obtained from amplification. In 1993, only "gold" profound losses were receiving implants in Israel. Even in the U.S., the stipulation that only "gold" hearing losses receive implants made our case somewhat controversial. We were a borderline case in the eyes of the Israeli establishment, as the girls had made "significant" progress in their first year using hearing aids.

We decided to have the surgery in New York — trusting the vast experience of the implant team, and the proximity to my family in Toronto. This was not a minor detail in light of the three months we were to spend in Toronto, commuting to New York eight times in that period. Without the support of my extended family, including my older children, this entire chapter of our lives could not have been written.

I moved into my parents' Toronto home with the four girls. Eli shuttled back and forth between Israel and Canada until we knew the surgery schedule. When we left Israel at the beginning of August, we had no idea when we would be back, when and if we would have a surgery date in New York, or how long we would have to stay close to New York following the implant, stimulation, and follow-up. The decision to have the cochlear implant was, however, a total family commitment.

When we met the surgeon on September 8, he told me that the girls appeared to be good candidates. I nonchalantly asked, "Could we take out our calendars?" "Yes," he replied, "What about next week?" Although he was a perfect stranger, my response was to give him a big hug. The date he gave us was the Jewish New Year. From that day, my brother coined a new blessing for the holiday: Happy New Ear! And it has been a Happy New Ear ever since.

"How do you implant twins?" I joked. "Simultaneously — one with the left hand and one with the right?" He assured me it wasn't quite that simple. But the operations went smoothly, and after a somewhat sleepless night in the hospital, we flew back to the family in Toronto. Michal and Noa were upset by the "baseball stitching" behind the twins' ears, but they got used to it. We knew that a new stage of our lives was about to begin.

Six weeks after the surgery, the implants were stimulated for the first time. The girls took the procedure beautifully. They had learned to perform excellently in hearing tests, and this was just another in the series. Two weeks later, we were back for more stimulation, enough for the girls to be able to detect many sounds.

Dana and Tamar were both responding with their new technology, but it took me some time to understand the parts of the system. One day at the playground, Dana came down the slide without the microphone or the magnet. I was sure that everything had been for naught until we found the pieces at the top of the slide, with the prongs of the short cable going every which way. I consulted an experienced family who allayed my fears, and we began learning more about this important device.

It is our good fortune to have a control group of implant users in our own home: two hearing children and two children who have implants. One of the twins has been doing remarkably well with her implant from the start. Her sister is doing... fine. I know parents are not supposed to compare their children, but even on the most inconsequential issues — it's difficult not to do.

Even the twin who is doing "fine" is a very auditory child. She enjoys listening to music and playing the piano, understands questions, responds appropriately, and expresses herself through speech with natural gestures. She has an inner sense of rhythm and enjoys dancing. She is learning all the time, and combined with reading, her language is beginning to flow. Her sister can process most language through listening alone; her speech is very intelligible, and her memory for vocabulary and idioms is excellent. She loves to play with her voice — acting out different characters, imitating her hearing sisters, singing, and making phone calls to her friends. Her sister has the same confidence, but less hearing.

I am an aggressive advocate for my children. When in doubt, I ask. When the answer doesn't satisfy me, I search for a second opinion. And when I feel unsure, I go for what I consider to be the very best, to give my children every chance to maximize their listening potential. I am in constant contact with our center in New York, while the girls receive maintenance care in Israel. We are investing a great deal in our auditory-verbal therapist, trying to arrange learning opportunities for her with outstanding professionals. Her professional excellence is to our children's advantage.

Looking Back

When I look back over the three years since the implant, I see how far we have come. I stopped keeping a "word list" almost a year ago when we reached about nine hundred words, but I remember how long it took to learn each word! I have kept journals from the beginning and videotaped the girls often. Whenever I feel I'm scraping the bottom of the energy barrel, I read a few words or watch a few moments of old video footage, and I see where we have come from and how hard we have worked, all of us: therapist, family, parents, and, especially, the girls.

Our house has become a language center — what better place is there to learn? The refrigerator is covered with magnets and word lists. The wall heaters are lost beneath work sheets and lesson materials. Items are labeled all over the house — the computer, the windows, the aquarium, the mirrors, doors, beds. This would be a good place for anyone interested in learning Hebrew!

Last year, while the girls were still in kindergarten, we focused our attention on preparing them for first grade. Though our therapist was not convinced that they would be ready, I was sure. We taught them to read and to do basic math, with the help of a teacher from the

Jerusalem Ministry of Education. We had chosen a mainstream school, thereby initiating a new system of remedial assistance! Until last year, everything had been done privately, at our expense. By kindergarten, when the twins were five, the newly passed special-education law in Israel authorized the provision of support services to children with special needs in mainstream educational environments. Finally, we appealed to the ministry and got what we needed, and the special-education teacher joined our intimate team of service providers. At the end of that year, Dana and Tamar were ready for school.

Into the Mainstream

The twins began first grade this past September. Michal is now in sixth grade, and Noa in fourth; all are at the same school. I take nothing for granted. Dana and Tamar have earned their desks at school. We are currently installing acoustic ceilings in their classrooms to reduce some of the noise, and there are plans to put up curtains. Throughout their preschool years, we put carpeting on the walls and throw rugs on the floor, and tried many other tricks to make their rooms more acoustically friendly. We continue to work with our therapist and now receive additional hours from the school's remedial teacher. I attend afternoon homework and language sessions to help the girls keep on top of the subjects learned at school.

Dana and Tamar's language skills are not at par with those of their friends. But in class, they try to listen, to ask for help when needed, to read all the cues to know what's going on, and to do their assignments. They participate in classroom discussions, and when the teacher doesn't understand their speech, friends who have been with them in kindergarten supply the translation. My girls have made genuine friendships. When I told one of the mothers how touched I was by her son's friendship with my daughter, she said, "He doesn't think he's doing any favor; he really likes her!"

Today... Tomorrow

I never imagined that it was possible to pass that dark period where I felt that the twins' cup was "half empty." Today, when I see and hear them talking to each other, whispering secrets into each others' ears, laughing with friends, enjoying piano lessons, reading their homework, bullying their big sisters, and being a bit "chutzpahdik" to Mom and Dad, I know that we are doing well! I will continue to be an advocate for my children until they can advocate for themselves.

I give thanks to those who invented and work with cochlear implant technology. Without cochlear implants, Dana and Tamar would not be who they are today. With the implant — the sky is the limit!

For all parents who are about to become part of the cochlear community, I have one wish: Happy New Ear!

Epilogue

As a professional who works in the field of auditory-verbal practice, I am extremely enthusiastic about cochlear implant technology and the scientific and artful habilitation required to foster children's ability to explore the colorful world of sound and speech.

As we enter the new century, technology will be more sophisticated, more user-friendly and more effective; the range of support services for children with cochlear implants will be much broader. The understanding of personal, social, and educational issues for children with cochlear implants will expand; knowledge of child development and the entire family system will be far more extensive than in earlier times.

Through the ongoing work of the medical, scientific, and educational communities and the commitment of parents and caregivers, there will be many more children, teenagers, and adults with cochlear implants, who will experience successful listening and spoken language communication.

It is time to celebrate!

— *Warren Estabrooks*

APPENDIX   A

Meaningful Auditory Integration Scale (MAIS)

Amy M. Robbins

Name _____   Date _____

Interval _____   Condition (device) _____

Examiner _____   Informant _____

1.   **Score item 1a if the child is younger than age 5 and item 1b if the child is older than age 5.**

1a.   Does the child wear the device all waking hours WITHOUT resistance?

Ask the parent, "What is your routine for putting on _____'s device each day?" Have the parent explain how long the child wears the device and determine if the child wears it all waking hours WITHOUT resistance or for only restricted periods of time. Ask, "If one day you didn't put the device on _____ would _____ show any indication that s/he missed wearing it (such as pulling or pointing to his/her ear, going over to where the device is kept when not in use, looking upset or quizzical, etc.)?" An additional query would be, "Does you child give any nonverbal indication that s/he is upset when the device is removed (such as crying or fussing)?"

❏	0 – Never	If parent seldom puts the device on the child because the child resists wearing it.
❏	1 – Rarely	If the child wears the device for only short periods of time but resists wearing it.
❏	2 – Occasionally	If child wears device for only short periods of time but without resistance.
❏	3 – Frequently	If the child wears the device all waking hours without resistance.
❏	4 – Always	If the child wears the device all waking hours and provides some indication if the parent forgets to put it on one day and/or some indication that s/he is upset or misses the device when it is not on.

Parent Report:

374   Cochlear Implants for Kids

1b. Does the child ask to have his or her device put on, or put it on him/herself WITHOUT being told?

Ask, "What is _____'s routine for putting on his/her device each day?"
Have parent explain if it is the parent or the child who takes responsibility
for it. Ask, "If one day, you didn't put the device on _____ and didn't mention it, would _____ ask to wear it and be upset by not having it?" An additional query would be, "Does your child basically wear it according to routine (such as all day at school and one hour at night) or does s/he want it
on all waking hours?" (for example, s/he puts it on at night even after
his/her bath). The latter would indicate a child who is more bonded and
dependent on his her device than the former.

- ❏   0 – Never   If the child resists wearing it.

- ❏   1 – Rarely   If the parent says child wears it without resistance,
                       but would never ask for it.

- ❏   2 – Occasionally   If child might inquire about it and is content to
                       wear it with a set time routine.

- ❏   3 – Frequently   If the child wears the device all waking hours
                       without resistance.

- ❏   4 – Always   Only if child wears it all waking hours and it's part
                       of his/her body (like glasses would be).

Parent Report:

2.   Does the child report and/or appear upset if his/her device is nonfunctioning for any reason?

Ask parent to give examples of what the child has done (verbally or nonverbally) when the device was not working. Ask also, "Have you ever
checked _____'s device and found it was not working (or headpiece had fall-
en off), but s/he had not noticed or had not told you?" In the case of the
younger child, ask, "Have you ever checked _____'s device and found it
wasn't working but s/he had not provided any nonverbal indication (such as
crying, reaching for the headpiece, etc.) that it was not working?"

- ❏   0 – Never   If child has no awareness as to whether the device is
                       working or not.

- ❏   1 – Rarely   If parent says child might only notice a malfunc-
                       tioning device (using verbal or nonverbal indica-
                       tion) once in a while.

- ❏   2 – Occasionally   If parents can give some examples of when the child would recognize a malfunctioning device (or if headpiece has fallen off) more than 50% of the time and may be beginning to distinguish some device problems from others.

❑   3 – Frequently   If parent gives examples and/or child can often distinguish different types of malfunction (e.g., bad cord vs. weak batteries).

❑   4 – Always   If child would never go without immediately detecting and reporting a problem with his/her unit and can easily identify what the problem is.

Parent Report:

3. **Does the child spontaneously respond to his name in quiet when called auditorially only with no visual cues?**

Ask, "If you called _____'s name from behind his back in a quiet room *with no visual cues,* what percentage of the time would he respond *the first time* you called?"

❑   0 – Never   If the child never does.

❑   1 – Rarely   If s/he has done it only once or twice or only with multiple repetitions.

❑   2 – Occasionally   If s/he does it about 50% of the time on the first trial or does it consistently but only when parent repeats his/her name more than once.

❑   3 – Frequently   If s/he does it at least 75% of the time on the first try.

❑   4 – Always   If s/he does this reliably and consistently, responding every time just as a hearing child would. Ask for examples.

Parent Report:

4. **Does the child spontaneously respond to his/her name in the presence of background noise when called auditorially only with no visual cues?**

Ask, "If you called _____'s name from behind his back with no visual cues in a noisy room, with people talking and the TV on, what percentage of time would s/he turn around and respond to you *the first time* you called?"

❑   0 – Never   If the child never does.

❏   1 – Rarely   If the child has done it only once or twice or only with multiple repetitions.

❏   2 – Occasionally   If s/he does it about 50% of the time on the first trial or does it consistently, but only when the parent repeats his/her name more than once.

❏   3 – Frequently   If s/he does it at least 75% of the time on the first try.

❏   4 – Always   If s/he does this reliably and consistently, responding every time just as a normal hearing child would. Ask for examples.

Parent Report:

5. Does the child spontaneously alert to environmental sounds (doorbell, telephone) in the home without being told or prompted to do so?

Ask, "Tell me about the kinds of environmental sounds _____ responds to at home and give me examples." Question parents to be sure that the child is responding *auditorially only* without any visual cues. Examples could be: the child asks about the telephone, doorbell, dog barking, water running, smoke alarm, toilet flushing, engines revving, horns honking, microwave bell, washer changing cycles, thunder, etc. The child must be responding *spontaneously* to three examples, and is not prompted by parent.

❏   0 – Never   If parent can give no examples or if child responds only after a prompt.

❏   1 – Rarely   If parent can give only one or two examples, or give several examples where the child's responses are inconsistent.

❏   2 – Occasionally   If child responds about 50% of the time to more than two environmental sounds.

❏   3 – Frequently   If child consistently responds to many environmental sounds at least 75% of the time.

❏   4 – Always   If child basically responds to environmental sounds the way a hearing child would. If there are a number of sounds that regularly occur to which the child does not react (even if s/he consistently responds to two sounds such as the phone and the doorbell), s/he would score no higher than *Occasionally*.

Parent Report:

6. Does the child alert to auditory signals spontaneously when in new environments?

Ask, "Does your child show curiosity (verbally or nonverbally) about new sounds when in unfamiliar settings, such as in someone else's home or a restaurant by asking, "What was that sound?" or saying, "I hear something!" A younger child may provide nonverbal indications that s/he has heard a new sound by widening his/her eyes, looking quizzical, searching for the source of the new sound, or imitating the new sound (such as when playing with a new toy). Examples parents have reported are children asking about clanging dishes in a restaurant, bells dinging in a department store, PA systems in public buildings, or an unseen baby crying in another room.

❏ 0 – Never   If parents can give no examples.

❏ 1 – Rarely   If parents can give only one or two examples.

❏ 2 – Occasionally   If child has done this numerous times and parents can give examples.

❏ 3 – Frequently   If parents can give numerous examples and this is a common occurrence.

❏ 4 – Always   If very few sounds occur without the child asking about them (or, in the case of the younger child, showing curiosity nonverbally).

Parent Report:

7. Does the child spontaneously RECOGNIZE auditory signals that are part of his/her school or home routine?

Ask, "Does _____ regularly recognize or respond appropriately to auditory signals in his/her classroom (e.g., school bell, PA system, fire alarm) or in the home (e.g., running to the window to see which family member is home when s/he hears the garage door opening; going to the table when the bell of the microwave goes off, signaling that the food is cooked and it is time to eat) with no visual cues or other prompts?"

❏ 0 – Never   If s/he never does it.

❏ 1– Rarely   If there are one or two instances.

❏ 2 – Occasionally   If s/he responds to these signals about 50% of the time.

❏ 3 – Frequently   If many examples are given and the child does it 75% of the time.

❏ 4 – Always   If s/he has clearly mastered this skill and does it all the time.

Parent Report:

8. **Does the child show the ability to discriminate spontaneously between two speakers, using audition alone (such as knowing mother's vs. father's voice, or parents' vs. sibling's voice)?**

Ask, "Can _____ tell the difference between two voices, like Mom or Dad's (or Susie's or John's) just by listening to them?"

❑   0 – Never   If parent can give no examples of the child discriminating between two speakers.

❑   1 – Rarely   If one or two examples are given.

❑   2 – Occasionally   If several examples are given and the child does this at least 50% of the time.

❑   3 – Frequently   If many examples are given and the child does this 75% of the time.

❑   4 – Always   If s/he always does this and shows no errors in doing this.

Parent Report:

9. **Does the child spontaneously know the difference between speech and nonspeech stimuli with listening alone?**

Ask, "Does _____ recognize speech as a category of sounds that are different from nonspeech sounds? For example, if you were standing behind your child and a noise occurred, would s/he ever say, "What was that noise?" In the case of the younger children, ask, "Would _____ever run into the next room to search for a family member's voice versus looking out the window for a dog or fire truck?"

❑   0 – Never   If parent can give no examples of the child dis-criminating speech from nonspeech.

❑   1 – Rarely   If one or two examples are given.

❑   2 – Occasionally   If several examples are given and the child does this at least 50% of the time.

❑   3 – Frequently   If many examples are given and the child does this 75% of the time.

❑   4 – Always   If s/he always does this and shows no errors in doing this.

Parent Report:

10. Does the child spontaneously associate vocal tone (anger, excitement, anxiety) with its meaning based on hearing alone?

Ask, "By listening only, can _____ tell the emotion conveyed in someone's voice such as an angry voice, an excited voice, etc.?" (e.g., Dad yells at child to "hurry up" through the bathroom door and the child responds, "Why are you mad?" and yells back at him. In the case of the younger child, the child starts to cry because of the angry sound in his/her voice). Another example is if the parent is reading a new book to a young child while s/he is sitting on the parent's lap and cannot see their parent's face (e.g., Mom says, "the boy yelled "Let's go!" and the child says, "The boy is happy to go to the park").

❏   0 – Never   If the parent can give no examples or if the child
                         has never had the opportunity to do this.

❏   1 – Rarely   If the child does it 25% of the time.

❏   2 – Occasionally   If the child does it about 50% of the time.

❏   3 – Frequently   If s/he does it 75% of the time.

❏   4 – Always   If s/he consistently can identify more than one
                         emotion in the listening alone condition.

Parent Report:

APPENDIX   B

Infant–Toddler: Meaningful Auditory Integration Scale (IT–MAIS)

S. Zimmerman-Phillips, M.J. Osberger, A. M. Robbins

1.   Is the child's vocal behavior affected while wearing his/her sensory aid (hearing aid or cochlear implant)?

The benefits of auditory input are often apparent first in the speech production skills of very young children. The frequency and quality of vocalizations may change when the device is put on, when it is turned off, or when it is not working properly.

Ask the parent, "Describe _____'s vocalizations when you first put his/her device on each day." Have the parent explain how and if the child's vocalizations change when the sensory aid is first turned on and auditory input is experienced at the start of each day. Ask, "If you forget to put the device on ____, or if the device is not working properly, do you and/or others notice that ____'s vocalizations are different in any way (e.g., quality, frequency of occurrence)?" Perhaps ask, "Does the child 'test' the device by vocalizing when the device is first turned on?"

❑   0 – Never   No difference in the child's vocalizations with or without the device.

❑   1 – Rarely   Slight increase in the frequency of the child's vocalizations (approximately 25% increase) with the device on (or similar decrease with the device off).

❑   2 – Occasionally   Child vocalizes throughout the day and there are increases in vocalizations (approximately 50% increase) with the device on (or similar decrease with the device off).

❑   3 – Frequently   Child vocalizes throughout the day and there are noticeable increases in vocalizations (approximately 75% increase) with the device on (or a similar decrease with the device off). Parent may report that individuals outside the home notice a change in the frequency of child's vocalizations with or without the device.

❑   4 – Always   Child's vocalizations increase 100% with the device on compared to the frequency of occurrence with the device off.

Parent Report:

2.   Does the child produce well-formed syllables and syllable-sequences that are recognized as "speech"?

This type of utterance is characteristic of the speech of developing infants. The utterances contain speech sounds and syllables that are recognized as "speech" by the parents (e.g., "mamama," "dadada," "bababa," or "yayaya"). Parents often assert the baby is "talking." Ask, "Does _____ 'talk' to you or to objects?" Ask, "As _____ plays alone, what kinds of sounds do you hear when the device is on?" Ask the parent, "Does _____ say sounds and words used in nursery rhymes or playing with toys?" (e.g., "hop hop," "moo," "baaa," "choo-choo," "mmmmm"). "Ask the parent to give specific examples of the types of utterances the child produces, as well as the frequency with which they are produced.

❑ 0 – Never Child never produces speech-like utterances; child only produces undifferentiated vocalizations; or the parent can give no examples.

❑ 1– Rarely Child produces speech-like utterances once in awhile (approximately 25% of the time), but only when provided with a model.

❑ 2 – Occasionally Child produces speech-like utterances 50% of the time when provided with a model.

❑ 3 – Frequently Child produces these utterances approximately 75% of the time; parents must give many examples. Child produces the syllable sequences *spontaneously,* but with a limited phonetic repertoire. The child can clearly and reliably imitate sequences *with a model.*

❑ 4 – Always Child produces syllable-sequences consistently and on a spontaneous basis (i.e., without a model). The utterances consist of a varied repertoire of sounds.

Parent Report:

3. **Does the child spontaneously respond to his/her name in quiet with auditory cues only (i.e., no visual cues)?**

Infants and toddlers demonstrate a variety of behaviors in response to sound. Examples of such responses in a very young child may be: momentary cessation of an activity (e.g., stops moving, playing, sucking, crying), searching for the sound source (e.g., infant looks up or around after hearing his/her name), eye-widening or eye-blink. Ask the parent, "If you called _____'s name from behind his/her back in a quiet room with no visual cues, what percentage of the time would s/he respond *the first time* that you called his/her name?" Many young children commonly demonstrate an "off-response" when auditory stimulation stops; any repeatable behavior is considered a response, provided the child demonstrates the behavior consistently. Ask for specific examples of the types of responses that the parent observes, especially to assign the highest ratings.

❑ 0 – Never Child never responds to his/her name, or the parent can give no examples.

❑ 1 – Rarely Child responds to his/her name only about 25% of the time on the first trial; or only with multiple repetitions.

❑   2 – Occasionally   Child responds to his/her name about 50% of the
time on the first trial; or does it consistently but only
after parent repeats the name more than once.

❑   3 – Frequently   Child responds to his/her name at least 75% of the
time on the first trial.

❑   4 – Always   Child responds to his/her name reliably and consistently on the first trial.

Parent Report:

4. **Does the child spontaneously respond to his/her name in the
presence of background noise with auditory cues only (i.e., no
visual cues)?**

Ask the parent, "If you called _____'s name from behind his/her back with
no visual cues in a noisy room (e.g., people talking, children playing, the TV
on), what percentage of time would s/he respond to you *the first time* that
you called his/her name?" Use the response criteria specified in Question 3
to score the parent's observations. Ask for specific examples of the types of
responses that the parent observes.

❑   0 – Never   Child never responds to his/her name in noise, or
the parent can give no examples.

❑   1 – Rarely   Child responds to his/her name in noise about 25%
of the time on the first trial; or only with multiple
repetitions.

❑   2 – Occasionally   Child responds to his/her name in noise about 50%
of the time on the first trial; or does it consistently
but only after parent repeats the name more than once.

❑   3 – Frequently   Child responds to his/her name in noise at least
75% of the time on the *first* trial.

❑   4 – Always   Child responds to his/her name in noise reliably
and consistently on the *first* trial.

Parent Report:

5. **Does the child spontaneously alert to environmental sounds (dog,
toys) in the home without being told or prompted to do so?**

Ask the parent, "Tell me about the kinds of environmental sounds to which
_____ responds at home and in familiar situations (e.g., grocery store,

restaurant, playground). Give me examples." Question parents to be sure the child is responding via audition, without visual cues. Ask the parent to provide specific examples, such as responding to the telephone, TV, a dog barking, the smoke alarm, toys that make sounds (e.g., music boxes, music mobiles "see-and-say" toys, horns honking, dishwasher, microwave bell). The child must be reacting spontaneously to the sound without prompting from the parent. Use the response criteria specified in Question 3 to score the parent's observations. The response behaviors may be demonstrated when the sound is first detected or when it ceases.

❏   0 – Never   Child never demonstrates the behavior; the parents can give no examples; or child responds only after a prompt.

❏   1 – Rarely   Child responds about 25% of the time to different sounds. Parents can give only one or two examples, or they give several examples of sounds that the child responds to on an inconsistent basis.

❏   2 – Occasionally   Child responds about 50% of the time to more than two environmental sounds. If there are a number of sounds that regularly occur to which the child does not respond (even if he consistently responds to two sounds such as the phone and the doorbell), assign a score no higher than *Occasionally.*

❏   3 – Frequently   Child consistently responds to many environmental sounds at least 75% of the time.

❏   4 – Always   Child basically responds to all environmental sounds reliability and consistently.

Parent Report:

6. Does the child spontaneously alert to environmental sounds in new environments?

Ask the parent, "Does _____ show curiosity (verbal or nonverbal) about sounds when in unfamiliar settings (e.g., such as in someone else's home, unfamiliar store, or a restaurant?)." Examples include: clanging dishes in a restaurant, bells dinging in a department store, PA systems in public buildings, a baby crying in another room, a smoke alarm, or an unfamiliar toy at a playmate's home. A younger child may provide nonverbal indications that s/he has heard a new sound with eye-widening, a frown or a smile, searching for the source of the new sound, imitation of the new sound (such as when playing with a new toy), starting to cry after a loud or unusual sound, or looking to a parent for information. The response behaviors may be demonstrated when the sound is first detected or when it ceases.

❏   0 – Never   Child never demonstrates the behavior or the
                      parent can give no examples.

❏   1 – Rarely   Child demonstrates the behavior but does so only
                      about 25% of the time; parent can give only one or
                      two examples of this behavior.

❏   2 – Occasionally   Child demonstrates the behavior numerous times
                      (about 50%) of the time and parents can give a
                      number of different examples.

❏   3 – Frequently   Child demonstrates the behavior about 75% of the
                      time; parents can give many different examples;
                      responses are a common occurrence.

❏   4 – Always   Very few new sounds occur without the child's
                      showing a response to or curiosity about them.

Parent Report:

7. Does the child spontaneously RECOGNIZE auditory signals that are part of his/her everyday routines?

Ask, "Does _____ regularly recognize or respond appropriately to auditory signals at daycare, preschool, or in the home with no visual cues or other prompts?" Examples of this may be: looking for a familiar toy that the child hears but cannot see; looking at the microwave when it goes off or the telephone when it rings; looking at the door when the dog is outside barking, wanting to come in the house; looking at the door upon hearing the garage door opening; putting hands over his/her eyes if you stand behind the child and verbally initiate an interactive play game such as "Peek-a-boo!" (Other games include "Pat-a-Cake" or "So Big!")

❏   0 – Never   Child never demonstrates the behavior or the
                      parent can give no examples.

❏   1 – Rarely   Parent can give one or two examples of the behav-
                      ior; child responds to these signals 25% of the time.

❏   2 – Occasionally   Parent can provide more than two examples. Child
                      responds to these signals about 50% of the time.

❏   3 – Frequently   Parent can give many examples. Child demonstrates
                      the response to these signals 75% of the time.

❏   4 – Always   Child clearly has mastered this skill and routinely
                      responds to auditory signals that are part of every-
                      day routines.

Parent Report:

8. **Does the child demonstrate the ability to discriminate spontaneously between two speakers with auditory cues only (i.e., no visual cues)?**

Examples of this behavior include discriminating between the voice of a mother or a father and that of a sibling, or discriminating between the voices of a mother and a father. Examples of this behavior may be attending/ responding to the parent who spoke when only auditory cues are present. Ask, "Can _____ tell the difference between two voices, like Mom or brother/ sister, just by listening to them?" At a more difficult level, ask "If _____ is playing with two siblings and one sibling spoke, would _____ look in the direction of the appropriate brother/sister?"

❑ 0 – Never — Child never demonstrates the behavior or the parent can give no examples.

❑ 1 – Rarely — Child can discriminate between two very different voices (adult/child) about 25% of the time.

❑ 2 – Occasionally — Child can discriminate between two very different voices (adult/child) about 50% of the time.

❑ 3 – Frequently — Child discriminates between two very different voices (adult/child) 75% of the time; sometimes discriminates between two similar voices (e.g., voices of two children).

❑ 4 – Always — Child always discriminates between two very different voices; discriminates between two similar voices very often.

Parent Report:

9. **Does the child spontaneously know the difference between speech and nonspeech stimuli with listening alone?**

The purpose of this question is to evaluate whether the child has categorical perception between speech and nonspeech stimuli. We address this by inquiring about instances where the child may confuse these two stimuli, or show that he is not confused. For example, if a child has an established response to certain stimuli (e.g. rocking in response to music), does s/he ever exhibit this behavior in response to speech stimuli?

Ask, "Does _____ recognize speech as a category of sounds that are different from nonspeech sounds?" For example, if you are in a room with your child and you called to him/her, would s/he look for you or for a favorite toy? Ask, "Does _____ ever search for a family member's voice versus looking for a familiar toy?"

☐   0 – Never   Child does not demonstrate the behavior or parent can give no examples.

☐   1 – Rarely   Child demonstrates the behavior about 25% of the time; parents can give only one or two examples.

☐   2 – Occasionally   Child demonstrates the behavior about 50% of the time; parents give a number of different examples.

☐   3 – Frequently   Child demonstrates the behavior 75% of the time; parents give many different examples.

☐   4 – Always   Child consistently and reliably demonstrates the behavior; child makes essentially no errors in discriminating speech from nonspeech stimuli.

Parent Report:

10. Does the child spontaneously associate vocal tone (anger, excitement, anxiety) with its meaning based on hearing alone?

In the very young child, does the child recognize changes in emotion conveyed by voice associated with the use of "motherese"? Examples of this include: laugh or coo in response to large fluctuations in the intonation or changes in voice, upset when scolding or told firmly "no-no," even with no substantial increase in the loudness of the voice. Ask the parent, "By listening only, can _____ tell the emotion conveyed in someone's voice such as an angry voice, an excited voice, etc.?" (e.g., mother yells and child startles and cries in response, or child laughs or smiles in response to changes in intonation and prosody in parents' voices without seeing their face).

☐   0 – Never   Child does not demonstrate the behavior; parent can give no examples; child has no opportunity to show the behavior.

☐   1 – Rarely   Child demonstrates the behavior about 25% of the time.

☐   2 – Occasionally   Child demonstrates the behavior about 50% of the time.

☐   3 – Frequently   Child demonstrates the behavior about 75% of the time.

☐   4 – Always   Child consistently and appropriately responds to a range of vocal tones.

Parent Report:

APPENDIX C

Auditory-Verbal Ages & Stages of Development

Listening (Levels I–VIII)

Level I Awareness of Sound

*✓ + –

- Responds to very low loud *gross* sounds, such as a drum, bell, or clacker presented within a 3-foot radius at ear level.
- Responds to music with a strong beat, such as a lively march.
- Responds to loud *inside* environmental sounds when attention is directed to the sound (blender, mixer, vacuum cleaner, TV, etc.)
- Responds to *outside* environmental sounds (car, airplane, fire engine, ambulance, police car, birds singing, etc. when attention is directed to the sounds).
- Indicates when something is heard by pointing to the ear, nodding head, vocalizing, or smiling.
- Shows an awareness of music, inside/outside meaningful environmental sounds or speech *without attention being directed to the sound.*
- Notices the *acoustic feedback* produced when the earmold of the hearing aid is partially out.
- Indicates when the hearing aid or cochlear implant is not working.

Level II Sound Has Meaning

✓ + – **Responds to:**
- Music by dancing, singing, or clapping.
- Some simple speech sounds accompanied by gesture (Sh!, Bye-bye, No-no, or Come).
- Own name

✓ + – **Associates:**
- A specific sound with an object in environment (I hear that; that's Mother's car).

*Legend:
✓ accomplished, + emerging, – not developed

Level I   Awareness of Sound (cont'd)

* ✓ + −

- A specific sound with a happening (That's Mother's car... Aha, Mother's home! Time to eat).
- *Learning to Listen Sound* with a toy, object, or happening.

Level III   Early Listening ↔ Talking Loop

✓ + −

- Imitates gross body movements appropriate to his age level (Pat-a-Cake, Peek-a-Boo, Follow the Leader, Simon Says, etc.).
- Responds to music by clapping, dancing, swaying or singing.
- Vocalization increases when hearing aid or cochlear implant is on.
- Imitates laughing, crying, coughing, or yelling.
- Imitates mother's vocal play (call to each other with stimulating rhythmic and inflectional patterns).
- Tests the hearing aid or cochlear implant with voice when turned on.
- Practices additional vocal play incorporating the vowel sounds ah, oo, and ee.
- Imitates mother's babble play, incorporating new inflectional/ rhythmic patterns
- Approximates new words or short phrase beginning with the babbled consonant practiced. (mu, mu, mu; Mama, more; That's mine! More milk, etc.)
- Imitates new babble sounds appropriate to listening age.
- Calls back and forth in calling games, such as Hide and Seek, incorporating inflectional patterns and vowel sounds.

Approximates:
- Temporal pattern of a short phrase.
- Temporal plus inflectional pattern of a short phrase.
- Temporal, inflectional, stress, and articulation of a short phrase.
- Imitates whispering.

Level IV   Discrimination

✓ + −

Responds to the presence or absence (on or off) of the following sounds (first inside, then outside):
- Clackers, noisemakers.
- Music.

Level IV
✓ + –

Discrimination (cont'd)

- Inside environmental sounds.
- Outside environmental sounds.
- Speech.

Discriminates:
- Loud and quiet sounds in above areas.
- High and low aspects of sound in above areas.
- Fast and slow sounds.
- A continuous or an abrupt sound.
- Angry or cheerful voice and responds appropriately.
- Daddy's and Mommy's voice.
- A man's, woman's or child's voice.
- Two gross sounds; later, 3 gross sounds (drum, bell whistle).
- Imitates the vowel sound ah and oo; later, ah, oo, and ee.
- Imitates the consonant and vowel sounds associated with trucks, cars, fire engines, planes, boats, motorbike, etc.
- Recognizes own name from the most different family name on the basis of the number of syllables, vowel and consonant differences.
- Detects the primary signal from other quiet background noise.
- Imitates a few familiar commands with natural gestures (Close your eyes, Don't touch it).
- Discriminates familiar words on the basis of syllable length (one vs. 3 syllables, one vs. 2 vs. 3 syllables).
- Familiar words on the basis of vowel and consonant differences (hat, shoe, coat) but the same number of syllables.
- Imitates a 2- to 3-word sequence.
- Imitates phrases on the basis of rhythmic structure and known words ("up the slide," " in the car," "to the store").
- Imitates various short familiar sentence patterns (exclamatory, statement, or question on the basis of inflectional and rhythmic patterns.
- Between words containing different vowels but the same initial or final consonant (bat, boat, bee).
- Imitates a 3- to 4-word sequence.

Level IV   Discrimination (cont'd)

✓ + −

- Discriminates similar phrases or sentences (a big blue truck, a little black car).
- Among rhyming words (shoe, blue, two).
- Important but minor differences in sentences (in/on; the/a; he/she).
- Between classes of consonants in syllables (sha, ma, ta, vs. see, knee, bee).
- Within classes of consonants (pa, ta, or ka) (bu, du, gu).
- Remembers and approximates sentence of 7–10 words.

Level V   Localization Skills

✓ + −

- Locates a sound presented at ear level within a 3-foot radius in front or on either side, but not behind.
- Locates a sound presented at ear level within a 3-foot radius behind them.
- Understands and verifies gross, environmental, music, or speech sounds within 6 feet, then 9 feet, 12 feet, and finally, within the same room in all directions.
- Understands sounds that come from a specific location or direction from another room.
- Understand sounds with a specific location or direction outside.

Level VI   Distance and Directional Listening

✓ + −

- Shows awareness of gross sounds in all directions at 3 feet, 6 feet, 9 feet.
- Discriminates between gross sounds in all directions in increasing 3-foot intervals.
- Discriminates other aspects of sound, high or low, loud or quiet, fast or slow, etc., in all directions at increasing 3-foot intervals.
- Responds to own name from increasing distances in all directions.
- Responds to a few short, familiar commands at increasing distances in all directions on the basis of rhythmic structure and inflectional patterns.
- Discriminates among familiar words of varying syllable lengths at increasing distances.

Level VI   **Distance and Directional Listening (cont'd)**

✓ + −

 • Discriminates familiar vocabulary on the basis of vowel and consonant differences (hat, coat, shoe) in all directions at increasing distances.

Level VII   **Listening in Background Noise**

✓ + −   **Recognizes the following with increasing distances in all directions with added background noise:**
 • Own name.

 • Familiar words (closed set → open set).

 • Short, familiar, descriptive phrases.

 • Short, familiar, descriptive sentences.

 • Follows familiar, simple one-step commands.

 • Follows more complicated 2-step and 3-step commands with background noise (Go outside; Bring me the paper).

Level VIII   **Auditory Memory and Sequencing**

✓ + −   **Short-term memory:**
 • Approximates 2- or 3-word phrase by echolalia (I want one).

 • Chooses correct picture names from choice of 2, then 3, then 4, then more (Where is the doggie?).

 • Selects 2 pictures or objects named correctly, but not necessarily in order.

 • Selects 2 pictures/objects named correctly, in correct sequence.

 • Tells which object/picture of 3 is missing.

 • Selects 3 objects or pictures correctly out of a choice of 5 or 6 in sequence.

 • Imitates a 4-word sequence (echolalia).

 • Repeats random numbers out of sequence (1, 4, 3, 2).

 • Imitates nonsense syllables.

 • Selects 4 or 5 cards' names out of a choice of 8 or 9.

Approximates a 6- or 7-word sequence by:
 • Breaking it into 2 natural phrases and repeating each one after a model.

 • Approximating the whole phrase.

Level VIII   Auditory Memory and Sequencing (cont'd)

✓ + − | **Long-term memory span:**
- Knows own first name, then last name.
- Knows names of other family members, including pets.
- Uses 2- or 3-word patterned sequence spontaneously.

Knows names of the following important people, places, and things:
- Family.
- Parts of the body.
- Clothes.
- Foods.
- Toys.
- Other things used.
- Rooms of the house.
- Basic furniture at home.
- Names of feelings (happy, sad, sick, tired, hungry, I like it, I don't like it, I love it, etc.).
- Common descriptive adjective phrases (It's pretty! Oh, icky! That's nice).
- Present progressive, tense of common verbs for the things s/he does (is, am, sleeping, eating, playing, working, etc.).
- Generates own 2-word sequence.
- Knows and supplies key words in favorite nursery rhymes or other repetitive children's stories.
- Rote counts 1, 2... then 1, 2, 3... etc., always adding new numbers.
- Generates own 3- or 4-word telegraphic language phrases or sentence.
- Singing the Alphabet Song.
- Singing Happy Birthday.
- Singing seasonal songs or poems.
- Generates 3-, 4-, or 5-word sequence (may not use adult syntax).
- Tells age, address, and/or telephone number.
- Knows mother's, father's and sibling's names, sibling's ages, and names of parents' occupations.
- Describes past event with fair degree of accuracy and sequence.

Age	✓ + −	Receptive Speech and Language
3 mo		• Anticipates feeding by voices and visual stimuli. • Looks at speaker's face. • Quieted by adult's voice. • Activity diminishes when approached by sound.
6 mo		• Recognizes tone and inflection of voice of known persons. • Locates source of sound. • Distinguishes between friendly and angry voices. • Turns to voice and will search for source.
9 mo		• May carry out simple commands, pleased with understanding. • Responds to verbal requests like "Wave bye-bye" or "Pat-a-cake." • Raises arms when mother says "Come up" and reaches toward child. • Listens to own vocalizations and those of others.
12 mo		• Words assist in discrimination of object classes: "up" is kite, etc. • Understands key words in association with object or situation. • Recognizes words as symbols. • Gives toy on request when accompanied by gesture.
15 mo		• Understands 10 simple words or phrases without objects present. • Points to familiar persons, animals, or toys on request. • Follows simple request ("Give me the…; Get me the…"). • Understands simple phrases and questions with key word: "Where's Daddy?"
18 mo		• Understand 50 words without cue. • Listens to rhymes and songs for 2–3 minutes. • Identifies 2 objects in a box. • Points to own nose, eye, mouth, and hair.
21 mo		• Understands following pronouns: I, me, mine, it, this, that. • Points to any 4 or 5 parts of doll or self. • Understand about 100 words. • Understands simple verbal explanations ("You can have some later").

Age	✓ + −	Receptive Speech and Language (cont'd)
2 yrs		• Understands the following question forms: What, Where. • Understands negatives: no, not, no more, don't fall. • Understands *on, in, under,* in response to *where* questions. • Will follow a short series of related directions.
2 yrs, 3 mo		• Understands some prepositional phrases (on the bed, under the table, to the store). • Enjoys hearing stories using known vocabulary, people and experiences. • Understands words such as hair, hands, feet, nose, eyes, mouth.
2 yrs, 6 mo		• Can identify the use of things (in pictures.) • Enjoys simple stories from picture books, wants repetition day after day. • Understands 2 prepositions of: *on, in, under, behind, in front of.* • Understands the use of things (What do your hear with?).
2 yrs, 9 mo		• Points to 6 body parts. • Understands concept of one. • Enjoys looking at books by self. • Accepts new story slowly.
3 yrs		• Understands *why* question forms (Why do we have stoves?). • Listens eagerly to stories and demands favorites over and over again. • Enjoys repetition of familiar tunes and stories. • Understands concept of boy or girl.
3 yrs, 3 mo		• Understands opposite analogies. • Some appreciation of past and present; follows discussion about past/future. • Understands the concept of 2.
3 yrs, 6 mo		• Understands which of 2 things is longer. • Understands which of 2 things is bigger. • Understands which of 2 things is smaller.
3 yrs, 9 mo		• Can point to neck, arm, knee, thumb. • Understands more complex language (Why... because; If... then). • Acquires new words in terms of known words (Run quickly, fast).

Age	✓ + −	Receptive Speech and Language (cont'd)
4 yrs		• Appreciates past, present, future. • Comprehends picture description. • Understands concept of heavy/light.
4 yrs, 3 mo		• Can compare 3 pictures (Which one is prettiest?). • Understands commands using 4 prepositions. • Has auditory memory for 9- to 10-word sentence.
4 yrs, 6 mo		• Has auditory memory for 4 digits. • Can follow 3 commands in order. • Understands of what material objects are made.
4 yrs, 9 mo		• Listens to *long* stories, sometimes confusing fact and fantasy. • Understands the question *How many?* up to concept of 4.
5 yrs		• Understands analogies (Milk is white, butter is _____ ?). • Has auditory memory for 11-word sentence.

Age	✓ + −	Expressive Speech and Language
3 mo		• Vocalizes for feelings of pleasure. • Vocalizes—babbles or coos in play when alone, or when talked to. • Makes single vowel sounds (ah, eh, uh). • Uses consonants (h, k, g). • Vocalizes other than crying, small throaty sounds — short and staccato.
6 mo		• Intersperses vowel sounds with more consonants. • Babbles at persons to gain attention. • Vocalizes moods of pleasure up to 30 minutes — giggles, grins, laughs aloud. • Sustains pitch-modulated cooing for 15–20 minutes.
9 mo		• Babbles phrases (4 syllables or more). • Imitates coughs, tongue clicks, and kisses. • Imposes adult intonation on babbling. • Uses two-syllable babble (da-da; bu-bu; or ma-ma) nonspecifically.
12 mo		• Uses jargon; may use one word to express a sentence (holophrastic). • Says first true words, usually babble or function word (bye-bye). • Imitates number of syllables after someone (echolalia). • Uses a few meaningful words (says Dada or Mama as specific names).

Age	✓ + −	**Expressive Speech and Language (cont'd)**
15 mo		• Names several objects. • Tries to sing. • Says 3 words other than mama or dada. • Babbles short sentences — babbles sounds with inflection.
18 mo		• Echoes prominent or last word spoken. • Uses 6–20 recognizable words and understands many more. • On one-word response, often gets the initial consonant plus vowel. • Speaks 4–7 words clearly.
21 mo		• Begins to use question forms; what, where, and why. • Combines 2 or more words into ideas: "Dada, bye-bye." • Refers to self by name. • Begins to use possessive modifiers: my, mine.
2 yrs		• Uses 50 or more recognizable words and understands many more. • Begins to use the pronouns *it, mine, this, that*. • Uses 3-word sentences: nouns, some verbs, few adjective or adverbs. • Begins to eliminate jargon: constantly asking names of objects.
2 yrs, 3 mo		• Uses some form of plural (2 book, dogs). • Has discarded jargon. • Gives full name on request. • Names common objects.
2 yrs, 6 mo		• Says a few nursery rhymes. • Gives the use of an object. • Uses the question forms: what, where, why, how, when. • Uses forms of negation: it is not, can't, don't, this not.
2 yrs, 9 mo		• Answers: What's your name? What does the doggie say? • Asks an unsolicited question (Where's Daddy? What that for?). • Uses negative statement (He doesn't, none, nobody). • Uses 200 or more recognizable words; speech not completely intelligible.
3 yrs		• Begins to use *-ing* verb forms. • Says several words in a group (predominantly noun phrases). • Uses pronouns: you, she, he, they and we. • Verbalizes sounds: w-, m-, n-, h-, -m-, b-, -b-, p-, -p-, d-, -d-.

Age	✓ + −	**Expressive Speech and Language (cont'd)**
3 yrs, 3 mo		• Uses basic grammar: subject... verb... object. • Repeats 5-, 6-, or 7-syllable sentence. • Uses well-patterned inflection. • Speaks in approximately 6-word sentences.
3 yrs, 6 mo		• Verbalizes sounds: -w-, -m, -n-, g-, -g-, k-, -k-, f-, -f, t-, -h. • Uses plurals appropriately. • Uses the question forms: Whose, who, what, when, why and how. • Begins to use model and auxiliary verbs: do, have.
3 yrs, 9 mo		• Carries out 4-step command within situational context. • Speaks intelligibly but has many phonetic substitutions. • Refers to self by pronoun. • Talks to self in long monologue, mostly about the present.
4 yrs		• Begins to use model and auxiliary verbs: be, can, will. • Recites poem from memory or sings a song. • Uses all commonly used pronouns. • Can tell about pictures.
4 yrs, 3 mo		• Can repeat a 12- to 13-syllable sentence correctly. • Counts to 5 in proper order. • Gives appropriate reply to *What do you do when you're sleepy? Cold?* • Identifies and points to pictures described.
4 yrs, 6 mo		• Asks questions: Why? When? and How? and the meaning of words. • Defines some words in terms of function of object. • Gives connected account of recent events and experiences. • Speaks in nearly complete sentences: errors of vocabulary, word order, grammar.
4 yrs, 9 mo		• Has a vocabulary of 1,500 words. • Can define some words. • Can answer: Why do we have houses, books, clock, eyes? • Listens to and tells long stories; may confuse fact and fantasy.
5 yrs		• Counts up to 10. • Uses *and* when referring to 2 objects, persons or actions. • Communicates freely with friends, family and strangers. • Verbalizes the sounds: y-, -ng, -ng-, -r-, l-, -mp, j-, -f-, s-.

Age	✓ + –	Cognitive Skills
3 mo		• Coordination between vision and hearing: discriminates between sounds. • Differentiation: rejects other objects placed in mouth if desires nipple. • Prefers complex visual stimuli.
6 mo		• Grasping and striking acts are repeated intentionally. • Looks for objects that have moved out of field of view. • Grasps and manipulates objects within reach.
9 mo		• Uses means to attain ends (moves pillow to reach toy hidden under it). • Distinguishes between mother's face and unfamiliar. • Will follow the path of a falling object.
12 mo		• Searches for objects that disappear (toy under cloth). • Associates properties with things (points up when sees bird, etc.). • Shows clear signs of anticipation of events (cries when sees person leaving).
15 mo		• Understands the meaning of up and down. • Hands a toy to parent when asked to do so. • Beginning interest in experimenting with objects — trial and error.
18 mo		• Objects beyond self seen as causes of actions (cries, calls, points). • Points to one body part of doll or self. • Begins to understand use of household objects.
21 mo		• Follows 2 or 3 directions (Put the doll in the chair). • Puts large pegs on a pegboard. • Names one picture of 5 common objects (cat, bird, dog, horse, man).
2 yrs		• Has a sense of time (recognizes cues for meals and bedtime). • Predicts cause-effect relationship (turns lights on/off, pushes buzzers). • Beginning sense of ownership: my.
2 yrs, 3 mo		• Says when something is heavy. • Imitates crayon strokes, both vertical and horizontal. • Completes 3-shape formboard (circle, square, triangle).
2 yrs, 6 mo		• Repeats 2 digits (2, 8, etc.). • Counts 2 objects. • Names any 5 objects (What's this?).

Age	✓ + –	Cognitive Skills (cont'd)
2 yrs, 9 mo		• Builds an 8- or 9-block tower. • Identifies at least one color correctly. • Knows concept of *one* when asked.
3 yrs		• Points to or names the bigger of 2 objects when asked. • Knows the meaning of same, different. • Can answer correctly, Are you a boy or a girl?
3 yrs, 3 mo		• Builds a bridge with blocks. • Repeats 3 digits in sequence (5-3-1, etc.). • Verbalizes opposites.
3 yrs, 6 mo		• Can put 2- to 5-piece puzzle together. • Can find pictures of animals that are alike (Lotto). • Can sort by color.
3 yrs, 9 mo		• Can point to tongue, neck, arm, knee thumb. • Knows how many fingers on each hand. • Asks the meaning of words.
4 yrs		• Tells what an object is made of. • Tells what he or she is going to draw before drawing it. • Draws a 2-part person: head and body.
4 yrs, 3 mo		• Matches many shapes (circle, square, triangle, hexagon, star, oval, moon). • Works on 7-piece puzzle. • Can respond correctly to *A hat goes on your head, shoes go* _____.
4 yrs, 6 mo		• Can follow 3 commands in proper order. • Listens to and tells long stories, sometimes confusing fact and fantasy. • Knows day and night and appropriate associated activities.
4 yrs, 9 mo		• Tells jokes or riddles. • Knows right hand from left. • Draws a 3-part man (head, body, legs etc.).
5 yrs		• Copies a square from a pattern. • Recognizes and names common coins. • Tells where he/she lives by street and number.

APPENDIX   D

Listening Skills Scale for Kids with Cochlear Implants (LSSKCI)*

Level I   Pre-Verbal

❑   Quiets when wearing cochlear implant.

❑   Noisy without cochlear implant.

❑   Quiets, stills or smiles upon hearing ❑ a loud sound, ❑ a quiet sound.

❑   Responds to noisemaking toys.

❑   Responds to environmental sounds (doorbell telephone, knocking, barking, car horns, airplanes, others).

❑   Explores environment for new sounds (bangs spoon on table, bangs blocks).

❑   Quiets, stills, or smiles to singing, humming or music.

❑   Quiets, stills, or smiles when spoken to.

❑   Tries to localize sounds, usually by head turning.

❑   Indicates something heard (by pointing to cochlear implant and/or looking puzzled).

❑   Turns to: ❑ loud speech, ❑ quiet speech, ❑ whispered speech.

❑   Turns when called from a distance.

❑   Reacts when noises suddenly stop.

❑   Looks from one speaker to another.

❑   Attends by listening for a few minutes.

Level II   Verbal

❑   Turns to name when called: ❑ 3 ft, ❑ 6 ft, ❑ 9 ft, ❑ far away

❑   Stops activity to "no."

Matches suprasegmental features.

❑ Duration	❑ long	❑ short	❑ varied
❑ Pitch	❑ rising	❑ lowering	❑ varied
❑ Intensity	❑ loud	❑ quiet	❑ whisper	❑ varied

* Based on: *Schedules of Development* by A.L. Phillips, *Auditory Training* by N. Erber, Foreworks Program, and *Learning to Listen: A Hierarchy* by C. Edwards & W. Estabrooks.

❑ Learning to Listen Sounds (Appendix F)

_____	_____	_____	_____
_____	_____	_____	_____
_____	_____	_____	_____

❑ Words varying in number of syllables (umbrella, car, ice cream, rhinoceros, hippopotamus):

_____	_____
_____	_____
_____	_____

❑ Familiar expressions (Don't touch! Let's go home! Mm that's good!)

_____	_____
_____	_____
_____	_____

❑ One-syllable words (different vowels and consonants; limited choice) (hat, comb, ball, shoe).

❑ Phrases based on known words (in the car, to the store, up the stairs).

❑ One-syllable words with different vowels but same initial or final consonant (bat, boat, bee, ball, bug, bin).

❑ Similar phrases (a big purple truck, a small purple truck).

❑ Words with same vowel but different consonants (blue, shoe, two; cow, pow, bow, now).

❑ Memory for 2 items, ❑ 3 items, ❑ 4 items.

❑ Minor differences in sentences (in/on; the/a; he/she).

❑ Memory for phrases.

❑ Memory for short sentences.

Level III   Comprehension

A. Structured set

❑ Familiar expressions.

❑ Single directions, e.g., close the door. ❑ 2 directions, ❑ 3 directions.

❑ Two critical elements (e.g., the big house, the green ball).

❑ Three critical elements (e.g., flowers on the table).

❑ Four critical elements (e.g., purple car on the road).

❑ Multielement directions.

B.   Sequencing

❑   Sequence a series of multielement directions.

❑   Make identification based on several related descriptions.

❑   Sequencing ❑ 2 events, ❑ 4 events, ❑ 4+ events.

❑   Recall details in a story, lesson or event, ❑ 2 details, ❑ 3 details,
❑ 4 details.

❑   Understand main idea of ❑ a story, ❑ lesson, ❑ conversation.

C.   Conversation

❑   Answer questions requiring comprehension of main idea of a short
conversation.

❑   Paraphrase ❑ stories, ❑ conversations.

❑   Spontaneous, pragmatically correct conversation skills.

Level IV   Figure Ground

All above skills need to be developed in figure ground through the following
hierarchy.

A.   Quiet → Regular Noise → Noisy Environment

❑   Next to the sound source.

❑   5–6 feet from source.

❑   Across the room.

B.   In the presence of :

❑   Fan-type noise.

❑   Classroom-type noise.

❑   Cafeteria-type noise.

❑   Four-speaker babble.

C.   In the presence of:

❑   Increased distances.

❑   Various background noises.